S0-ANG-720

Clinical Management of Dysarthric Speakers

Clinical Management of Dysarthric Speakers

Kathryn M. Yorkston, Ph.D.
Rehabilitation Medicine
University of Washington
Seattle, Washington

David R. Beukelman, Ph.D.
Special Education
& Communication Disorders
University of Nebraska
Lincoln, Nebraska

Kathleen R. Bell, M.D.
Rehabilitation Medicine
University of Washington
Seattle, Washington

pro·ed

8700 Shoal Creek Boulevard
Austin, Texas 78757

Printed in the United States of America

ISBN 0-89079-316-6

Library of Congress Cataloging in Publication Data
Main entry under title:

Yorkston, Kathryn M., 1948–
Clinical management of dysarthric speakers.

Includes bibliographies and index.
1. Articulation disorders. I. Beukelman, David R., 1943– . II. Bell, Kathleen R., 1953– . III. Title [DNLM: 1. Speech Disorders—diagnosis. 2. Speech Therapy. WL 340 Y65c]
RC424.7.Y67 1987 616.85'5 87-3380

pro·ed

8700 Shoal Creek Boulevard
Austin, Texas 78757

5 6 7 8 9 10 95

Dedicated to the Speech/Language Pathologists
of University Hospital and Harborview Medical Center,
whose commitment to clinical service
has created a wonderful setting in which
to learn about dysarthria

Contents

Preface

Clinical Management of Dysarthric Speakers was written for graduate students and practicing speech/language pathologists interested in neurogenic communication disorders. A recent survey by the Washington Speech Language and Hearing Association indicated that management of dysarthric speakers is an important part of the caseload of those speech/language pathologists who work in hospitals, private practice and home health agencies. The survey revealed that of the communication disorders treated in hospitals and medical centers, dysarthria ranked second only to adult aphasia, with dysarthria accounting for 12 percent of the clinical revenue generated and aphasia accounting for 17 percent. Although individuals with dysarthria due to a variety of neurological disorders are served by speech/language pathologists, individuals with dysarthria due to head injury represent an increasing percentage of clinical caseloads. In this text, we summarize the basic neurological and medical information associated with the various diseases, disorders, and syndromes that cause the dysarthrias. In addition, we review and organize the available literature about the dysarthrias and relate it to the clinical management of speakers with this disorder. Finally, the clinical management chapters contain discussions of clinical practice that the authors have developed or adopted while treating dysarthric speakers in a hospital-based speech/language service.

The first several chapters contain general information. Chapter 1, "Perspectives on Dysarthria: A Clinical Point of View," reviews the perspectives from which the dysarthrias can be viewed, including the viewpoints of the neurologist, the speech physiologist, and the rehabilitationist. Dysarthria is defined within the framework of a model of chronic disorders as an impairment, a disability, and a handicap. Chapter 2, "Neuromotor Aspects of Speech Production and Dysarthria," was written by Dr. Michael D. McClean. This chapter provides an overview of the neural basis of normal speech production, the neuromotor disorders seen in dysarthria, and physiological approaches to the measurement of those disorders. Chapter 3, "Differential Diagnosis," reviews approaches for distinguishing motor speech disorders from language disorders and apraxia of speech from dysarthria. This chapter also summarizes the research literature concerned with distinguishing among the various dysarthrias.

Individuals with dysarthria frequently have serious underlying neurological diseases and syndromes. Therefore, speech/language pathology services are often delivered in conjunction with other medically related services. Chapters 4, 5, and 6 are provided as a resource guide to speech/language pathologists serving individuals with neurological disorders. Dr. Kathleen Bell provides a review of medical issues related to those neurological conditions that are frequently associated with dysarthria. The dysarthrias have been grouped according to their age of onset and the natural course of the disorder, because these two aspects of dysarthria are so important in clinical management. Chapter 4, "Congenital Dysarthrias," contains a discussion of cerebral palsy and Moebius syndrome. Chapter 5, "Adult-Onset, Non-Progressive Dysarthrias," contains a discussion of stroke and traumatic brain injury. Chapter 6, "Degenerative Dysarthrias," contains a discussion of those dysarthrias with a progressive course, including Parkinson's disease, progressive supranuclear palsy, dystonia, Huntington's disease, Wilson's disease, amyotrophic lateral sclerosis, Friedreich's ataxia, multiple sclerosis, and myasthenia gravis. A summary of research describing the speech characteristics related to selected neurological conditions is included. These chapters provide a summary of the literature and are not intended to critically review that literature.

Chapter 7, "Assessment and Treatment Planning," provides an overview of evaluation including both perceptual and instrumental approaches to measurement. The remainder of the chapters in this text provide detailed discussion of specific areas of intervention. Chapter 8, "Transition to Speech With Severely Dysarthric Individuals," reviews techniques for establishing early communication and physiological support for speech. Chapter 9, "Respiration," outlines approaches for assessment and training of the respiratory aspects of speech, including establishing respiratory support, stabilizing respiratory patterns, and increasing respiratory flexibility. Chapter 10, "Phonation," outlines the phonatory characteristics of a number of types of dysarthria, describes approaches to assessment, and reviews such management topics as treating the aphonic individual, increasing loudness, improving voice quality and improving phonatory coordination. Chapter 11, "Velopharyngeal Function," reviews the assessment and intervention of velopharyngeal dysfunction in dysarthria, including behavioral, prosthetic, and surgical methods. Chapter 12, "Oral Articulation," reviews the research literature related to articulatory aspects of dysarthria and presents management techniques designed to normalize function or to compensate for the impairment. Chapter 13, "Rate Control," reviews topics including candidacy for rate control and selection of appropriate techniques. Included is a discussion both of the rigid rate control techniques used with the severely impaired and those techniques that attempt to preserve prosody. Chapter 14, "Maximizing Speech Naturalness," provides a discussion of assessment and management of the prosodic aspects of dysarthric speech.

A project such as *Clinical Management of Dysarthric Speakers* reflects the contributions of many individuals. The work of numerous colleagues is referenced throughout the text. We are indebted to those clinicians and researchers who have been disciplined enough to record their observations, insights, and conclusions. Unfortunately, space and confidentiality do not permit a listing of clients who have served as our "teachers." We also acknowledge the pervasive influence of the speech pathology staff of University Hospital and Harborview Medical Center. Although their contributions are rarely referenced directly in this text, they have encouraged us, challenged us, listened to seemingly endless audio recordings of dysarthric speakers, critiqued early versions of tests and software, and provided a wonderful setting in which to learn about dysarthria. Finally, Laura McDaniel and Mary Rowan have assisted us by spending long hours managing the manuscript of this text.

CHAPTER 1

Perspectives on Dysarthria: A Clinical Point of View

Clinical issues: Family conferences in which the patients and their families have the opportunity to meet with the entire team are frequent occurrences on our rehabilitation unit. After one such conference, which began on a particularly discordant note, our student asked, "How do you prepare yourself for such a confrontation?" Our advice was to try to understand the interaction from the viewpoints of the various participants. In this particular case, Sam was diagnosed as having Parkinson's disease over 12 years ago. He was being discharged from a two week hospitalization for adjustment of his medication. The physician considered the hospitalization a success in that Sam's rigidity, together with the excessive movements that were a side effect of his former medication schedule, were reduced. The occupational therapist also considered it successful because Sam could more safely perform some activities of daily living. His speech was considered functional if the family modified their communication style. This required that his partners be face to face with Sam when he was attempting to speak, that they clearly signaled when they were not understanding, and that they took an active role in resolving communication breakdowns. However, Sam's wife and son were less positive. They concluded that Sam had not changed in any important ways and that the hospitalization was a waste of time and money. Sam still required a wheelchair for mobility, he needed some supervision when carrying out many activities of daily living, and his speech was still extremely difficult to understand. The family's disappointment with the intervention was clear. Sam could not return to work or even to an independent life-style.

- *How could people observe the same events and interpret them so differently?*
- *Was the family less observant than the rehabilitation staff?*
- *Was the rehabilitation staff exaggerating the changes that had occurred?*

Perspectives are standpoints from which a problem may be viewed. They provide a means for understanding or judging observations and for showing those observations in relationship with one another. This chapter presents a number of perspectives from which the speech/language clinician can view and understand the dysarthrias. Each perspective is valid for its own purposes. Before proceeding, an overview of some characteristics of the dysarthrias is discussed.

CHARACTERISTICS OF THE DYSARTHRIAS

Dysarthria is a neurogenic motor speech impairment which is characterized by slow, weak, imprecise, and/or uncoordinated movements of the speech musculature. Literally, the term comes from the Greek *dys* + *arthroun*, which means "inability to utter distinctly." Rather than being described by a single set of characteristics, different types of dysarthria vary along a number of dimensions:

- Age of Onset. The dysarthrias can be either congenital or acquired.
- Cause. The origin of the underlying neuromotor problem can be vascular, traumatic, infectious, neoplastic, metabolic, etc.
- Natural Course. The course of the dysarthria may follow a number of patterns, including developmental (as in cerebral palsy in children), recovering (as in early post onset traumatic head injury and stroke), stable (as in cerebral palsy in adults), degenerative (as in amyotrophic lateral sclerosis), or exacerbating—remitting (as in some cases of multiple sclerosis).
- Site of Lesion. The neuroanatomic site of lesion may be either the central or peripheral nervous system or both, including the cerebrum, cerebellum, brain stem, and cranial nerve.
- Neurological Diagnosis of Disease. A number of diagnoses may be associated with dysarthria, including cerebral palsy, Parkinson's disease,

multiple sclerosis, amyotrophic lateral sclerosis, brain stem CVA, and bilateral cortical CVA. See Table 1-1 for a more complete listing.

- Pathophysiology. One of a combination of pathophysiological processes may be involved, including spasticity, flaccidity, ataxia, tremor, rigidity, and dysmetria.
- Speech Components Involved. All or several of the speech components may be involved to varying degrees. These include the respiratory, phonatory, velopharyngeal, and oral articulatory (lip, tongue, and jaw) components.
- Perceptual Characteristics. The various dysarthrias have unique perceptual features. See Chapter 3 for a description of the perceptual characteristics of the various dysarthrias.
- Severity. Dysarthria may range in severity from a disorder so mild that it is just noticeable during connected speech, to a disorder so severe that no functional speech is present.

Differences among the dysarthrias have an impact on nearly every aspect of clinical management, for example, different medical courses influence sequence for treatment. In recovering or developmental dysarthria, an extended period of intervention may be appropriate. Degenerative disorders, on the other hand, usually warrant a different approach involving short, intensive periods of intervention at critical points during the course of the disorder. Different underlying pathophysiological problems may dictate quite different intervention techniques, for example, the reduction of habitual speaking rate which brings about an important increase in intelligibility for certain ataxic or hypokinetic dysarthric speakers may be counterproductive for individuals with flaccid dysarthria. Biofeedback programs designed to reduce overall muscle tone may be appropriate for those dysarthric individuals with increased spasticity but are counterindicated for those with weakness. Knowing the pattern of speech component breakdown is critical in knowing where to intervene, for example, when developing a management program for velopharyngeal incompetency, the appropriateness of palatal lift may be dependent on the level of function of other speech components, including respiration and oral articulation. Thus, appreciation of the diversity of the dysarthrias is critical for management. Rather than developing a generic dysarthria treatment, the field is very rightfully developing specific interventions for specific patterns of impairment.

The Neurologist's Point of View

Historically, the dysarthrias have been viewed by neurologists as signs or symptoms of disease. The term *disease* has been defined (Wood, 1980) as a "disruption of normal body processes" that results in changes in the structure or functioning of the body. For the dysarthric speaker, the disease may

TABLE 1-1.
Characteristics of the Dysarthrias

Type	Etiology	Location	Neuromuscular Condition
Flaccid dysarthria	Poliomyelitis CVA Congenital conditions Myasthenia gravis Bulbar palsy Facial palsy Trauma	Lower motor neuron	Flaccid paralysis Weakness Hypotonia Muscle atrophy Fascisulations
Spastic dysarthria	CVA Tumor Encephalitis Trauma Spastic cerebral palsy	Upper motor neuron	Spastic paralysis Weakness Limited range of motion Slowness of movement
Ataxic dysarthria	CVA Tumor Trauma Ataxic cerebral palsy Friedreich's ataxia Infection Toxic effects (e.g., alcohol)	Cerebellar system	Inaccurate movement Slow movement Hypotonia
Hypokinetic dysarthria	Parkinson's disease Drug induced	Extrapyramidal system	Slow movements Limited range of movement Immobility Paucity of movement Rigidity Loss of automatic aspects of movements

(continued)

TABLE 1-1 *(continued)*

Type	Etiology	Location	Neuromuscular Condition
Hyperkinetic dysarthria			
Predominately quick	Chorea Infection Gilles de la Tourettes's syndrome Ballism	Extrapyramidal system	Quick involuntary movements Variable muscle tone
Predominately slow	Athetosis Infection CVA Tumor Dystonia Drug induced Dyskinesia	Extrapyramidal system	Twisting & writhing movements Slow movements Involuntary movements Hypertonia
Mixed dysarthria			
Spastic-Flaccid	ALS Trauma CVA	Upper & lower motor neuron	Weakness Slow movement Limited range of movement
Spastic-ataxic-hypokinetic	Wilson's disease	Upper motor neuron, cerebellar & extra-pyramidal	Intention tremor Rigidity Spasticity Slow movement
Variable (Spastic-ataxic-flaccid)	Multiple Sclerosis	Variable	Variable

Based on work of Darley, F.L., Aronson, A.E. & Brown, J.R. (1975). *Motor Speech Disorders.* Philadelphia: W.B. Saunders.

Cited in Wertz, R.T. (1985). Neuropathologies of speech and language: An introduction to patient management. In D.F. Johns (Ed.), *Clinical management of neurogenic communicative disorders*. Boston: Little, Brown & Company.

be multiple sclerosis, Parkinson's disease, amyotrophic lateral sclerosis, cerebral palsy, or stroke. At times these neurological changes result in signs and symptoms. The signs of a disease are those characteristics observed by others, including professionals examining the patient. The symptoms of a disease are those characteristics perceived by the disordered individuals themselves.

For nearly 120 years, the characteristics of speech have been used to describe neurological disease. For example, in 1877 Charcot described a triad of symptoms that were characteristic of disseminated sclerosis, now known as multiple sclerosis. These symptoms included tremor, nystagmus, and scanning speech. In 1929 Hiller studied the dysarthria of Friedreich's ataxia and concluded that the primary speech problem of patients with cerebellar lesion is one of respiratory control. In 1937 Zentay classified the dysarthric speech resulting from cerebellar lesions as ataxic speech, adiadochokinesis, explosive speech, and scanning speech.

Early descriptions of dysarthria were associated with impairments of the nervous system that were diagnosed by medical professionals. Therefore, the illness or disease model, which is frequently employed in the medical field, has been applied to the dysarthrias. According to the illness model, the severity of the dysarthria is associated with the severity of the illness or disease process, and the dysarthria is managed by treating the disease. Thus, dysarthria has been used as an index of disease severity through the years, although little attention has been focused on remediation of the speech disorder itself.

As shown throughout this text, the practice of describing neurological disease in terms of speech characteristics continued in a rather unsystematic fashion until the late 1960s. It was then that Darley and colleagues (1969a, 1969b, 1975) studied the perceptual speech characteristics associated with a wide variety of neurological conditions. This work is referenced throughout this text with a detailed discussion of differential diagnosis in Chapter 3 and a summary of the characteristics associated with various neurological conditions in Chapters 4, 5, & 6.

At times, speech/language clinicians need to take the point of view that suggests dysarthria is a sign or symptom of a neurological disease or condition. This leads them to seek answers to specific types of questions:

- Is dysarthria present or are the signs or symptoms characteristic of some other communication problem? This line of questioning will eventually lead to a differential diagnosis of dysarthria from other neurogenic communication problems, including aphasia, apraxia, and dementia.
- If dysarthria is present, are the features consistent with those typically observed in speakers with the proposed diagnosis? This line of questioning will lead to a differential diagnosis among the dysarthrias and may contribute eventually to a differential diagnosis of the neurological disorder.
- How severe are the signs and symptoms of dysarthria and are they changing? Answers to these questions will eventually lead to an index of the severity of the neurological disease and a means of monitoring the course of the disease or response to medication.

The Speech Physiologist's Point of View

The viewpoint adopted by speech physiologists in their attempt to understand the dysarthrias is equally valid but quite different from the one taken by neurologists. They view dysarthria as a motor speech problem. Speech is a wonderfully complex phenomenon: consider the rapid, precise, well-coordinated movements required to produce understandable speech. Speakers use approximately 100 different muscles and produce recognizable sounds at a rate as high as 14 per second. Each of these sounds requires specific respiratory, laryngeal, and oral articulatory postures. Sound productions are not based on fixed patterns, rather, speakers appear to have the ability to produce a sound acceptable to the listener in a number of different ways. And, perhaps most remarkably, the speech motor activity is almost completely automatic. Although speakers may be consciously aware of formulating a message, they devote almost no conscious effort to planning motor speech activities. Given the complexity of motor speech, one would expect that impairment in motor control would have negative consequences in the form of reduced intelligibility, naturalness, and articulatory adequacy.

During the 1960s a new, physiological perspective on dysarthria appeared. Perhaps this position was most completely articulated by Hardy (1967) when he wrote the article "Suggestions for physiological research in dysarthria" to demonstrate the value of studying dysarthric speakers using the principles of experimental phonetics. In developing a research orientation, Hardy highlighted principles that continue to guide dysarthria research. Included among these are the following:

1. The physiology of one mechanism (respiratory, phonatory, or articulatory) interacts with all others to produce the speech signal.
2. Study of physiological aberrations of only one of these mechanisms without regard to the role of the others, or their compensatory capabilities for speech production, will allow only limited conclusions about speech problems of interest.
3. Many of the speech disorders that result from neuromuscular deficits may be studied advantageously by viewing the entire speech production system as an aerodynamic-mechanical system.

Through the years, the clinical speech pathology community has focused its attention on the speech process. During the 1970s and 1980s an effort has been made to study the observations of Darley and colleagues and to examine the conclusions and assumptions using physiologic and acoustic observational techniques. For example, Darley and colleagues reported that persons with dysarthria due to Parkinson's disease produced imprecise consonants. Subsequently, many researchers have concluded that persons with Parkinson's disease have reduced articulatory displacements compared to normal speakers and incoordination of agonist and antagonist muscle groups (Hirose, Kiritani, Sawashima, 1982; Hunker, Abbs, & Barlow, 1982; Leanderson, Meyerson, & Persson, 1971). Another example of the viewpoint on dysarthria as a reflection of physiologic dysfunction can be found in the work of Hunker (1986). These researchers studied the relationship between the tremor and movement initiation problems of dysarthric speakers with Parkinson's disease, and concluded that these speakers may delay initiating movements until the movement coincides with the phase of the tremor. Many examples of research from the speech physiologist's viewpoint are included in this text.

At times, especially when developing specific intervention plans, the speech/language clinician must take the speech physiologist's viewpoint. This leads to questions quite different from those posed from the neurological perspective.

- How can aspects of speech mechanism performance be objectively measured during speech production activities? Answers to this question have led to the development of techniques for measuring physiologic aspects of speech and for comparing the performance of the various aspects of speech production. In addition, this approach has allowed for comparison of the performance of dysarthric speakers to that of normal individuals.
- Are there means of compensating for the abnormal performance of the speech mechanism? Answers to this question have led to the development of a series of behavioral or prosthetic approaches to intervention.
- What malfunctions of the speech mechanism contribute substantially to reduced intelligibility? Answers to this question may form part of the strategy for sequencing of intervention tasks.

The Rehabilitationist's Point of View

It is obvious that a speech/language clinician managing a caseload of dysarthric individuals must be familiar with a number of perspectives for understanding the disorder. Clinicians must be thoroughly familiar with the viewpoint of the neurologist in order to plan intervention that is compatible with the underlying neuropathology, and is appropriate considering the natural course of the disorder. In addition, this viewpoint is required to participate in the differential diagnosis process. Likewise, the clinician must have an understanding of speech physiology in order to select and sequence intervention tasks appropriately. The viewpoint taken by the speech/language clinician planning rehabilitation programs is somewhat different from the one taken by either the neurologist, who wishes to identify the disease or disorder and to treat that condition, or the speech physiologist, who wishes to understand both the normal and abnormal motor speech process. The following are among the types of questions asked by the clinician in the rehabilitation setting:

- How is the dysarthria affecting the individual's life style?
- How can that effect be lessened?
- What are reasonable goals for intervention?
- What are important measures of successful intervention?
- How can these goals be achieved? Does this individual need an augmentative communication system, or a palatal lift, or an amplifier, etc?

DYSARTHRIA AS A CHRONIC DISORDER

Almost without exception, dysarthria is associated with diseases and conditions that are chronic or long-term. Therefore, models of the consequences of chronic disorder (Bettinghaus, 1980; Nagi, 1965, 1969, 1976, 1977; Wood, 1980) are helpful in developing a clinical perspective for management of dysarthric individuals. Frey (1984) reviewed a number of models of chronic disability and presented a series of definitions which he adapted from Bettinghaus (1980). The term *impairment* refers to "any loss or abnormality of psychological, physiological, or anatomical structure or function." The term *disability* is any "restriction or lack (resulting from an impairment) of the ability to perform an activity in the manner or within the range considered normal for the human being." Although an impairment is reflected in the functions of organs, body parts, and body systems, disability is reflected in integrated functioning required to perform and complete skills or tasks. The term *handicap* refers to a "disadvantage for a given individual (resulting from an impairment or a disability) that limits or prevents the fulfillment of a role that is normal (depending on age, sex, social, cultural factors) for that individual."

Impairment

According to the model of chronic disorder, dysarthria can be defined on at least three levels (see Table 1-2). The first of these levels relates to the impairment. Dysarthria is a neurogenic motor speech impairment that is characterized by abnormalities in movement rate, precision, coordination, and strength. When attempting to describe the impairment of a dysarthric individual, measures of physiological control and support are needed. These measures may include those that supply information about the speech mechanism as it functions in nonspeech activities and information about respiratory, phonatory, and articulatory components of speech tasks. Many of the measures of impairment are instrumental, physiological measures. However, certain aspects of the impairment, such as voice quality, may also be measured perceptually with, for example, perceptual judgments of voice quality. Approaches to the measurement of specific aspects of impairment will be described throughout this text. To date, a large part of the research literature in dysarthria has focused on the impairment. Although it is beyond the scope of this chapter to review this extensive literature, references to research focusing on the underlying motor dysfunction of the various dysarthrias is included in many of the chapters that follow.

Disability

Dysarthria can also be defined as a disability. The disability resulting from the motor speech impairment is characterized by reduced speech intelligibility and rate and by abnormal prosodic patterns. When attempting

TABLE 1-2.
Dysarthria as a Chronic Disorder

	A Consequence of Chronic Disorders	Dysarthria	Measures
Impairment	Any loss or abnormality of psychological, physiological or anatomical structure or function.	A neurogenic motor speech impairment that is characterized by slow, weak, imprecise, and/or uncoordinated movements of the speech musculature.	Respiratory control Phonatory function Velopharyngeal function Oral articulation
Disability	Any restriction or lack (resulting from an impairment) of ability to perform an activity in the manner or within the range considered normal for a human being.	The disability resulting from the motor speech impairment is characterized by reduced speech intelligibility and rate and by abnormal prosodic patterns.	Speech intelligibility Speaking rate Articulatory adequacy Naturalness
Handicap	A disadvantage for a given individual (resulting from an impairment or disability) that limits or prevents the fulfillment of a role that is normal (depending on age, sex, social, cultural factors) for that individual.	The handicap resulting from the motor speech disability involves the reduced ability to function in communication situations which require understandable, efficient, and natural-sounding speech and involves the reactions or persons who impact the social, educational, and vocational opportunities and experiences of the dysarthric individual.	Speech & speaker adequacy

Adapted from Frey, W.D. (1984). Functional assessment in the '80s: A conceptual enigma, a technical challenge. In A.S. Halpern & M.J. Fuhrer (Eds.), *Functional assessment in rehabilitation*. Baltimore: Paul H. Brookes.

to describe the disability, a number of overall measures of dysarthric performance are available. These will be discussed in more detail in Chapter 7. Briefly, these measures include speech intelligibility and rate, perceptual judgments of overall articulatory adequacy, and prosody. The majority of these measures are perceptually derived, however, certain aspects of prosody lend themselves to acoustic analysis.

Reduction or stabilization of the disability is the primary goal of intervention. Therefore, measures of disability are frequently considered the outcome measures of dysarthria treatment, and also serve as an overall index of the severity of the disorder. The relationship between impairment and disability is not always simple or straightforward. Unfortunately, this relationship has received little systematic attention in the research literature. Our clinical experience suggests relatively severe impairment of single components of speech may not result in severe disability. For example, severely restricted lip movement in the presence of adequate functioning of other speech components may not result in a severe disability. However, even moderate impairment in multiple speech components may result in severe disability. Clinical experience also suggests that severe impairment of certain speech components may be particularly devastating in terms of their impact on the disability. For example, severe respiratory timing and coordination problems may result in severe disability.

Handicap

Dysarthria may be defined as a handicap. The handicap resulting from a motor speech disability involves the reduced ability to function in communication situations that require understandable, efficient, and natural-sounding speech, and involves the reactions of persons who impact the social educational and vocational opportunities and experiences of the dysarthric individual. As defined here, the level of handicap depends on at least two factors—the severity of the disability and societal attitudes. An individual can be prevented from participating in desired roles because of the severity of the disability. An unintelligible speaker cannot function adequately in the role of a telephone operator. However, an individual may also be prevented from participating in a desired role because of the biases and attitudes of those in the environment. An intelligible speaker who does not sound natural might not be hired in an occupation involving extensive public contact, even though that individual possesses all of the skills required for the job. No standard technique is currently available to the clinician for measurement of handicap. Until a more systematic approach is developed, clinical interviews and informal questionnaires about speech adequacy and acceptability will continue to be used. The extent of the handicap is determined by multiple factors, including the severity of the impairment and the communication needs determined by the lifestyle of the individual. For example, an individual who is regularly involved in public speaking, such as a teacher, attorney, minister, or salesperson would be more handicapped by symptoms that may not be handicapping to a person with minimal public communication requirements.

Although documentation of the handicap associated with dysarthria is rare, a few examples of such efforts can be found in recent literature. For example, Hooks (1985) explored the impact of societal biases toward dysarthric speakers. He demonstrated that vocational counselors discriminated against dysarthric speakers by suggesting that these individuals would not only be unsuccessful at jobs with high speaking requirements, but would also be unsuccessful at jobs with minimal speaking requirements. This handicap was imposed by the vocational counselors despite the fact that the personnel files of the dysarthric individuals contained information showing them to be qualified to successfully perform the work described for the jobs with minimal speech requirements. Gies-Zaborowski and Silverman (1986) used a semantic differential scale to document the impact of mild dysarthria on peer perceptions of an 11 year old girl with mild cerebral palsy. Their results indicated that "her speech caused her to be perceived as frightened, nervous, tense, and unlovable."

THE CLINICAL PROCESS

For the speech/language pathologist, the clinical intervention may be thought of as a process of observing behavior, gathering pertinent information, and making decisions about the management of the communication problems of the dysarthric individual. The decisions made by speech/language pathologists in the clinical setting can be characterized by three features. First, they are individualized. Almost without the exception, the clinician is faced with decisions that relate to a single individual. This individual may or may not exhibit a classic pattern of impairment, disability, and handicap which is associated with a particular neurological disorder. It is usually the case in clinical management that complicating factors or special considerations make each dysarthric individual unique. Second, there is almost always an urgency to clinical decisions. Rather than waiting until research has provided better measurement techniques or a more complete understanding of the disorder, the clinician is forced to do the best job with the knowledge and tools that are available at the moment. Third, the clinician must make decisions based on the broadest possible perspective. The dysarthria researcher may quite rightfully choose to focus on a limited aspect of this complex disorder and to study that aspect both systematically and in great detail. The clinician usually does not have this option. Viewing dysarthria as a chronic disorder serves a number of clinical purposes. We will close this chapter by identifying some pressing clinical issues and discussing how the perspective of the chronic disorder model may help to resolve these issues.

Identifying Perspectives

The model of chronic disorders provides a vocabulary for communicating with other professionals and with dysarthric speakers and their families. It allows the clinician to identify the perspectives of others. In the introduction to this chapter, we described a family conference where there was an apparent disagreement about the outcome of intervention. Reviewing that situation from the perspective of a model of chronic disorder suggests that each of the participants in the family conference may have been viewing dysarthria from a different perspective. The physician was viewing it as an impairment. Thus, demonstrable changes in rigidity were a signal of successful intervention. The rehabilitation clinicians, including the occupational therapist and the speech/language pathologist, viewed the dysarthria as a disability. Thus, the patient's ability to perform more activities of daily living signaled successful intervention. On the other hand, the family was viewing the dysarthria as a handicap. Thus, the fact that the parkinsonian individual was no longer able to return to his former occupation or to carry out his role as husband and father as he had before signaled to the family that intervention had fallen short of its target. Although it may be true that recognizing the viewpoints of others may not change the reality of the outcome, the level of discontent may have been reduced if communication had been clearer. The lack of close relationship between impairment, disability, and handicap makes it manditory for professionals to communicate clearly the point of view from which they are discussing the disorder.

Obviously, changes in component performance do not always result in immediate changes in the disability. At times, improvement in the performance of several components is required before a reduction in the disability can be observed. Nevertheless, the ultimate goal of intervention is either stabilization or reduction in disability, depending on the natural course of the individual's disorder.

Identification of the perspectives of others is also important when attempting to read, understand, and interpret the dysarthria literature. Students given the task of reviewing research literature in this area are quickly impressed with the diversity of approaches to measurement. Any number of physiologic, acoustic, and perceptual measures have been used to understand the nature of the disorder. This diversity may at first give the impression that there is little agreement as to the single best way of understanding dysarthria, so writers simply choose the measures they prefer. We do not believe that this is the case. Rather, the diversity of approaches to measurement may simply reflect the differing perspectives from which the problem is being viewed. The vocabulary used in the model of chronic disorders may enable the reader to critically evaluate the adequacy of the measures employed in research. In other words, are the measures well-suited to their intended purpose? For example, aerodynamic measures of velopharyngeal resistance are frequently used as an indicator of velopharyngeal impairment. However, these measures alone without corroborating measures of disability such as speech intelligibility may not be sufficient to document the effectiveness of an intervention program. Because the ultimate goal of intervention is not better velopharyngeal performance but more intelligible speech, the measures of change in disability must accompany the measures that reflect a change in the impairment.

Identifying Treatment Candidates

Presence of dysarthria can be easily documented by listening to the speaker or by obtaining any number of measures of motor performance of the various speech components. However, merely knowing that dysarthria is present does not help the clinician decide how important it is to treat the individual. The model of dysarthria as a chronic disorder may provide some assistance in this area. Consider the case of two dysarthric speakers each having moderately severe impairment and disability. The urgency of treatment for these individuals does not depend entirely on the impairment or the disability, but on the handicap. Suppose that the first speaker was a retired individual living at home with his wife. His intelligible but slow speech may be sufficient to support his conversational needs. His level of handicap may be mild because he only has occasion to speak with those who are familiar with him and rapid, efficient, and natural-sounding speech is not manditory. However, suppose the second speaker was a minister whose duties required extensive public speaking. Intelligible speech is of course required, but rapid, efficient, natural-sounding speech is also manditory. Thus, even a moderate level of disability would be extremely handicapping for this individual. The severity of the impairment, disability, and handicap are not as closely correlated as they may first appear. An individual with minimal communication needs may experience a substantial impairment or disability before the disability becomes a handicap. For other individuals, even the mildest of impairment may be of real concern.

Setting Treatment Goals

There are many different approaches to goal setting in treatment. One of the most common is to set goals in relation to normal performance. This approach to goal setting is not appropriate in dysarthria intervention for at least two reasons. First, because of the nature of underlying neuropathology, normal performance can almost never be achieved. Second, some of the specific treatment techniques described in this text actually move at least some aspects of performance in a direction that is away from normal. An example of such a technique is rate reduction in which dysarthric speakers learn to slow their already slower than normal speech in order to increase intelligibility.

One alternative to setting normalcy as a general goal for dysarthric speakers is to set highly specific task-related goals for performance. For example, when attempting to intervene with severely dysarthric speakers, a treatment goal might be to sustain five centimeters of water pressure for five seconds. Unfortunately, specific goals may not be functionally important. Although setting treatment goals such as these is necessary to document recovery or learning rates, achieving these goals is only important clinically if they are also associated with some reduction of overall disability. Using the vocabulary of this model of chronic disorders, the goals of intervention are to decrease or stabilize the disability, thus improving such overall aspects of speech as intelligibility, rate, and naturalness. Setting goals related to disability may be an acceptable compromise between the general goals of normalcy which may not be achievable and the specific goals of changing a single component of speech production which may not be functionally important.

Assessing Treatment Efficacy

The model of chronic disorder may also be applied when studying treatment efficacy. A review of the literature reveals many articles describing various aspects of dysarthria and relatively few articles outlining treatment approaches. Still fewer articles document efficacy of treatment. This is not surprising in a field where attention has only recently turned to intervention. Documentation of treatment effectiveness progresses through a number of phases as a field of therapy matures. In the first phase, possible approaches to intervention are described. These descriptions are usually based on theoretical models of the disorder which suggest that a series of approaches "should work" if the understanding of the disorder is adequate. Darley and colleagues (1975), Rosenbek and LaPointe (1985), Perkins (1983), and Hardy (1984) have described approaches that have been used with dysarthric individuals. Although these descriptions are an important first step, they are being joined in the literature by an important second step, case studies that document treatment outcomes. For example, Netsell and Daniel (1979) reported the outcome of treatment of an individual with flaccid dysarthria, and Netsell and Clelland (1973) reported an EMG biofeedback study with lip retraction during speech. Hanson and Metter (1980, 1983) reported on the effectiveness of DAF on the speech of individuals with hypokinetic dysarthria. Yorkston and Beukelman (1981) reported the performance of four individuals with ataxic dysarthria. Helm (1979) reported a case study using a pacing board to control excessive speaking rate. A review of the literature shows a steady increase in the number of case studies being reported. This phase of efficacy studies is more specific than the first phase because, by describing the cases in detail, readers are provided some general guidelines for candidacy that are for the most part absent in the first phase of treatment outcome studies. Because of the heterogeneous nature of the dysarthric population, single case design research such as that described in McNeil and Kennedy (1984) and McReynolds and Kearns (1983) hold great potential for documenting the impact of treatment on dysarthric speakers.

The third phase of efficacy studies involves those that examine groups of individuals. There have been almost no group studies investigating the efficacy of dysarthria treatment. As is obvious to those familiar with the aphasia literature, well-constructed group efficacy studies are difficult to carry out. One of the most challenging aspects of this type of study is to separate factors that are related to the natural course of the disorder from those that relate specifically to the impact of treatment. For example, spontaneous recovery in an aphasic individual following stroke frequently prevents a clear interpretation of data describing the treatment outcomes. The model of chronic disorder may provide some guidelines for clearly interpreting treatment outcome data. The potential for independent measurement of the impairment and the disability provides some intriguing opportunities for documenting the impact of treatment. For example, consider the speaker with a degenerative disorder. In this case, increasing impairment is an inevitable consequence of the disease. However, if the clinician can document a stable disability in the face of increasing impairment, treatment effectiveness may be suggested. Likewise, a decrease in disability in the presence of a stable impairment would imply that intervention was effective. The important implications for efficacy studies provide another reason to encourage research investigating the relationship between impairment and disability in dysarthric speakers.

REFERENCES

Bettinghaus, C.O. (1980). *International standards for a system of disability classification.* Paper presented at the Annual Meeting of the American Psychological Association, Montreal.

Charcot, J.M. (1877). *Lectures on the diseases of the nervous system* (Vol. 1). London: The New Sydenham Society.

Darley, F.L., Aronson, A.E., & Brown, J.R. (1969a). Differential diagnostic patterns of dysarthria. *Journal of Speech & Hearing Research, 12,* 246–269.

Darley, F.L., Aronson, A.E., & Brown, J.R. (1969b). Cluster of deviant speech dimensions in the dysarthrias. *Journal of Speech & Hearing Research, 12,* 462–496.

Darley, F.L., Aronson, A.E., & Brown, J.R. (1975). *Motor speech disorders.* Philadelphia: W.B. Saunders.

Frey, W.D. (1984). Functional assessment in the '80s: A conceptual enigma, a technical challenge. In A.S. Halpern & M.J. Fuhrer (Eds.), *Functional assessment in rehabilitation.* Baltimore: Paul H. Brookes.

Gies-Zaborowski, J., & Silverman, F.H. (1986). Documenting the impact of a mild dysarthria on peer perception. *Language, Speech, & Hearing Services in Schools, 17*(2), 143.

Hanson, W., & Metter E.J. (1980). DAF as instrumental treatment for dysarthria in progressive supranuclear palsy: A case report. *Journal of Speech & Hearing Disorders, 45,* 268–276.

Hanson, W., & Metter, E.J. (1983). DAF speech rate modification in Parkinson's disease: A report of two cases. In W. Berry (Ed.), *Clinical dysarthria.* Austin, TX: PRO-ED.

Hardy, J. (1967). Suggestions for physiological research in dysarthria. *Cortex, 3,* 128–156.

Hardy, J. (1984). *Cerebral palsy.* Englewood Cliffs, NJ: Prentice Hall, Inc.

Helm, N.A. (1979). Management of palilalia with a pacing board. *Journal of Speech & Hearing Disorders, 44,* 350–353.

Hiller, H. (1929). A study of speech disorders in Friedreich's ataxia. *Archives of Neurology & Psychiatry, 22,* 75–90.

Hirose, H., Kiritani, S., & Sawashima, M. (1982). Velocity of articulatory movements in normal and dysarthric subjects. *Folia Phoniatrica, 34,* 210–215.

Hooks, D. (1985). *The effects of dysarthria on judgments of employability by vocational counselors.* Unpublished dissertation, University of Washington.

Hunker, C. (1986, February). *The nature and functional significance of parkinsonian resting tremor in the orofacial motor subsystem.* Paper presented at the Third Biennial Clinical Dysarthria Conference, Tucson.

Hunker, C., Abbs, J., & Barlow, S. (1982). The relationship between Parkinson rigidity and hypokinesia in the orofacial system: A quantitative analysis. *Neurology, 32,* 749–756.

Leanderson, R., Meyerson, B.A., & Persson, A. (1971). Effect of L-dopa on speech in parkinsonism: An EMG study of labial articulatory function. *Journal of Neurology, Neurosurgery & Psychiatry, 34,* 679.

McNeil, M.R., & Kennedy, J.G. (1984). Measuring the effects of treatment for dysarthria: Knowing when to change or terminate. *Seminars in Speech and Language,* 4(4), 337–358.

McReynolds, L.V., & Kearns, K. (1983). *Single subject experimental design in speech pathology.* Baltimore: University Park Press.

Nagi, S.Z. (1965). Some conceptual issues in disability and rehabilitation. In M.D. Sussman (Ed.), *Sociology and rehabilitation.* American Sociological Association, in cooperation with the Vocational Rehabilitation Administration. Washington, DC: U.S. Department of Health, Education, & Welfare, 1965.

Nagi. S.Z. (1969). *Disability and rehabilitation: Legal, clinical and self concepts and measurement.* Columbus: Ohio State University Press.

Nagi, S.Z. (1976). An epidemiology of disability among adults in the United States. In Health and Society. *Milback Memorial Fund Quarterly, 54,* 439–467.

Nagi, S.Z. (1977). The disabled and rehabilitation services: A national overview. *American Rehabilitation,* 2(5), 26–33.

Netsell, R. (1973). Speech Physiology. In F. D. Minifie, T.J. Hixon, & F. Williams (Eds.), *Normal aspects of speech, hearing and language.* Englewood Cliffs, NJ: Prentice-Hall, Inc.

Netsell, R. & Clelland, C. (1973). Modification of lip hypotonia in dysarthria using EMG feedback, *Journal of Speech & Hearing Disorders, 38,* 131–140.

Netsell, R., & Daniel, B. (1979). Dysarthria in adults: Physiologic approach to rehabilitation. *Archives of Physical Medicine & Rehabilitation. 60,* 502–508.

Perkins, W.H. (Ed.) (1983). *Dysarthria and apraxia: Current therapy of communication disorders.* New York: Thieme-Stratton, Inc.

Rosenbek, J.C., & LaPointe, L.L. (1985). The dysarthrias: Description, diagnosis, and treatment. In D.F. Johns (Ed.), *Clinical management of neurogenic communication disorders*. Austin, TX: PRO-ED.

Wertz, R.T. (1985). Neuropathologies of speech and language: An introduction to patient management. In D.F. Johns (Ed.), *Clinical management of neurogenic communicative disorders*. Boston: Little, Brown & Company.

Wood, P.H.N. (1980). Appreciating the consequences of disease—The classification of impairments, disability and handicaps. *The WHO Chronicle, 43,* 376–380.

Yorkston, K.M. & Beukelman, D.R. (1981). Ataxic dysarthria: Treatment sequences based on intelligibility and prosodic considerations. *Journal of Speech & Hearing Disorders, 46,* 398–404.

Zentay, P.J. (1937). Motor disorders of the nervous system and their significance for speech. Part I. Cerebral and cerebellar dysarthria. *Laryngoscope, 47,* 147–156.

CHAPTER 2

Neuromotor Aspects of Speech Production and Dysarthria

Michael D. McClean

We recently had the opportunity to participate in the third biennial Clinical Dysarthria Conference in Tucson, Arizona. On the last morning of the conference, an open period of discussion was scheduled. Somewhat to our surprise, the discussion did not focus on any of the papers that had been presented during the two previous days or on controversial topics of the field. Rather, the discussion turned to the issue of what clinicians need to know in order to work most effectively with individuals with neuromotor communication problems. No matter what the level of training or experience, there appeared to be a concensus within the group that clinicians need in-depth training in the neurophysiological basis of speech movement control, in consequences of pathological conditions affecting the central or peripheral nervous system, and in how individuals compensate for impairment.

Clinical management of dysarthria is changing. A number of trends are apparent in this change. The first is a growing appreciation that dysarthria is more than an oral articulation problem. Thus, in order to design appropriate intervention programs, clinicians must have a basic understanding of speech at all levels of production. The second trend is toward specificity of treatment.

Clinicians can no longer justify a "general" intervention program to be applied to any dysarthric speaker no matter what the type or severity of the underlying problem. Designing individualized treatment programs requires an understanding of the nature and implications of the underlying pathologies. Finally, we are seeing reports of a growing number of successful interventions with individuals who are apparently learning to compensate for their impairments. Many of these techniques are based on instrumental measures that provide various types of physiological feedback to the speaker. These biofeedback techniques require that clinicians be aware of recent advances in measurement of the physiological aspects of speech production. In short, the practicing clinician simply cannot know too much about the basics of neuroscience.

We have asked Michael McClean, a speech physiologist and Associate Professor in the Graduate Department of Speech Pathology at the University of Toronto, to write this chapter and include a review of the neural basis of normal speech production, the neuromuscular disorders seen in dysarthria, and physiological approaches to the measurement of those disorders. It is intended to provide an overview bringing together information about normal as well as disordered movement control. Dr. McClean has also provided extensive references to direct the interested clinician to more detailed studies in topics of interest.

The purpose of this chapter is to review basic aspects of the neural control of speech production and neuromuscular dysfunction in dysarthria. For the speech clinician, the material dealing directly with dysarthria may have the most obvious appeal; however, the conceptual framework or paradigm for this work is derived primarily from more general studies of normal and disordered movement control. The rich history and rapidly expanding knowledge in the area of neural control of movement has considerable potential for enhancing the quality of clinical practice in dysarthria. This has become apparent through general advances in the area of clinical neurophysiology and the results of recent studies of the physiological aspects of dysarthria.

NEUROMUSCULAR BASIS OF SPEECH MOVEMENT CONTROL

Levels of Speech Production

Speech involves the production of sequences of movement which are controlled by several regions of the nervous system. Given its extreme complexity, the speech production process is usefully conceptualized in terms of its different physical levels. These levels are illustrated in Figure 2-1.

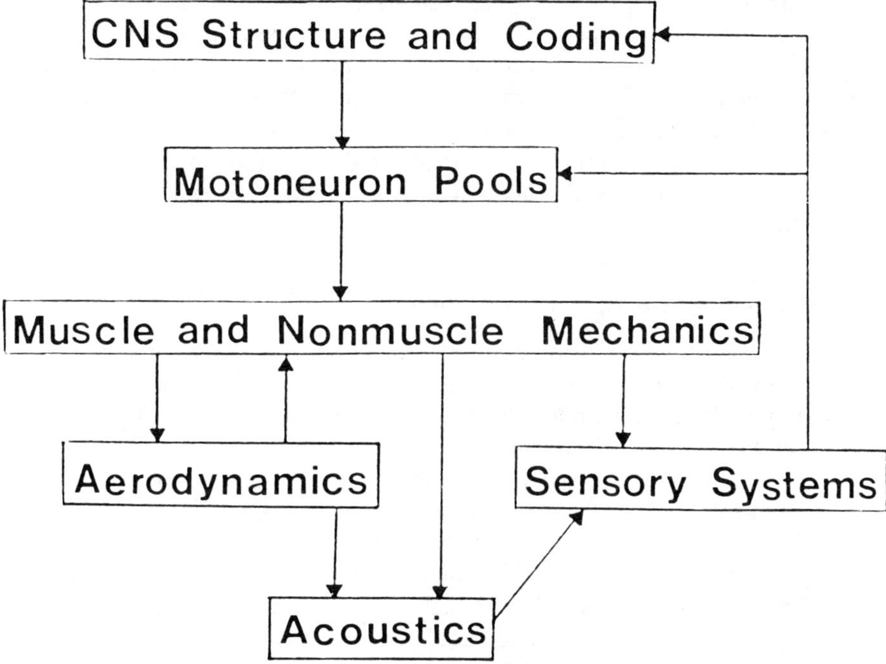

Figure 2-1. A schematic diagram of the major levels of speech production, showing primary lines of interaction and communication.

Certain brain centers and neural pathways are consistently involved in the neural processes underlying the control of speech movements. The net result of these processes is a highly organized discharge of the motoneurons innervating the speech muscles. Motoneuron discharge results in muscle fiber shortening and the generation of muscle forces. These muscle forces interact with the mechanical properties of muscular and nonmuscular tissue (e.g., elasticity and inertia). In some cases, speech muscle forces result directly in structural displacements, as in tongue movements for consonant and vowel production. In other cases, muscle forces function primarily to change the mechanical properties of a structure, as in regulation of the vibratory mass and tension of the vocal folds.

Movements of structures such as the chest wall, vocal folds, and tongue produce the precise changes in upper and lower respiratory airway pressure and flow required for normal speech (Warren, 1982, 1986). Vocal tract pressure and flow changes result in the transient, turbulent, and periodic sound sources of speech. These sound sources are modified by the resonance or filter properties of the vocal tract to produce the rapid changes in acoustic spectra characteristic of human speech production. Such changes are lawfully related to vocal tract position and movement (Fant, 1960; Lindblom & Sundberg, 1971; Minifie, 1973).

A number of different sensory systems may make significant contributions to the control of motoneuron discharge during speech production. These include the auditory system and a wide range of mechanoreceptors (e.g., muscle spindles and Pacinian corpuscles), which can sense the effects of speech muscle action. The influence of sensory system input on motoneuron discharge in speech may be relatively direct, occurring at the spinal and brain stem levels, or indirect, via higher level centers such as the cerebral cortex, basal ganglia, and cerebellum.

Functional Stages of Speech Production

Individuals who study the neurophysiology of movement often distinguish between different stages of the movement control process. Those stages most commonly identified are planning, programming, and execution. Before considering the brain centers involved in movement, it will be helpful to review these stages, as they are often used to interpret data bearing on the physiology of movement control. Consideration of these stages may also aid in the categorization of speech movement disorders.

According to Paillard (1983), motor planning involves selection of an appropriate movement strategy in light of intended goals and prevailing physical conditions. The intended goals of speech production may logically be thought of as linguistic units such as phonemes, words, or phrases (Abbs, in press). In the planning of speech utterances, such units may be represented or coded in terms of spatial, aerodynamic, or acoustic targets. A general strategy for the achievement of such targets may also be a component of the speech motor plan.

A second stage in movement control is called motor programming. This entails provisional specification of precisely how the motor plan is to be achieved, for example, which muscles are to contract, how much, and when. Programming is also likely to involve pretuning the excitability of various sensory and motor pathways to be involved in the ensuing movement process. This can provide for the optimal use of sensory information during movement execution.

The execution stage involves the direct activation of motoneurons, muscle contraction, and movement. Through the course of the execution process, the discharge of motoneurons may be influenced to varying degrees by numerous brain centers and sensory pathways.

The neural correlates of motor planning, programming, and execution are likely to vary with the type of movement and degree of learning. The nature of these processes in speech motor control is by no means well understood. However, the concepts do provide a logical framework for interpreting neurophysiological data. Some general examples of such interpretation are provided in the next section.

Brain Centers Regulating Speech Movements

The review presented in this section focuses on the functional aspects of the major brain centers involved in speech movement control. For additional discussion on this subject, the reader is referred to a recent paper by Gracco and Abbs (in press). Additional information on the relevant neuroanatomy can be found in Carpenter (1976).

Cerebral Cortex

The cerebral cortex is recognized as a major structure for speech/language processing. In right-handed and most left-handed individuals the left hemisphere is specialized for the speech/language function. Conceptualization of the physiological organization of the cerebral cortex for speech movement control has been greatly influenced by observations on the effects of cortical surface electrical stimulation (Penfield & Roberts, 1966; Sessle & Wiesendanger, Sequin, & Kunzle, 1982; Woolsey, 1958). This work resulted in maps delineating the cortical regions most directly involved in movement control. These regions, illustrated in Figure 2-2, include the primary motor cortex (area 4), the premotor cortex (lateral area 6), the supplementary motor area (medial area 6), Broca's area (area 44), and the somatosensory cortex (areas 3, 1, and 2).

Stimulation procedures involving the use of very low current strengths within the cortex are now providing a more detailed view of the spatial relationship of cortical areas to muscles (cf. Asanuma, 1975, Wiesendanger, 1981). For example, it is now known that cortical area 4 projections to individual muscles arise from multiple discontinuous sites. Abbs and Welt (1985) have recently suggested that such multiple representation may provide a partial basis for the control of diverse speech gestures in a single structure, for example, lip movements for rounding and closure.

Primary Motor Cortex

Various characteristics of the primary motor cortex indicate that it is a major point of sensorimotor integration immediately prior to the lower motoneurons. In primates, some area 4 neurons have monosynaptic projections to lower motoneurons (Kuypers, 1958), that is, individual axons are linked directly to the motoneurons with one synapse. Primary motor cortex activity is well correlated with muscle force changes in learned movements (Evarts, 1969; Hoffman & Luschei, 1980), and lesions in this area result in muscle weakness. Area 4 neurons are also most responsive to sensory input from regions for which they provide motor innervation. This sensory input projects over the somatosensory cortex (areas 3, 1, & 2).

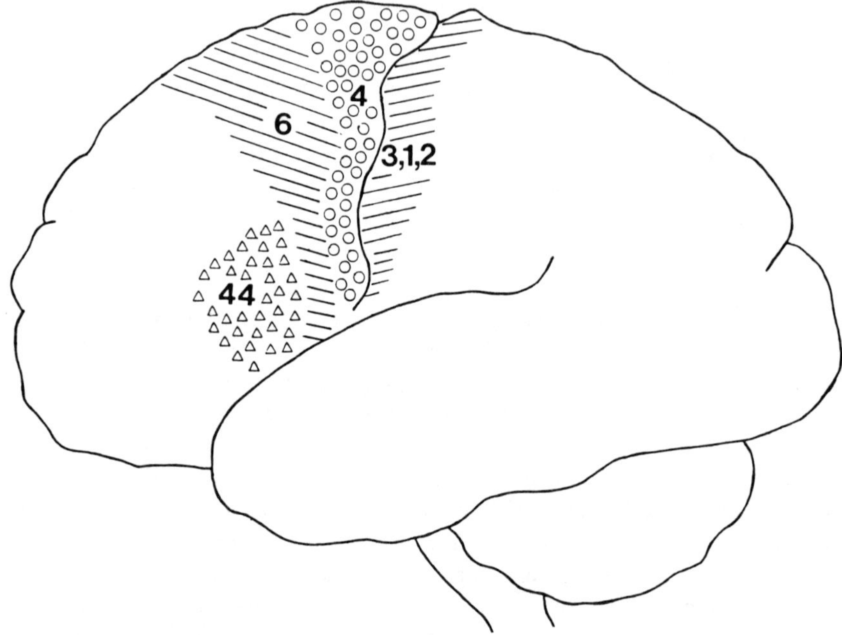

Figure 2-2. An illustration of the cortical regions involved in speech movement control; area 4 (primary motor cortex), areas 3, 1, & 2 (somatosensory cortex); area 44 (Broca's area); and area 6 (premotor cortex and supplementary motor area).

Area 4 is very much involved in the execution stage of movement control. Area 6, on the other hand, is more involved in movement planning and programming (cf. Porter, 1983). This is suggested by the fact that area 6 neurons show more complex activation patterns in relation to movement and an absence of short-latency responsiveness to peripheral stimulation. Area 6 has extensive projections to area 4 neurons, and it appears to be very important in shaping the pattern of motor output from area 4.

Cerebellum

The cerebellum has long been recognized as a highly developed and specialized center for movement control, and it is likely to be involved in several stages of the speech movement process. The cerebellar cortex receives sensory input from the tongue, lips, jaw, larynx, and auditory system (cf. Larson & Pfingst, 1982), and it rapidly integrates this information in contributing to speech motor processing. Two distinct corticocerebellar pathways are now seen to be important in the regulation of motor cortex output for speech

(Eccles, 1977; Kent & Rosenbek, 1982; Kornhuber, 1977; Neilson & O'Dwyer, 1984; Netsell, 1982). The important lines of communication are summarized in Figure 2-3A.

One pathway involves neural projections from area 6 to the lateral cerebellar hemispheres (LH) via pontine nuclei. A return pathway to areas 4 and 6 occurs via deep cerebellar and ventral thalamic nuclei. Animal studies suggest that this corticocerebellar loop is important in the planning and programming of learned movements (Brooks, 1979; Thach, 1980).

A second major corticocerebellar pathway involves collateral projection of descending corticospinal and corticobulbar fibers to the intermediate cerebellar hemispheres (I.H.). This pathway provides the cerebellum with immediate information on descending cortical motor output. There is a return pathway to cortical area 4 from the intermediate hemispheres via deep cerebellar and ventral thalamic nuclei. The intermediate hemispheres also have descending projections to brain stem and spinal motor centers via the red

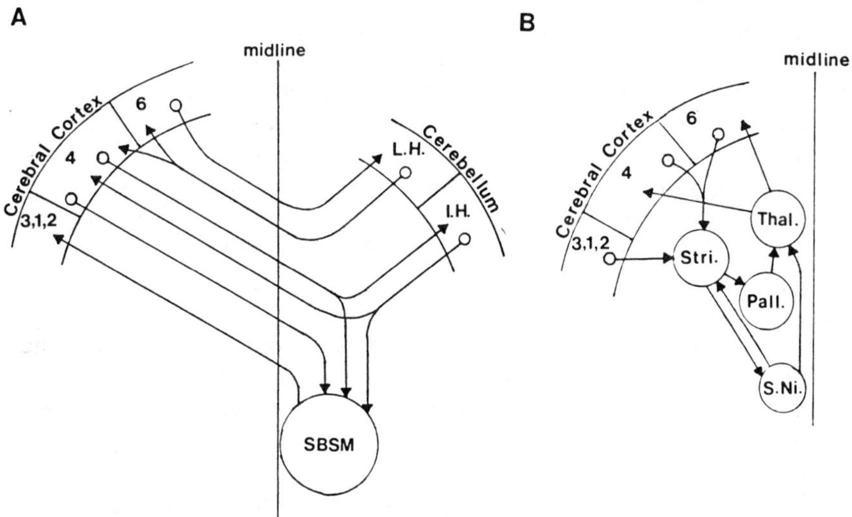

Figure 2-3. Schematic illustration of the motor system pathways interconnecting the cerebral cortex, cerebellum, and basal ganglia. Circles indicate output, and arrows indicate input. (A) Cortical-cerebellar pathways. L.H. and I.H. refer respectively to the lateral and intermediate cerebellar hemispheres. The projection from L.H. to the cerebral cortex occurs via ventral thalamic nuclei. SBSM refers to spinal and brain stem sensorimotor centers. (B) Pathways interconnecting regions of the cerebral cortex with various basal ganglia structures; striatum (Stri.), which includes the caudate nucleus and putamen, globus pallidus (Pall.), substantia nigra (S.Ni.). Basal ganglia communication to the cortex occurs via pathways projecting over the ventral nuclei of the thalamus (Thal.). (Adapted from Eccles, 1977.)

nucleus. The characteristics of these various pathways support the general view that the intermediate cerebellum utilizes sensory input to effect rapid modifications of cortical motor output during movement execution.

Basal Ganglia

The basal ganglia are a collection of large subcortical nuclei which comprise a major portion of the "extrapyramidal" motor system. It is likely that they make specialized contributions to speech movement control. This is suggested by the relatively distinct nature of dysarthric speech in individuals with Parkinson's disease, a basal ganglia disorder.

Major projections to the basal ganglia arise in the frontal cortex and converge on the caudate nucleus and putamen (i.e., the striatum). These pathways form the initial segment of a loop that projects back to the motor cortex via the globus pallidus and thalamic nuclei (see Figure 2-3B). The cortical-putamen pathway appears to be especially important for motor control processes, as it is composed of fibers projecting from the premotor cortex, whereas the caudate nucleus receives primary inputs from the more anterior regions of the frontal lobe. Neural output from the putamen projects to the globus pallidus and substantia nigra, then to the primary motor cortex via ventral thalamic nuclei. Thus, a multisynatpic pathway is formed between the premotor cortex and primary motor cortex over the basal ganglia and thalamus. Apparently, the segregation of body parts presented within the primary motor cortex is maintained in this pathway (DeLong, Georgopoulos, & Crutcher, 1983). With respect to the oral-facial system, there is a major pathway projecting from substantia nigra to supplementary motor cortex and then to area 4 (cf. Gracco and Abbs, in press).

In general, the basal ganglia are seen to be important in the planning and programming of learned movements. One important function may involve setting the kinematic parameters of movements, for example, recent electrophysiological studies of limb control in monkeys suggest that output from the globus pallidus is particularly important in regulating the direction and amplitude of movement (Anderson & Horak, 1985; DeLong & Georgopoulis, 1981).

Motor Units

Descending pathways from various brain centers converge on lower motoneurons within the brain stem and spinal cord. Motoneurons directly innervate muscle fibers, and thus, they represent an important interface between the rest of the nervous system and the mechanical systems involved in movement. Each motoneuron innervates a unique set of muscle fibers, and taken together, they comprise what is known as a motor unit.

Understanding the basic properties of motor units can have practical significance for the assessment and management of dysarthric speech. For example, such information is important in interpreting how different types of motor unit disease or trauma are manifested in speech motor performance. Some understanding of motor unit physiology is also important for effective use and interpretation of electromyography, a technique to be discussed that can have direct application in dysarthria assessment and therapy.

Motoneuron pools

The motoneuron cell bodies associated with a muscle tend to be grouped together in cell aggregates or pools within the brain stem or spinal cord. The motoneurons within a given pool innervate the muscle fibers of a single muscle (Henneman, 1980).

Various cranial nerve nuclei and the ventral regions of the spinal cord contain groups of motoneuron pools that innervate speech muscle systems. For example, the nucleus ambiguus is a collection of motoneuron pools within the medulla which innervate the intrinsic muscles of the larynx. Other cranial nerve motor nuclei of particular importance in speech motor control are the facial nucleus, the motor trigeminal nucleus, and the hypoglossal nucleus. Motoneuron axons project to their associated speech muscle fibers over the trigeminal, facial, hypoglossal, vagus, accessory, glossopharyngeal, and respiratory nerves.

Like any neuron, when a motoneuron's transmembrane potential is driven to its threshold by synaptic input, it produces an action potential which propagates the length of the axon. This results in the release of acetylcholine at the motor endplate. A muscle action potential then traverses through the associated muscle fibers, causing the release of calcium ions which then bind to muscle protein filaments. This results in the sliding action of the protein filaments, which is the basis for muscle shortening and the generation of brief forces or muscle twitches underlying whole muscle contraction (cf. Stein & Lee, 1981).

Types of Motor Units

The existence of different types of motor units is an important concept in motor physiology (Burke & Edgerton, 1975). Examination of muscle tissue reveals that some muscle fiber is white, some is red, and some is intermediate in color. These obvious differences in color have histochemical, mechanical, and electrophysiological correlates. Red muscle fiber has a high mitochondrial and capillary supply, and an oxidative or aerobic metabolism. White muscle fiber has a reduced blood supply, few mitochondria, and an anaerobic metabolism.

Electrical stimulation of motor unit axons and recording of their mechanical twitches has revealed some major differences in the physiology of motor unit types. On repeated electrical stimulation at low rates, red muscle motor units show low level twitch forces with slow rise or contraction times, and they tend to maintain their force levels over long periods of stimulation. In the same procedure, white muscle motor units show larger twitch force levels with faster contraction times, and their peak force levels are much reduced after prolonged stimulation, that is, they fatigue. Based on these results, which have been replicated many times (cf. Burke & Edgerton, 1975; Lewis, 1981), red muscle motor units are referred to as slow-twitch fatigue-resistant (type S), white muscle motor units as fast-twitch fatiguable (type FF), and intermediate muscle motor units as fast-twitch fatigue-resistant (type FR). In general, FF units tend to have larger motoneurons, axons, and muscle fibers, with larger muscle fibers partially accounting for their larger twitch forces.

It is known that type S motor units are the first and most frequently recruited under a number of different conditions of activation (Desmedt, 1981; Henneman, 1980). Because most activity requires low force levels to be sustained for a long time, for example, postural adjustment, this represents an effective adaptation of neuromuscular systems to the normal demands of animal movement. When rapid and/or large changes in muscle force are reqired, FF type units are recruited.

The wide range of motor unit properties are apparently utilized in different muscle systems to achieve their unique demands (Clamman, 1981). For example, the small extraocular muscles have very short contraction times to accommodate rapid eye movements, whereas leg muscles have much longer contraction times and generate large twitch tensions that are better matched to the more massive structures to be moved. Within muscle systems, however, there is further specialization; for example, the anterior tibial muscle is composed of a mixture of S, FF, and FR type units, whereas the soleus muscle is composed exclusively of S type units. Netsell (1982) has suggested that the muscles used in speech production tend to have motor units with properties that are intermediate to those for the eyes and the limbs. Among the lip muscles, there is considerable variability; for example, orbicularis oris has muscle fiber composition typical of S and FF type units, whereas platysma is an equal mix of fibers consistent with S, FF, and FR type units (Schwarting, Schroder, Stennert, & Goebel, 1982).

Electromyography

By placing extracellular electrodes in the vicinity of muscle fiber and amplifying the voltage across the electrodes, it is possible to record the propagated action potentials associated with one or more motor units. This technique is known as electromyography or EMG. EMG recording of a single motor unit will show a single brief-duration voltage with a constant waveshape. Figure 2-4A illustrates the action potentials of a pair of distinct motor units recorded from the platysma muscle. The other sections of the figure display the activation patterns of these two motor units during different gestures with

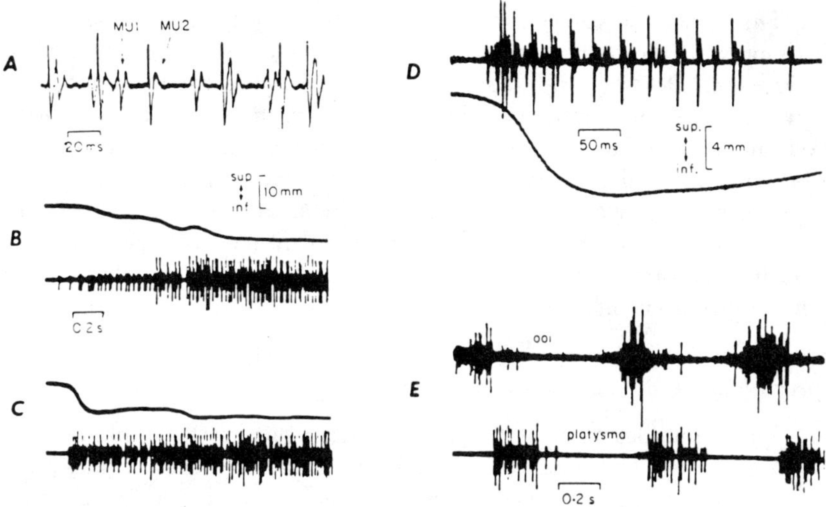

Figure 2-4. An illustration of electromyographic (EMG) recordings of two single motor units (MU1 and MU2) in the platysma muscle as they are activated for various speech and nonspeech behaviors. Lower lip displacement in the superior-inferior dimension was recorded with a strain gauge and is shown in B, C, and D. Platysma motor unit activation is shown during (A) sustained isometric contraction, (B) a very slow rounding-retraction movement associated with a gradual change in vowel production from /u/ to /ae/, (C) same as B, only performed rapidly, (D) production of the syllable /wae/, and (E) EMG recordings of the platysma and orbicularis oris inferior (ooi) muscles during repeated productions of /wae/. (From McClean & Sapir, 1981).

the lower lip. It may be seen in Figure 2-4B, C, and D that as velocity of lip displacement increases, the time between activation of the two motor units (i.e., the recruitment interval) decreases. This change in recruitment interval with movement velocity is a general characteristic of motor units in different muscles, and it reflects the requirement that more motor units must be activated together to achieve higher velocity movements (Desmedt, 1981).

The time of motor unit recruitment also varies systematically with changes in the movement direction of a structure (Desmedt & Godaux, 1981; Schmidt & Thomas, 1981). For example, motor units in the orbicularis oris inferior muscle will be activated earlier for anteriorly directed lower-lip movements than for superiorly directed lower-lip movements, whereas the converse applies to the mentalis muscle motor units (McClean, 1984).

EMG recordings typically include the contribution of several motor unit potentials which summate to produce complex-wave or interference patterns. Such patterns are illustrated in Figure 2-4E, which shows EMG recordings from the platysma and the orbicularis oris inferior muscles during three productions of the syllable /wae/.

The force of muscle contraction is determined by the rate of motor unit discharge and the number and type of motor units that are recruited or activated (cf. DeLuca, 1978; Stein and Lee, 1981). How the force output of a given muscle affects structural displacement will depend on the activation levels and relative timing of other muscles. For example, in Figure 2-4E the orbicularis oris and platysma muscles were activated in a reciprocal manner to produce the lip elevation and depression required for production of the syllable /wae/. If they had coactivated at equivalent levels, in the absence of other muscle force changes, the lower lip would have a negligible or much reduced displacement.

Speech Muscle Biomechanics

Speech muscles may be thought of as mechanical systems that respond to neural input and produce movement. To appreciate how neural signals affect speech structure movements we need to briefly consider the mechanical characteristics of muscle.

Mechanical Elements of Muscle

Figure 2-5A presents a simplified model depicting the mechanical characteristics of muscle. As individual motor units discharge, they produce single twitch-like forces. The twitch forces of different motor units summate to produce whole muscle contractile force (F). This force acts to displace a tissue mass (M). In actual muscle systems, the configuration of this mass is quite complex, and muscle tissue itself often comprises the bulk of the mass, as in the case of the tongue.

Muscle tissue is spring-like and has an elastic component (E). This causes tissue to resist displacement beyond its resting length and to generate a mechanical restoring force when stretched. Muscle systems also have internal fluid friction or viscosity (V), which requires additional forces in order for tissue layers to move across one another. The magnitudes of viscous and elastic forces can change significantly during the course of a movement, and their relationships to parameters of movement, such as displacement and velocity, tend to be nonlinear. Thus, movement characteristics are not simply dependent on the strength and timing of muscle contraction, but also the current mechanical state of the muscle and surrounding tissue (cf. Lewis, 1981).

An example of the importance of nonmuscular forces in speech motor control is provided by the interaction of respiratory muscle activation with chest wall tissue mechanics. The primary task of the rib cage and abdominal musculature during speech is to maintain a relative constant subglottal air pressure of 3–10 cm H_20. At high lung volume levels, the passive forces of the thoracic and abdominal tissue can generate subglottal pressure well in excess of that required for speech, but at low lung volumes, the passive forces

A

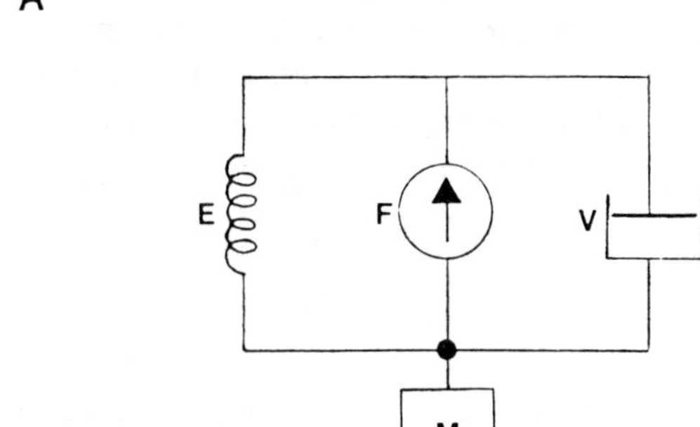

B

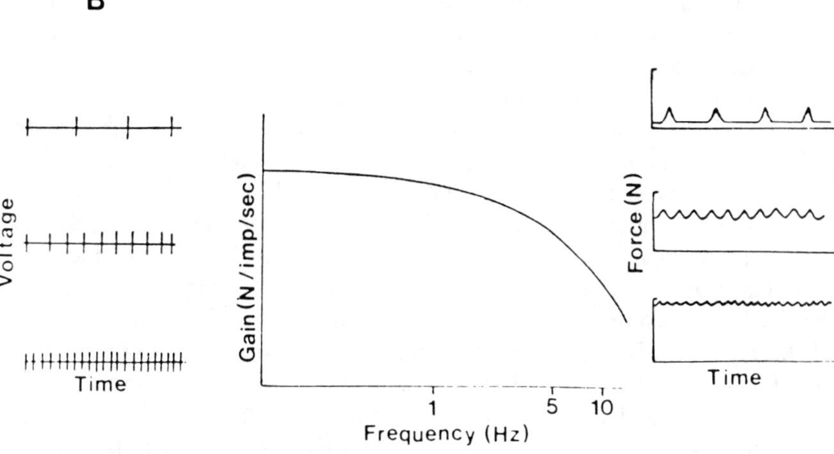

Figure 2-5. (A) Biomechanical elements of muscle systems. Abbreviations: E - elasticity, F - force, V - viscosity, M - mass. (B) Summary description of low-pass filter characteristics of muscle. The three waveform displays at the left refer to three rates of electrical stimulation applied to motor nerve innervating a muscle. The three force traces on the right indicate the corresponding changes in force output (in Newtons) recorded from the muscle. The middle plot summarizes the results of this type of experiment, showing the change in gain (Newtons divided by stimulation rate, impulses/sec) as a function of the frequency of stimulation. Reduced displacements during rapid movements are probably due in part to this mechanical characteristic of muscle.

generate pressures much less than that required for speech. Thus, the timing and magnitude of inspiratory and expiratory muscle activation must be coordinated in relation to the continuous changes in passive tissue mechanics of thoracic and abdominal structures (Draper, Ladefoged, & Whitteridge, 1959; Hixon, 1973).

Muscle as a Low-Pass Filter

In considering the relationship between motoneuron activity and movement, motor physiologists have found it very useful to conceptualize muscle as a low-pass filter, that is, a system that transfers energy at low but not high frequencies. Motor units can discharge at sustained rates of about 20 to 35 Hz (Freund, 1983). However, the mechanical properties of muscle fiber prevent motor units from generating distinct muscle-twitch forces at such high rates. This point is illustrated by some hypothetical data in Figure 2-5B. Such data could be obtained by electrically stimulating the motor nerve of a whole muscle at varying pulse rates while the muscle force is recorded. Waveforms of three stimulation rates are shown on the left in Figure 2-5B, and the corresponding force waveforms are shown on the right. It may be seen that at the lowest stimulation rate, relatively large muscle twitch curves result from each stimulus pulse. As stimulation rate increases, the twitch curves tend to fuse until there is almost complete fusion of the individual twitch curves. The peak force output does not increase in proportion to stimulation rate. In fact, there is an upper limit in all muscle at which there is no increase in force with increased stimulation rate. The input-output relationship in this experiment may be depicted by a gain or frequency response curve like that shown in the middle of the Figure 2-5B. This plots the ratio of force output to stimulation rate as a function of frequency. The general form of the curve is like that of a low-pass filter, and it is typical of all muscle. In the speech muscles the frequency-response curve tends to fall off markedly above 3 to 4 Hz (Cooker, Larson, & Luschei, 1980; Muller, Milenkovic, & McLeod, 1984).

Conceptualizing muscle as a low-pass filter can be of use in evaluating aspects of both normal and dysarthric speech. For example, when movement rates are increased beyond a certain point, there is invariably a reduction in the structural displacement which is most apparent at maximal diadokokinetic rates. This may be due to the mechanical properties of muscle as well as a tendency for antagonistic muscles to be coactivated at rapid movement rates (cf. Freund, 1983).

An important point with respect to dysarthria is that reductions in speech rate may be related to abnormalities of speech muscle mechanics as well as neural control. This is most likely in muscular dystrophy, and it might be expected generally in instances where muscle has atrophied due to disuse associated with neural impairment.

Sensory System Contributions to Speech Motor Control

The issue of how sensory input contributes to the coordination of speech muscle actions is intrinsic to the problem of how speech movement control is coded in the nervous system, and thus, it has considerable significance for study of the dysarthrias. Basic information on the anatomy and physiology of the human nervous system indicates that sensory afferents have strong diverse synaptic input to the numerous brain centers involved in the control of speech movement (Carpenter, 1976; Larson & Pfingst, 1982). Cutaneous, muscle, and auditory receptors have short-latency projections to the motoneurons innervating the speech muscles. This is readily demonstrated by means of reflex experiments in which EMG responses are recorded in speech muscles at short latencies following stimulation of different sensory systems (Bratzlavsky, 1976; Sapir, McClean, & Larson, 1983; Smith & Luschei, 1983).

Spatial Targets

An important feature of speech movement control is that relatively constant spatial targets are consistently achieved with structures that are continually changing their position and biomechanical states (MacNeilage, 1970). For example, consider how intelligible speech patterns are produced in an automatic fashion with changes in body position, simultaneous occurrence of other behaviors, variations in speed of locomotion, and the presence of objects in the mouth. This type of performance suggests that the brain routinely integrates sensory information from peripheral mechanoreceptors in controlling speech movements. Experimental evidence for this is provided by the observation that with controlled changes in jaw opening, as produced with bite blocks, the spectral pattern of the first periodic waveform of a vowel is relatively invariant (Lindblom, Lubker, & Gay, 1979). Thus, the neuromotor control processes underlying tongue positioning effectively integrate sensory information on jaw position and muscle state to produce an invariant formant structure.

The muscle actions associated with the production of individual speech sounds vary widely as a function of phonetic environment (cf. Fromkin, 1966; MacNeilage & DeClerk, 1969; Ohman, 1967). It is also known that the movement parameters of individual articulators vary widely across repetitions of constant phonetic sequences involving the same overall system output. For example, Hughes and Abbs (1976) noted that with repetitions of the same bilabial consonant and vowel sequence there was a trade-off in the relative contribution of upper-lip, lower-lip, and jaw displacement in achieving a consistent amount of lip opening. Although other explanations are plausible, it seems likely that these features of speech movement control are partially dependent on the use of sensory information in the organization of input to speech muscle motoneurons.

Studies of Sensory Function

The principal technique used to study sensory function in speech production has involved observations of speech motor output following controlled alteration of the normal pattern of sensory input during speech (cf. Borden, 1979). In many cases, sensory alteration results in adaptive or compensatory motor responses. For example, presentation of masking noise is followed by increased vocal intensity (Lane & Tranel, 1971) or application of force perturbations to the jaw result in rapid compensations by the lips (Folkins & Abbs, 1975).

Sensory alteration experiments in speech research have often involved predictable presentation of large-magnitude intrusive stimuli. Although this approach may tell us about how sensory information is utilized to adapt to background environmental or biomechanical conditions, it is not particularly revealing as to how sensory information is utilized during normal movement execution. The use of unpredictable stimuli at levels within the physiological range of the system is likely to be more informative in this regard. It has recently been observed that small force perturbations (10-55 grams) applied unpredictably to the lower lip during speech result in rapid compensatory responses by the upper and lower lips (Abbs & Gracco, 1984; Gracco & Abbs, 1985). The magnitudes of the compensations are in proportion to lower lip displacement and are adequate to ensure a normal production of the speech utterance. These findings strongly suggest that perioral mechanoreceptor information is integrated on a continuous or rapid-intermittent basis within the neuromotor systems controlling speech movement.

Efferent Control of Sensory Information

An important concept in motor physiology is that sensory processing at the spinal and brain stem levels may be under efferent or descending control by higher centers in the brain. This is most obviously manifested in the gamma motoneuron system which regulates muscle-spindle receptor sensitivity. It is now recognized that alpha and gamma motoneurons are coactivated during movement. This provides for continuous response of muscle spindles during muscle shortening.

Another type of efferent control of sensory information involves direct descending input to the primary afferent neurons and interneurons within brain stem and spinal sensory pathways. Recent experiments on cat locomotion suggest that the sensitivity of peripheral reflex pathways are dynamically modulated during movement execution (Forssberg, 1979). For example, a tactile stimulus delivered to a cat's paw during locomotion will elicit very different patterns of flexor and extensor muscle contraction in the hind limb depending on the phase of the movement cycle where the stimulus is applied. This suggests that for some behaviors, the brain actively controls how and when particular forms of sensory input will influence motoneuron discharge.

Continued research is required to determine whether this is an important aspect of speech motor control.

Recent discussions of the neural mechanisms underlying dysarthria have emphasized the potential significance of abnormal processing of sensory information (Abbs, Hunker, & Barlow, 1983; Neilson & O'Dwyer, 1984; Netsell, 1982). For example, Neilson and O'Dwyer (1984) suggest that the disordered movement processes associated with cerebral palsy speech are due to a sensory deficit resulting from congenital deformity of the neural pathways projecting over the ventral thalamic nuclei. They indicate that these nuclei are very likely to be involved in cases of brain damage associated with premature birth. The ventral thalamic nuclei represent a major relay for cerebellar and basal-ganglia projections to the motor and premotor cortex. In addition, the thalamus is the primary input relay for projection of somatosensory information to the postcentral gyrus. This includes mechanoreceptor input from tongue, perioral, jaw, laryngeal, and respiratory systems (Bowman, 1982; Dubner, Sessle, & Storey, 1978).

PATHOLOGIC NEUROMUSCULAR CONDITIONS ASSOCIATED WITH DYSARTHRIA

The dysarthrias tend to be associated with various pathologic neuromuscular conditions, for example, spasticity, athetosis, rigidity, tremor, hypokinesis, and flaccidity. Each of these conditions is relatively distinct within clinical neurophysiology, and the nature of their associated neural mechanisms is undergoing continued in-depth study (cf. Desmedt, 1973-1982). In some cases, we are beginning to understand how a specific neuromotor pathology is related to the symptoms of dysarthria. For example, the effect of flaccid paralysis of the spinal musculature on respiratory function during speech has been studied by Putnam and Hixon (1984). In other cases, the relationship between neuromotor pathology and dysarthric speech patterns is not well understood. The association between basal ganglia dysfunction and variability in speaking rate in Parkinson's disease is such a case (Netsell, Daniel, & Celesia, 1975). In either instance, an understanding of current views on the mechanisms of pathologic neuromuscular conditions is important for research and clinical practice with the dysarthrias.

In considering the mechanisms of various pathologic motor signs, clinical neurologists often distinguish between primary or negative symptoms and secondary or positive symptoms. Negative symptoms are those resulting directly from functional loss of certain neurons, and positive symptoms are seen as release phenomena resulting from disinhibition of healthy neurons. Thus, paralysis due to alpha motoneuron dysfunction is considered a negative symptom, whereas hyperactive reflexes associated with cortical damage are considered a positive symptom.

Adams (1973) suggests that different types of neuromuscular dysfunction are appropriately classified as paralysis, disorders of muscle tone, or forms of involuntary movement. This tripartite distinction is useful; however, motor disorders are generally discussed in relation to those parts of the nervous system that are primarily involved in a disease process or that constitute the site of lesion. Modern textbooks in neurology typically consider disorders of movement in relation to lower motoneurons, upper motoneurons, cerebellar, and basal ganglia dysfunction (cf. Adams & Victor, 1985). This general organization is used here in reviewing pathologic neuromuscular conditions associated with dysarthria.

Lower Motoneuron and Motor Unit Dysfunction

The alpha motoneurons within the brain stem motor nuclei and within the anterior horns of the spinal cord are known as lower motoneurons. These cells and the muscle fibers they innervate comprise the different motor unit types discussed earlier.

Various types of trauma or disease state may affect selected portions of the motor unit and thereby produce characteristic signs of neuromotor dysfunction (Woodbury, Gordon, & Conrad, 1965). Destruction of the motoneuron cell body or axon results in the abolition of muscle contraction in the affected motor units. Because the motor unit is the final common pathway for muscle contraction, both reflex and voluntary movements are impaired. Destruction of lower motoneurons results in a condition of flaccidity or muscle softness, reduced reflex magnitudes, and muscle atrophy. Reduced muscle tone or hypotonia, a lack of resistance to passive movement, is also often noted, and is believed to result in part from the absence of reflex contributions from muscle spindle and other mechanoreceptors. In some muscle systems, gamma motoneurons are likely to be affected by the lesion, and these are essential in maintaining appropriate levels of muscle spindle sensitivity, which in turn contribute to normal muscle tone.

Particular diseases may affect other portions of the motor unit and result in characteristic motor signs. For example, the muscle endplate is selectively affected by myasthenia gravis, which is characterized by weakness and heightened fatigability. Myotonia is a condition of the muscle fiber membrane which prevents muscle from relaxing normally and thus impairs voluntary control. The contractile mechanism of the muscle fiber may be affected by progressive muscular dystrophy which is manifested primarily in weakness.

In lower motoneuron disorders, small spontaneous visible contractions known as *fasciculations* sometimes may be observed. Fasciculations are triggered by events intrinsic to the motoneuron rather than synaptic input. Their presence in amyotrophic lateral sclerosis and progressive muscular atrophy is believed to result from disease processes attacking the motoneuron.

Upper Motoneuron Dysfunction

The term *upper motoneuron* encompasses the concepts of pyramidal tract, corticospinal neurons, and corticobulbar tract (Adams & Victor, 1985). The pyramidal tract includes only those neurons of cortical origin that descend over the internal capsule and decussate at the medullary pyramids. The corticospinal neurons include the pyramidal tract and more indirect pathways such as the corticorubrospinal and corticoreticulospinal tracts. The corticobulbar tract includes fibers that descend along with the corticospinal tracts and project to the motor nuclei of the brain stem, the reticular formation, and sensory relay nuclei. The cell bodies of upper motoneurons are found in several areas of the cerebral cortex, the primary ones being area 4, area 6, and the parietal lobe.

Upper motoneuron lesions can occur at several levels of the nervous system, and they seldom involve strictly corticospinal or corticobulbar pathways. For example, the close anatomical association of the ventral thalamic nuclei and the internal capsule makes it likely that lesions at that level will affect both upper motoneuron pathways and ascending thalamocortical projections from the basal ganglia and cerebellum. This point was discussed earlier in relation to the suggestion of Neilson and O'Dwyer (1984) that the characteristics of dysarthria in athetoid cerebral palsy may be due in large part to inappropriate sensory processing over ascending thalamic pathways.

Upper motoneuron lesions tend to be characterized by a condition of excessive muscular tone known as spasticity. In the limbs this is most notable in leg extensor muscles and arm flexors, which also show increased excitability to stretch stimuli. This increased reflex excitability is most likely due to both the removal of inhibitory influences and the increase of faciliatory drive to lower motoneurons. The neural mechanisms underlying spasticity are undergoing continued study by clinical neurophysiologists (cf. Feldman, Young, & Koella, 1980).

Recently Barlow and Abbs (1984) studied cranial-muscle fine motor control in a group of adult spastic dysarthrics. They were particularly interested in the contribution of muscle-spindle dysfunction to disorders of fine motor control, and they analyzed performance of three muscle systems known to have differing numbers of muscle spindles: the lips, tongue, and jaw. They did not observe greater deficits in motor control with the jaw and tongue, which are known to contain muscle spindles. This led Barlow and Abbs to suggest that deviant muscle-spindle activity is not a major cause of motor performance deficit in spastic dysarthria.

Basal Ganglia Dysfunction

The principal structures of the basal ganglia are the caudate nucleus, putamen, globus pallidus, substantia nigra, and subthalamic nucleus. These structures and their associated pathways have a distinct distribution of neurotransmitters that is an essential aspect of their function in motor control. Understanding in this area was greatly advanced by studies of Parkinson's disease, a basal ganglia disorder involving loss of biogenic-amine neurotransmitters, particularly dopamine. Dopamine is normally found in high concentration in the substantia nigra, but postmortem examination of the brains of parkinsonian patients shows low concentrations of dopamine and other biogenic amines.

Dopaminergic neurons project from the substantia nigra to the striatum and thalamus (see Figure 2-3), and their action is inhibitory. Thus, the loss of such neurons results in disinhibitory effects (i.e., reduced inhibition) on striatal and thalamic neurons. This has led to the view that pathologic motor symptoms in Parkinson's disease represent a type of release phenomenon, in which excitatory neuronal activity, normally held in check by basal ganglia input, are allowed to exert an abnormal level of influence.

Diseases of the basal ganglia typically involve involuntary movements, disorders of muscle tone, and both reductions and exaggerations in the extent of movement. Hypokinesia or reduced activity is a prevalent symptom in some basal ganglia disorders, particularly Parkinson's disease. It is distinguished from paralysis in that it can occur without significant weakness. Another motor symptom that may have an origin similar to hypokinesia is bradykinesia. Bradykinesia refers to a reduced velocity of movement and a slowed speed of reaction.

Rigidity is a disorder of muscle tone, which unlike spasticity, shows a uniform amount of stiffness in response to passive movements. It is often present in the oral-facial musculature of parkinsonian individuals, and it may contribute to bradykinesic speech movements. A recent investigation of this issue by Hunker, Abbs, and Barlow (1982) is discussed in a later section of this chapter.

Another prominent sign of Parkinson's disease is tremor. Generally, tremor refers to an involuntary oscillatory movement. A distinction is made between normal and pathologic tremor; the former typically occurs at frequencies of 8 to 12 Hz, and the latter at frequencies of 3 to 6 Hz, although there can be overlap in these ranges. For example, on prolonged sustained activation of a muscle, nonimpaired subjects will show a downward shift in tremor frequency to approximately 4 Hz and an increase in tremor amplitude (Gottlieb & Lippold, 1983; Stiles, 1976). The mechanisms of tremor have been associated with reflex, central oscillatory, and mechanical factors (Stein & Lee, 1981).

Three types of pathologic tremor are usually distinguished: resting, postural, and action. Resting tremor is quite characteristic of Parkinson's disease, and as the name implies, is present when a structure is not maintaining a fixed posture or executing a movement. Postural tremor occurs during maintenance of a fixed posture, and action tremor during volitional movement. Recently, Hunker and Abbs (1984) performed spectral analyses of these various forms of tremor in the oral-facial muscles of parkinsonian subjects. A prominent oscillation or spectral peak was observed at 4 to 5 Hz during resting tremor and at 9 Hz in postural and action tremor. They suggest that this fluctuation in tremor frequency with muscle task may contribute to a dynamic variation in disruption of speech control, since different speech components are undergoing continuous changes between resting, postural, and action states during speech.

Basal ganglia disorders are sometimes characterized by exaggerated or hyperkinetic movement. Three major forms of hyperkinesia are chorea, athetosis, and dystonia. Chorea refers to rapid, unpredictable movements which may be simple or complex in form. Athetosis refers to an inability to maintain a fixed posture due to slow involuntary movements. Chorea and athetosis are sometimes seen in combination in individuals with Huntington's chorea, a condition involving degeneration of the striatal neurons. The concept of dystonia is closely related to athetosis, and generally refers to a postural exaggeration of an athetoid-like movement.

Cerebellar Dysfunction

Lesions of the cerebellum in humans result primarily in conditions of ataxia and hypotonia. Ataxia refers to a disorder of volitional movement that involves errors in rate, range, force, and direction of movement (Holmes, 1979, Thatch, 1980). The ataxic individual often overshoots spatial targets with the limbs and then produces excessively large corrective movements. When these corrective movements become rhythmic, they are termed *intention tremor*, which is most marked at the end of movements. Other terms used to describe ataxic behavior are *asynergia*, a lack of muscle coordination, and *dysmetria*, errors in the range of movement.

The cerebellum is believed to be responsible for much of the automatic nature of motor behavior. This is strongly suggested by the observations of Holmes (1979) on individuals having ipsilateral cerebellar lesions. One of his patients who had a lesion in the right side of the cerebellum commented that, "the movements of my left hand are done subconsciously, but I have to think out each movement of my right arm." The loss of automaticity is reflected in a "decomposition of movement, or the performance of actions in successive parts rather than as a whole" (Thach, 1980, p. 847).

The decomposition of movement is borne out in the speech patterns of individuals having dysarthria in association with cerebellar lesion. For example, it has been observed in cases of cerebellar ataxia that syllable durations are lengthened and that the durations of unstressed syllables are disproportionately long (Kent, Netsell, & Abbs, 1979; Kent & Rosenbek, 1982). Kent and Rosenbek note that individuals with left-hemisphere lesions show similar prolongations of syllabic duration. This implies involvement of common corticocerebellar circuitry in cerebellar ataxia and cortically based dysarthria and apraxia.

Hypotonia, or a reduced resistance to passive movement, is another symptom common in human cerebellar disorders. It is believed to result from reduced activity of both alpha and gamma motoneurons (Gilman, 1970). It has been suggested by some that hypotonia is the primary deficit or negative symptom in cerebellar dysfunction and that ataxic symptoms are a secondary or positive symptom. Others suggest that the principal function of the cerebellum is coordination and that ataxic symptoms are primary in cerebellar disorders. Thach (1980) indicates that this dispute is largely semantic, as "none of the observed deficits provides an unmistakable clue to the nature of cerebellar function" (p. 849).

PHYSIOLOGICAL ANALYSIS OF DYSARTHRIC SPEECH

Physiological analysis of the peripheral aspects of speech production can provide both an indirect means of studying the neuromotor mechanisms underlying dysarthria and an improved basis for clinical assessment of individual cases of dysarthria. In this section, research involving electromyographic, movement, aerodynamic, and acoustic analysis is reviewed. The primary goal of this review is to illustrate the current approaches toward the physiological study of dysarthria, and to indicate the relevance of certain types of data for research and clinical practice with the dysarthrias. Some of the described measurement techniques can be used to provide feedback to dysarthric speakers during treatment, or for research into the efficacy of different biofeedback procedures (Rubow, 1984).

Electromyographic Studies

Electromyography (EMG) has considerable potential as a tool for describing speech muscle function in dysarthria. However, because of their small size and complex geometry, many of the speech muscles are difficult to isolate in EMG recording, and interpretation of speech muscle EMG data should be carefully considered in relation to the operational criteria used to associate EMG signals with particular muscles (Blair & Smith, 1986). For some research problems, correct association of EMG signals with a particular muscle may be of secondary importance. For example, in group comparison studies, it may be acceptable to record from more than one muscle with an electrode, provided one ensures that the electrode pick-up fields are equivalent in the two subject populations (e.g., Neilson & O'Dwyer, 1984). However, studies that address aspects of function such as cocontraction of antagonist muscles may require the use of more restricted electrode pick-up fields and operational criteria that greatly limit the potential for contribution of more than one muscle to the recording (e.g., McClean, Goldsmith, & Cerf, 1984).

Several descriptive analyses of lip muscle activity in parkinsonian dysarthria have been performed (Hunker, Abbs, & Barlow, 1982; Leanderson, Meyerson, & Persson, 1972; Netsell, Daniel, & Celesia, 1975). Consistent observations in these studies are that background or resting EMG levels are heightened and that reciprocal actions of antagonist muscles are reduced. These EMG characteristics may underly the rigidity and hypokinesia typical of parkinsonian dysarthria.

Recently, Neilson and O'Dwyer (1984) reported a quantitative analysis of EMG signal-to-noise ratios in the oral-facial muscles of athetoid cerebral palsy and nonimpaired speakers. Their method involves signal averaging the reproducible component and noise in 20 repetitions of the same utterance. As expected, they observed greater EMG levels and variability in the athetoid group; but surprisingly, the signal-to-noise ratios were equivalent in the two groups (see Figure 2-6). Neilson and O'Dwyer interpret this latter finding in relation to possible sensory deficits in motor programming, rather than pathological muscle states such as rigidospasticity, spasm, and involuntary movement.

One approach to quantitative EMG analysis which may be effectively applied to the study of speech motor disorders involves analysis of reflex responses to imposed structural displacements. Studies of this type on limb muscles in parkinsonian subjects indicate that long-latency reflexes, which are assumed to be mediated over the sensorimotor cortex, have exaggerated magnitudes (Mortimer & Webster, 1978; Tatton, Beddingham, Verrier, & Blair, 1984). It is suggested that this heightened reflex sensitivity contributes to muscle rigidity. In the future, EMG reflex testing paradigms may be applied to the study of speech muscle systems in dysarthric individuals in order to address similar issues relative to speech motor control.

Speech Muscle Function in Nonspeech Tasks

A standard approach to dysarthria assessment has been to obtain measures of speech muscle function during nonspeech tasks (cf. Darley, Aronson, & Brown, 1975; Enderby, 1983; Rosenbek & LaPointe, 1985). This technique permits observation of speech-mechanism structures such as the tongue and jaw in relative isolation during tasks that are less complex and interactive than during contextual speech. Darley and colleagues identified features of neuromuscular function that they believed to be "most influential upon the adequate production of motor speech" (p. 69). These include muscle strength, speed of movement, range of excursion, accuracy of movement, motor steadiness, and tone. An important issue for future research in dysarthria concerns the extent to which features such as these are more or less salient for speech motor control.

Quantitative analyses of nonspeech movement in dysarthria have been undertaken only recently (Barlow & Abbs, 1984; Dworkin, Aronson, &

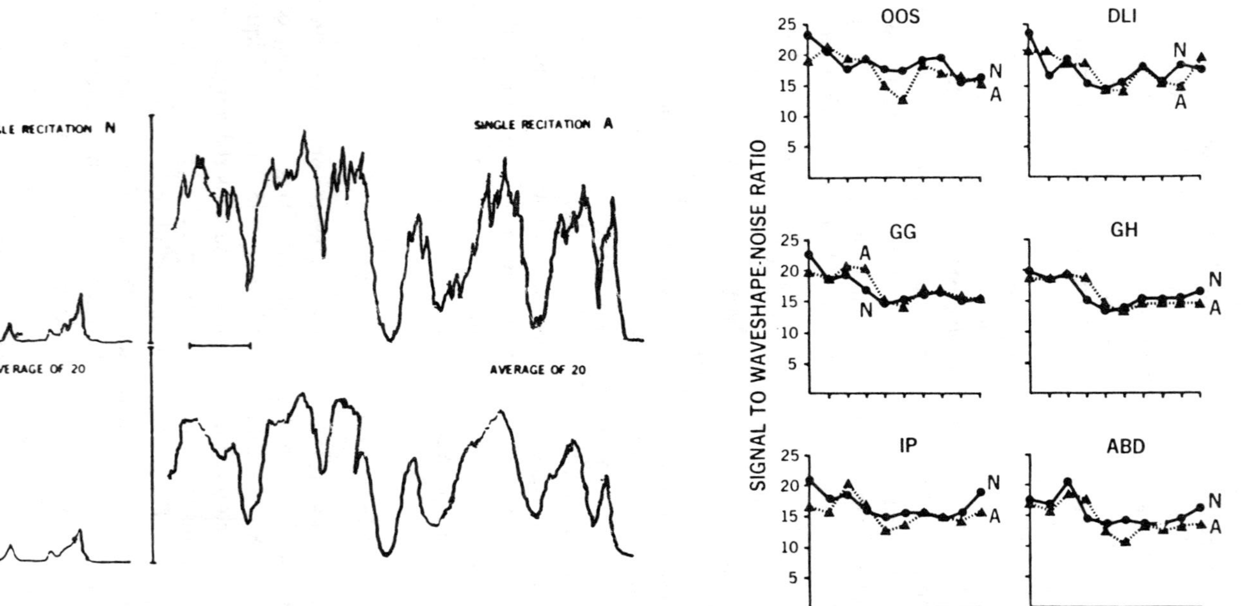

Figure 2-6. Comparison of oral-facial muscle EMG activity in normal subjects, N, and athetoid subjects, A, during repetitions of the test sentence, "Do all old rogues abjure weird ladies?" (A) Waveforms recorded from the orbicularis oris inferior muscle for a single recitation and after signal averaging 20 repetitions. The calibrations are 1 second and 0-100% maximum voluntary contraction. (B) The signal to noise-waveshape ratios for the two subject groups for various muscles as derived from the type of data shown in (A). Abbreviations: OOS - orbicularis oris inferior, DLI - depressor labii inferior, GG - genioglossus, GH - geniohyoid, IP - internal pterygoid, ABD - anterior belly of digrastric. (From Neilson & O'Dwyer, 1984, with permission.)

Mulder, 1980; Hunker et al., 1982; Hunker & Abbs, 1984; McClean, Beukelman, & Yorkston, 1987; Putnam & Hixon, 1984). These studies involve the use of force and/or displacement transducers which are coupled to the muscle systems of interest. Subjects are instructed to execute a well-defined nonspeech task, and objective measures are obtained on the recorded signals.

The potential value of this approach is well illustrated by the studies of Barlow and Abbs (1983; 1984), who have used force transducers to evaluate the motor performance of the lips, jaw, and tongue in adult spastic and parkinsonian dysarthrics. In their procedure, subjects are presented with step-like changes in a visual target and asked to generate matching changes in tongue, jaw, or lip force as quickly as possible. Level of performance is measured in terms of variability in the force signal. In general, they have observed marked differential impairment across the various speech muscle systems within and between subjects. Typical data are illustrated in Figure 2-7. Panel A in this figure illustrates differences in tremor magnitude of three muscle systems of a subject with Parkinson's disease. Panel B shows differences in force stability in an individual with spastic symptoms. In spastic subjects, Barlow and Abbs have noted the greatest levels of force instability at low force levels which correspond to those used in speech production. An important aspect of their work is that it demonstrates the feasibility of evaluating different speech muscle systems with the same procedures and quantitative techniques.

The degree of learning and goals of output associated with speech and nonspeech movement are quite different. Thus, one might reasonably question the value of nonspeech testing for assessment and remediation with the dysarthrias. However, if the speech-nonspeech distinction is viewed as a continuum (cf. Netsell, 1983), then it becomes an important area of study that may lead to useful refinements in procedures for assessing muscle system function for speech. A logical approach to work in this area is to obtain concurrent speech and nonspeech movement control data on the same individuals.

To date, few studies of dysarthria have involved quantification of speech muscle system performance in speech and nonspeech tasks. A notable exception is an investigation of lip rigidity and speech hypokinesia in a group of adult parkinsonian subjects (Hunker et al., 1982). Rigidity was quantified as a stiffness coefficient derived by applying specified forces independently to the upper and lower lips, and measuring the magnitude of lip displacement. Lip displacement during speech was transduced in the superior-inferior dimension by means of a head-mounted strain gauge transducer system. A strong positive association was noted between degree of resting rigidity and degree of hypokinesia during speech. The hypokinesia may have resulted in part from the rigidity, but both the hypokinesia and rigidity could represent positive symptoms having a common neural mechanism.

Rather than being a positive or negative neurological symptom, a sign of neuromotor dysfunction during speech production may represent a compensation to an impaired neural mechanism (cf. Hixon, Putnam, & Sharp,

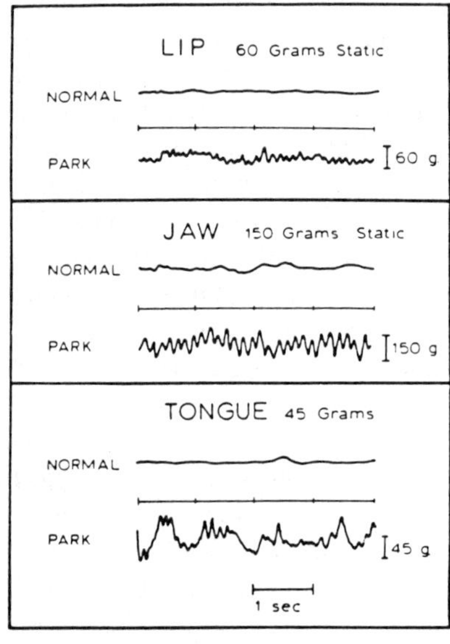

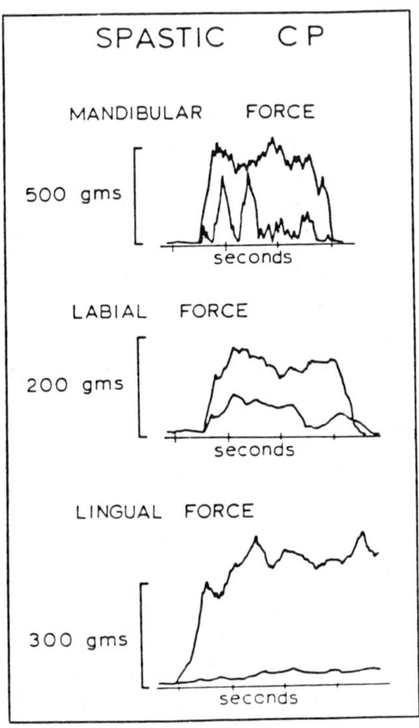

Figure 2-7. Records of lip, jaw, and tongue fine-force control in normal, parkinsonian, and spastic subjects. Panel A illustrates differences in tremor magnitude and frequency across the three muscle systems of a parkinsonian subject. Panel B shows evidence of differential impairment across different muscle systems in an individual with spastic symptoms. For the jaw, there also appeared to be a more marked impairment in force control at low static force levels. (From Barlow & Abbs, 1983, with permission.)

1983; Kent et al., 1979). This possibility points up the extreme difficulty of inferring the nature of neural mechanisms underlying disordered muscle function for speech. Quantitative assessment of speech-muscle function in both speech and nonspeech tasks may provide a valid approach to this problem with some forms of dysarthria.

Speech Structure Movement

Deviant movements of the speech structures underly the various acoustic events that we identify as dysarthric speech. Fortunately, it is now quite practical with electronic transducers to obtain records of lip, jaw, and chest wall displacements during speech. The tongue, velum, larynx, and pharyngeal walls are less accessible and require ultrasound, cineradiography, or endoscopic techniques.

A widely used method for recording lip and jaw movements for speech involves the use of resistive-wire strain gauges (Abbs & Gilbert, 1973). A recent head-mounted version of this type of system is illustrated in Figure 2-8 (Barlow, Cole, & Abbs, 1983). This system has particular promise for work with the dysarthrias, because it eliminates possible signal contamination due to involuntary head movements which are likely to occur in association with some forms of dysarthria.

Figure 2-9 illustrates the type of records obtained from a head-mounted strain gauge system (Barlow & Abbs, 1983). These data were recorded in an adult cerebral-palsied individual under two speaking conditions: (1) with the jaw free to move, and (2) with the jaw fixed. Clearly, a more stable pattern of lip displacement and oral pressure variation was achieved with the jaw fixed. This suggests that quantification of speech structure movement during different remediation or management conditions has some promise as a clinical technique with the dysarthrias.

Chest wall movements during speech may be recorded with mercury strain gauges (Baken, 1977), inductive coil systems (Hunker, Bless, & Weismer, 1981),

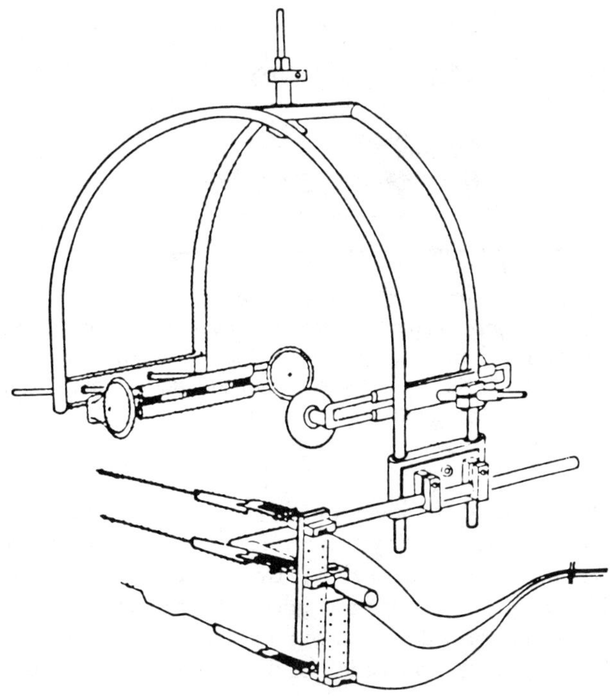

Figure 2-8. Line drawing of a head-mounted strain gauge transducer system (From Barlow, Cole, & Abbs, 1983, with permission.)

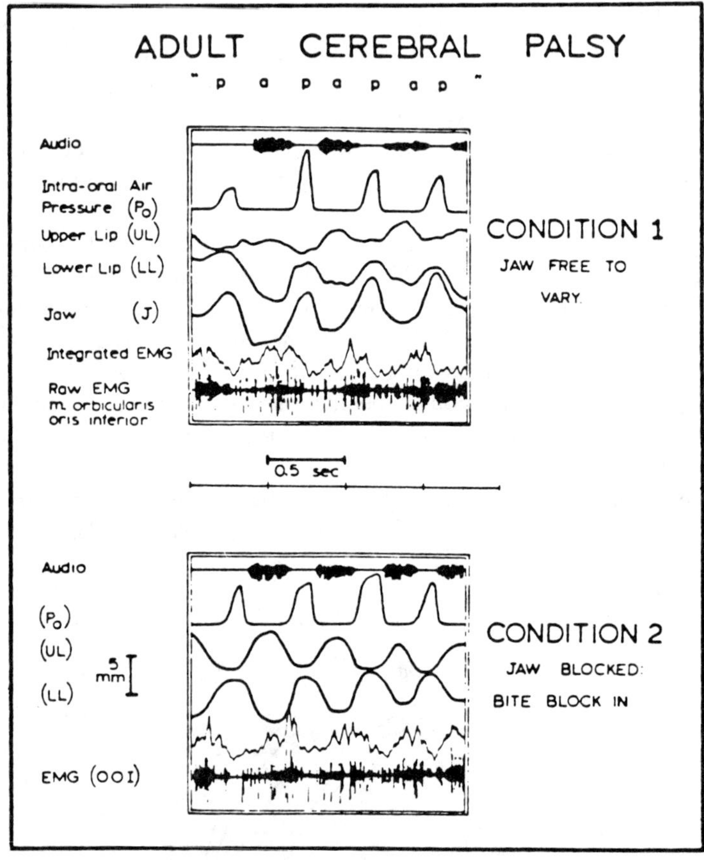

Figure 2-9. Oscillographic plots of audio and various physiologic signals associated with repetitions of the syllable /pɑ/ by a cerebral palsied subject under jaw-free and jaw-fixed conditions. The lip and jaw displacement records were obtained with the type of system illustrated in Figure 2-8. (From Barlow, Cole, & Abbs, 1983, with permission.)

or magnetometers (Hixon, Goldman, & Mead, 1976). The magnetometer has been the most extensively used system for describing displacements of the rib cage and abdominal wall during speech in dysarthric individuals (Hixon, 1982; Putnam & Hixon, 1984). The magnetometer system consists of pairs of electromagnetic coils that provide a voltage proportional to the distance between the coils. Effective clinical application of this system is illustrated by a recent case study involving assessment of the chest wall movement patterns of an individual with acute poliomyelitis (Hixon et al., 1983). The individual had no control of the thoracic and abdominal musculature normally used to regulate lung volume changes required for speech. In spite of this loss, he generated perceptually normal speech through the judicious use of clavicular and glossopharyngeal breathing. Careful description of successful compensation strategies such as this may have benefit in the remediation efforts with individuals having similar types of impairment.

During speech production various muscle groups function in a highly unified and synergistic manner to achieve intended aerodynamic and acoustic targets (cf. Grillner, Lindblom, Lubker, & Persson, 1982). From this perspective it may be especially important to obtain simultaneous measures on the movements of several speech structures in the description of dysarthria. Such data are illustrated in Figure 2-10, which shows the vertical motions of four articulators during two repetitions of the same utterance as produced by a 59 year old lady with progressive ataxic dysarthria (Kent & Netsell, 1975). These data were obtained from cineradiographic films shot at 28 frames/sec. A striking feature of the data is the consistency of coordination in the two productions. Kent and Netsell interpret these data "to mean that this ataxic speaker often was capable of coordinated, synergistic movements for speech, despite an abnormally slow speaking rate" (p. 122).

A new radiological method known as X-ray microbeam now permits tracking of several points along the vocal tract with the use of very minimal levels of radiation. Hirose, Kiritani, and Sawashima (1982) have applied the X-ray microbeam in describing the articulatory velocity patterns of the lips, jaw, tongue, and soft palate in a diverse group of dysarthric subjects. Their observations suggest that variability of structural velocity during syllable repetition may be a useful indicator of dysarthria type. In the future, the X-ray microbeam may be of particular value in describing compensatory trade-offs among speech muscle systems in individual cases of dysarthria.

The concept of motor compensation is especially important in the area of dysarthria. Individuals may suffer differing degrees of impairment among various speech muscle systems (cf. Abbs et al., 1983), and develop compensatory movement patterns with their more intact systems. Although it seems likely that muscle system synergy and compensation is a fundamental feature of the speech production mechanism, it has yet to be widely studied in a manner that would permit its optimal use in remediation of dysarthria.

Speech Aerodynamics

The immediate result of speech structure movements are precise changes in air pressure and airflow rates within the upper and lower respiratory airways. These processes are briefly discussed here; however, the reader is referred to Chapters 6 and 8 on respiration and velopharyngeal function for more detailed descriptions of speech aerodynamics.

Sustained phonation and conversational speech require relatively constant subglottal pressures of 3 to 10 cm H_20. The capacity of the respiratory pump to generate such pressures may be readily assessed in cases of dysarthria

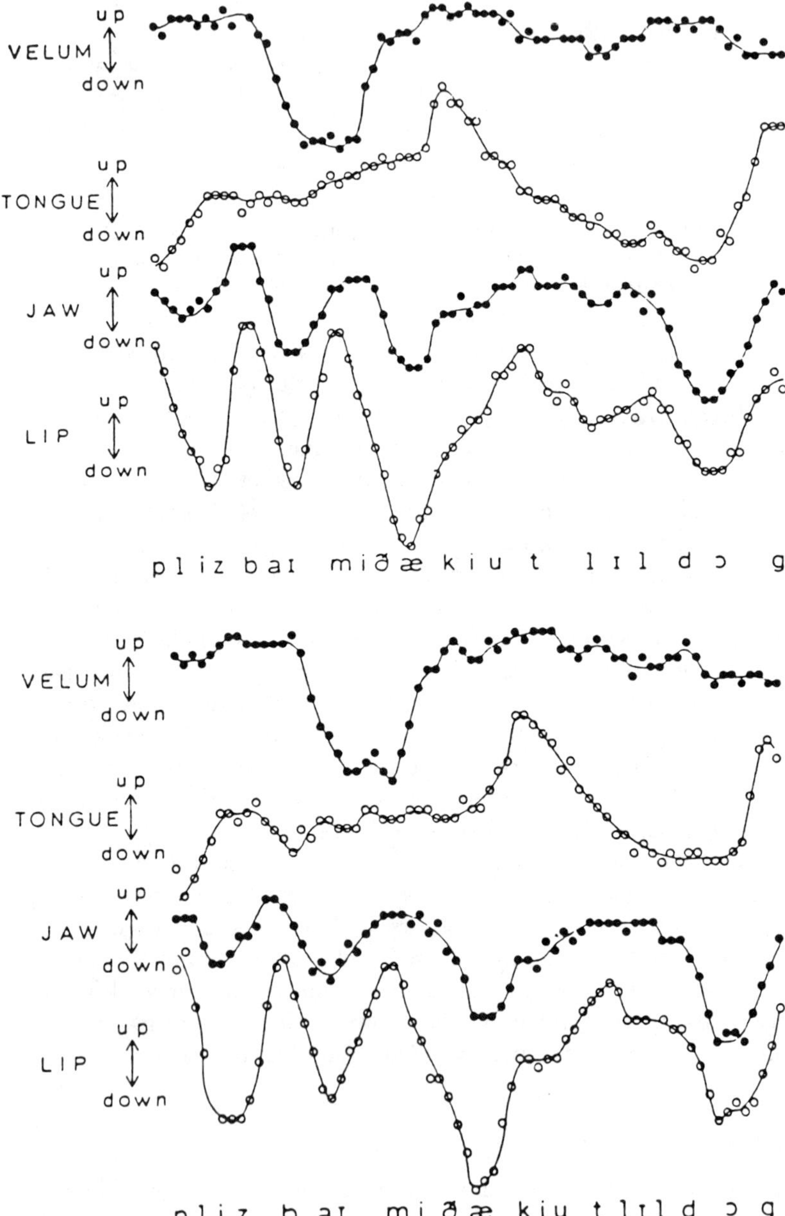

Figure 2-10. Vertical motion plots of four articulatory points as derived from lateral cineradiographic films of an ataxic speaker producing the same sentence twice (top and bottom of figure). The film speed was 28 frames/sec, and each data point is separated on the ordinate by approximately 37 msec. (From Kent & Netsell, 1975, with permission.)

by means of a U-tube manometer fitted with a leak tube simulating glottal resistance (Netsell & Hixon, 1978; Rosenbek & LaPointe, 1985). Maintenance of relatively constant subglottal pressures must occur against rapid changes in laryngeal and supralaryngeal valving. This process may involve elaborate neurophysiological mechanisms (e.g., reflexive load compensation) acting on rib cage and abdominal musculature (Hixon, 1973).

Major speech sound classes are normally associated with unique patterns of oropharyngeal pressure, oral airflow rate, and nasal airflow rate (cf. Netsell, 1973; Warren, 1982). The general value of aerodynamic measures for evaluating dysarthric speech patterns is illustrated by various descriptive studies of the dysarthrias (Gracco & Muller, 1981; Netsell, 1969). It is now practical, with modern electronic transducers, to obtain records of vocal tract pressures and airflows during speech in dysarthric individuals. An example from Gracco and Muller (1981) of oral pressure and airflow records from a normal and a dysarthric speaker is illustrated in Figure 2-11. These records were obtained during production of /ɑpɑ/. Increased oral pressure with neglible airflow may be noted during the occlusion phase of the /p/. It may be seen that the peak pressure values are equivalent in the two speakers; however, the time-varying aspects of the pressure wave are quite different. Gracco and Muller emphasize the value of measuring pressure waveform parameters other than just peak amplitude.

Computer modeling of speech mechanism biomechanics may provide a valid basis for inferring the nature of kinematic events underlying the pressure and flow patterns in speech (Muller & Brown, 1980). Gracco and Muller (1981) utilized this approach in analyzing stop consonant production in spastic dysarthria. Using the type of pressure and airflow data shown in Figure 2-11, they matched individual aerodynamic profiles with computer-simulated outputs to explain the likely patterns of abnormal respiratory, laryngeal, and articulatory control among individual dysarthric speakers. This approach has considerable promise for aerodynamic analysis of dysarthric speech.

Speech Acoustics

The acoustic speech signal is a very important source of information for objective description of aspects of speech movement control in dysarthria. Rapid changes in manner of articulation are often reflected by clear boundaries in spectrographic and oscilloscopic acoustic records. This makes it practical to obtain objective measures of speech sound segments in dysarthria (Kent et al., 1979; Kent & Rosenbek, 1982; Lehiste, 1965; Ludlow & Bassich, 1984; Weismer, 1984a, 1984b; Yorkston, Beukelman, Minifie, & Sapir, 1984). However, the acoustic features classically used to identify speech-segment boundaries may be distorted in dysarthric speech, thus requiring more qualitative approaches to describing the acoustic speech signal. In an analysis of voiceless stop consonants, Weismer (1984b) recently noted a high frequency of stop closure intervals with significant voicing or spirantization, that is, presence of aperiodic noise. This was most prominent in parkinsonian subjects,

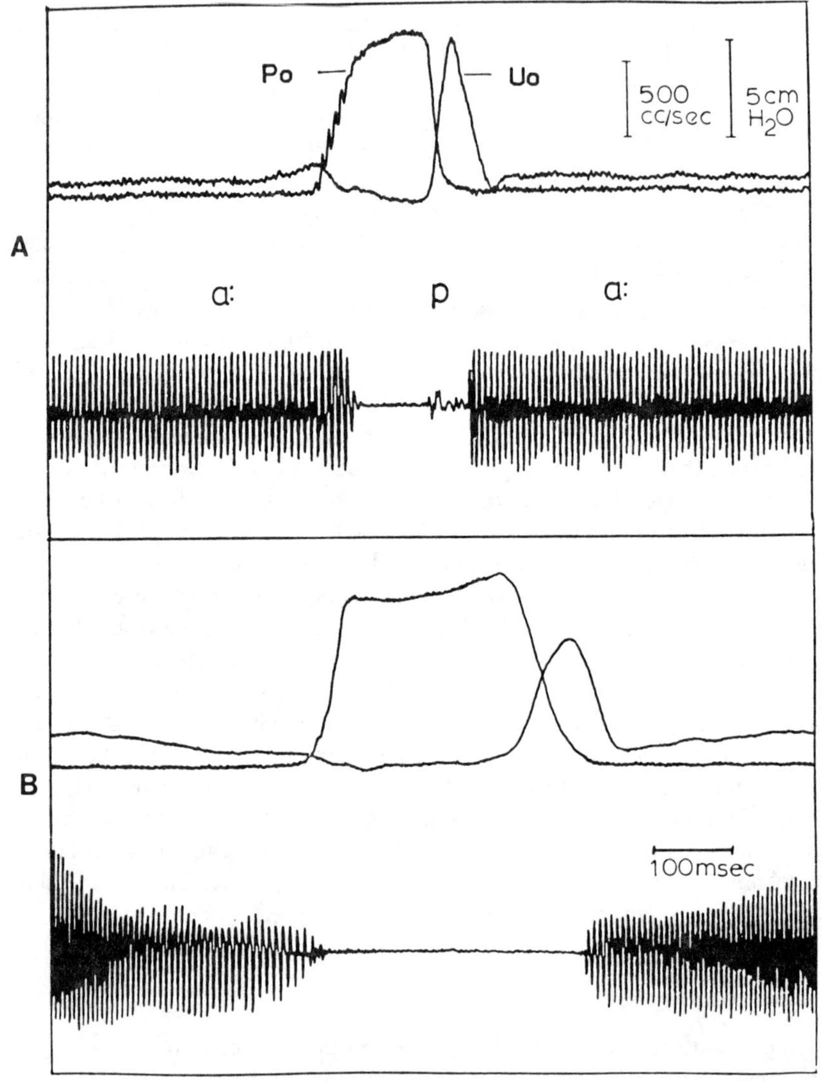

Figure 2-11. Aerodynamic and audio signal records obtained during productions of /ɑpɑ/ by a nonimpaired and dysarthric speaker. P_0 refers to oral pressure in centimeters of water and U_0 to oral airflow rate in cubic centimeters per second. (From Gracco & Muller, 1981, with permission.)

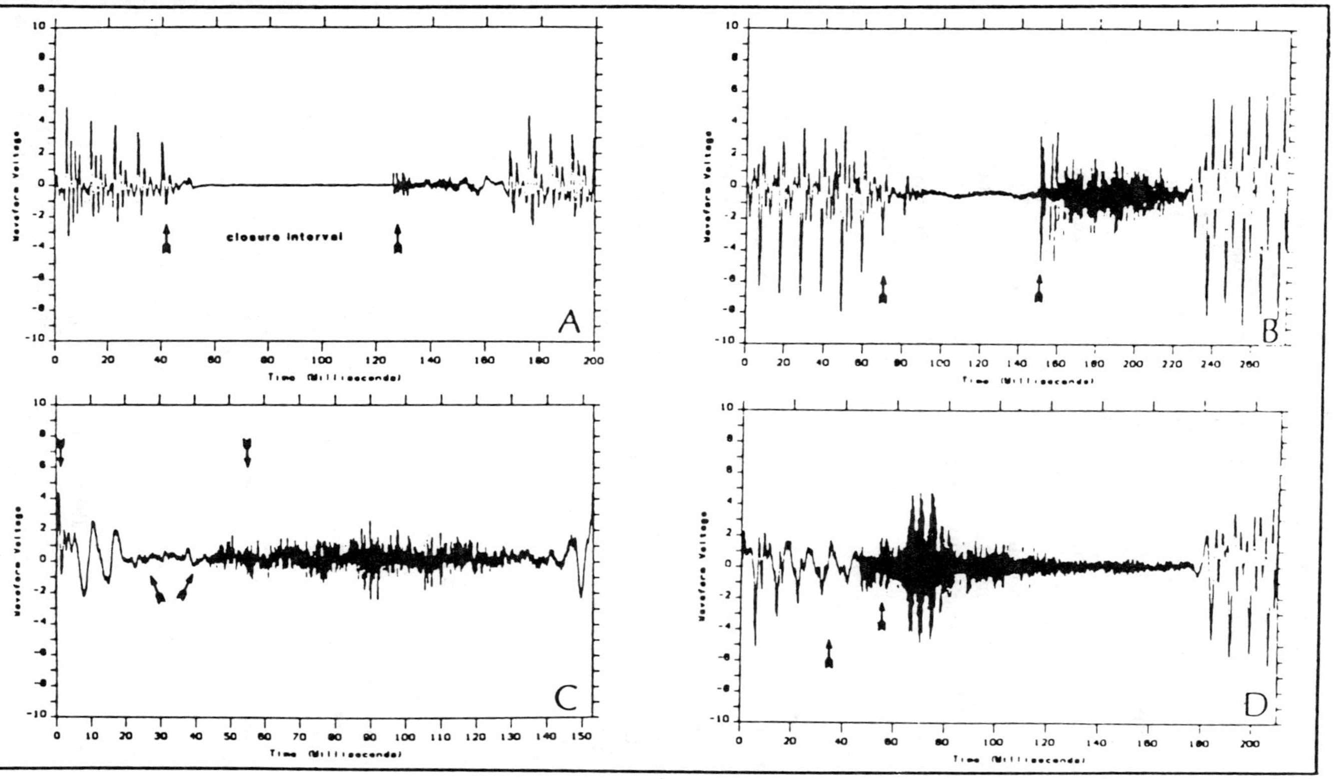

Figure 2-12. Oscilloscopic records illustrating various forms of spirantization on the stop consonants. The waveform in panel A was judged to be "nonspirantized" and the others "spirantized." In each panel the bottom arrow on the left indicates the onset of the closure interval, and in panels A and B the right arrows indicates indicate the stop burst. The raised arrows in C and D indicate spirantized portions of the waveforms. (From Weismer, 1984, with permission.)

but it was also seen in geriatric subjects, and to a lesser degree, in young adults. Figure 2-12 illustrates oscillographic plots from Weismer's research showing different patterns of spirantization on stop consonants. Panel A shows a "nonspiratized" stop closure interval, and the three remaining panels illustrate "spiratized" closure intervals. This analysis was performed with a storage oscilloscope, an instrument well-suited for efficient measurement of sound segment durations and provision of acoustic feedback during treatment.

In addition to segmental duration measures, a wide range of acoustic parameters related to laryngeal control may be extracted by means of spectrographic, oscillographic, or computer-based analysis; for example, fundamental frequency range, glottal amplitude and period perturbation (Ludlow & Bassich, 1984), and harmonic-to-noise ratio (Yumoto, Sasaki, & Okamura, 1984). It is also possible to approximate the temporal and spatial aspects of vocal tract area in dysarthric speech patterns from measures of vowel formant frequency (Kent et al., 1979) or fricative-consonant spectral pattern (Weismer, 1984a).

Given the vast literature on normal aspects of speech acoustics and the relative ease with which acoustic recordings can be obtained, it seems appropriate that more extensive use be made of acoustic analysis of dysarthric speech patterns. As noted by Weismer (1984a), the acoustic speech signal provides information about both the speech production process and its likely effects on the listener. Improved acoustic descriptions of the various dysarthrias should provide important direction for aerodynamic, movement, and EMG studies, since the acoustic signal contains the essential target information of the speech production process.

REFERENCES

Abbs, J. (in press). Invariance and variability in speech production: A distinction between linguistic intent and its neuromotor implementation. In J. Perkell & D. Klatt (Eds.), Invariance and variability of speech processes. Hillsdale, NJ: Lawrence Erlbaum Associates.

Abbs, J., & Gilbert, B. (1973). A strain gage transduction system for lip and jaw motion in two dimensions: Design and calibration data. *Journal of Speech & Hearing Research, 16,* 248–256.

Abbs, J., & Gracco, V. (1984). Control of complex motor gestures: Orofacial muscle responses to load perturbations of the lip during speech. *Journal of Neurophysiology, 52,* 705–723.

Abbs, J., Hunker, C., & Barlow, S. (1983). Differential speech motor subsystem impairments with suprabulbar lesions: Neurophysiological framework and supporting data. In W. Berry (Ed.), *Clinical dysarthria.* Austin, TX: PRO-ED.

Abbs, J., & Welt, C. (1985). Structure and function of the lateral precentral cortex: Significance for speech motor control. In R. Daniloff (Ed.), *Speech science: Recent advances.* San Diego: College-Hill Press.

Adams, R. (1973). Muscular hypertonia—the clinical viewpoint. In J. Desmedt (Ed.), *New developments in electromyography and clinical neurophysiology.* Basel: Karger.

Adams, R., & Victor, M. (1985). *Principles of neurology.* New York: McGraw-Hill.

Anderson, M., & Horak, F. (1985). Influence of globus pallidus on arm movement-related information. *Journal of Neurophysiology, 54,* 433–448.

Asanuma, H. (1975). Recent developments in the study of the columnar arrangement of neurons within the motor cortex. *Physiological Reviews, 55,* 143–156.

Baken, R. (1977). Estimation of lung volume change from torso hemicircumferences. *Journal of Speech and Hearing Research, 20,* 808–812.

Barlow, S., & Abbs, J. (1983). Force transducers for the evaluation of labial, lingual, and mandibular motor impairments. *Journal of Speech and Hearing Research, 26,* 616–621.

Barlow, S., & Abbs, J. (1984). Orofacial fine motor control impairments in congenital spasticity: Evidence against hypertonus related performance deficits. *Journal of Neurology, 34,* 145–150.

Barlow, S., Cole, K., & Abbs, J. (1983). A new headmounted lip-jaw movement transduction system for the study of motor speech disorders. *Journal of Speech and Hearing Research, 26,* 283–288.

Blair, C., & Smith, A. (1986). EMG recording from human lip muscles: Can single muscles be isolated? *Journal of Speech and Hearing Research, 29,* 256–265.

Borden, G. (1979). An interpretation of research on feedback interruption in speech. *Brain and Language, 7,* 307–319.

Bowman, J. (1982). Lingual mechanoreceptive information I. An evoked-potential study of the central projections of hypoglossal nerve afferent information. *Journal of Speech and Hearing Research, 25,* 348–356.

Bratzlavsky, M. (1976). Human brainstem reflexes. In M. Shahani (Ed.), *The motor system: Neurophysiology and muscle mechanism.* New York: Elsevier North Holland.

Brooks, V. (1979). Control of intended movements by the lateral and intermediate cerebellum. In H. Asanuma & V. Wilson (Eds.), *Integration in the nervous system.* Tokyo: Igaku-Shoin.

Burke, R., & Edgerton, V. (1975). Motor unit properties and selective involvement in movement. In J. Wilmore & J. Keogh (Eds.), *Exercise and Sports Sciences Reviews* (Vol. 3). New York: Academic Press.

Carpenter, M. (1976). *Human neuroanatomy.* Baltimore: Williams & Wilkins.

Clamman, H.P. (1981). Motor units and their activity during movement. In A. Towe & E. Luschei (Eds.), *Handbook of neurobiology: Motor coordination.* New York: Plenum Press.

Cooker, H., Larson, C., & Luschei, E. (1980). Evidence that the human jaw stretch reflex increases the resistance of the mandible to small displacements. *Journal of Physiology, 308,* 61–78.

Darley, F., Aronson, A., & Brown, S. (1975). *Motor speech disorders.* Philadelphia: W.B.Saunders.

Delong, M., & Georgopoulous, A. (1981). Motor control functions of the basal ganglia. In V. Brooks (Ed.), *Handbook of physiology: Section 1. The nervous system: Vol. 2, Motor Control* (pp. 1017–1061). Bethesda, MD: American Physiological Society.

DeLong, M., Georgopoulos, A., & Crutcher, M. (1983). Cortico-basal ganglia relations and coding of motor performance. *Experimental Brain Research,* (Suppl. 7), 30–40.

DeLuca, C. (1978). Towards understanding the EMG signal. In J. Basmajian, *Muscles alive.* Baltimore: Williams & Wilkins.

Desmedt, J. (1973-1982). Progress in clinical neurophysiology, (Vols. 1–10). Basel: Karger.

Desmedt, J. (1981). The size principle of motoneuron recruitment in ballistic or ramp voluntary contractions in man. In J. Desmedt (Ed.), *Progress in clinical neurophysiology* (Vol. 9). Basel: Karger.

Desmedt, J., & Godaux, E. (1981). Spinal motoneuron recruitment in man: Rank deordering with direction but not with speed of voluntary movement. *Science, 214,* 933–936.

Draper, M., Ladefoged, P., & Whitteridge, D. (1959). Respiratory muscles in speech. *Journal of Speech & Hearing Research, 2,* 16–27.

Dubner, R., Sessle, B., & Storey, A. (1978). *The neural basis of oral and facial function.* New York: Plenum Press.

Dworkin, J., Aronson, A., & Mulder, D. (1980). Tongue force in normals and in dysarthric patients with amyotrophic lateral sclerosis. *Journal of Speech and Hearing Research, 23,* 828–837.

Eccles, J. (1977). *Understanding the brain.* New York: McGraw-Hill.

Enderby, P. (1983). *Frenchay dysarthria assessment.* Austin, TX: PRO-ED.

Evarts, E. (1969). Activity of pyramidal tract neurons during postural fixation. *Journal of Neurophysiology, 32,* 375–385.

Fant, G. (1960). *Acoustic theory of speech production.* The Hague: Mouton.

Feldman, R., Young, R., & Koella, W. (1980). *Spasticity: Disordered movement control.* Chicago: Yearbook Medical Publishers.

Folkins, J., & Abbs, J. (1975). Lip and jaw motor control during speech: Responses to resistive loading of the jaw. *Journal of Speech and Hearing Research, 18,* 207–220.

Forssberg, H. (1979). Stumbling corrective reaction: A phase dependent compensatory reaction during locomotion. *Journal of Neurophysiology, 42,* 936–953.

Freund, H. (1983). Motor unit and muscle activity in voluntary motor control. *Physiological Reviews, 63,* 387–436.

Fromkin, V. (1966). Neuromuscular specification of linguistic units. *Language and Speech, 9,* 170–199.

Gilman, S. (1970). The nature of cerebellar dysynergia. In D. Williams (Ed.), *Modern trends in neurology.* London: Butterworths.

Gottlieb, S., & Lippold, C. (1983). The 4-6 Hz tremor during sustained contraction in normal human subjects. *Journal of Physiology, 336,* 499–509.

Gracco, V., & Abbs, J. (1985). Dynamic control of the perioral system during speech: Kinematic analyses of autogenic and nonautogenic sensorimotor processes. *Journal of Neurophysiology, 54,* 418–432.

Gracco, V., & Abbs, J. (in press). Programming and execution processes of speech movement control: Potential neural correlates. In E. Keller & M. Gopnik (Eds.), *Symposium on motor and sensory language processes.* Hillsdale, NJ: Lawrence Erlbaum Associates.

Gracco, V., & Muller, E. (1981). *Analysis of supraglottal air pressure variations in spastic dysarthria.* Paper presented at the Convention of the American Speech-Language-Hearing Association, Los Angeles, CA.

Grillner, S., Lindblom, B., Lubker, B., & Persson, A. (1982). *Speech motor control.* Oxford: Pergamon Press.

Henneman, E. (1980). Organization of the motoneuron pool: The size principle. In V. Mountcastle (Ed.), *Medical physiology.* St. Louis: C.V. Mosby.

Hirose, H., Kiritani, S., & Sawashima, M. (1982). Velocity of articulatory movements in normal and dysarthric subjects. *Folia Phoniatrica, 34,* 210–215.

Hixon, T. (1973). Respiratory function in speech. In F. Minifie, T. Hixon, & F. Williams (Eds.), *Normal aspects of speech, hearing, and language.* Englewood Cliffs, NJ: Prentice-Hall

Hixon, T. (1982). Speech breathing kinematics and mechanism inferences therefrom. In S. Grillner, B. Lindblom, J. Lubker, & A. Persson (Eds.), *Speech motor control.* Oxford: Pergamon.

Hixon, T., Goldman, M., & Mead, J. (1976). Dynamics of the chest wall during speech production: Function of the thorax, rib cage, diaphragm, and abdomen. *Journal of Speech and Hearing Research, 19,* 297–356.

Hixon, T., Putnam, A., & Sharp, J. (1983). Speech production with flaccid paralysis of the rib cage, diaphragm, and abdomen. *Journal of Speech and Hearing Disorders, 48,* 315–327.

Hoffman, D., & Luschei, E. (1980). Responses of monkey precentral cortical cells during a controlled jaw bite task. *Journal of Neurophysiology, 44,* 333–348.

Holmes, G. (1979). The cerebellum of man. In C. Phillips (Ed.), *Selected papers of Gordon Holmes.* New York: Oxford University Press.

Hughes, O., & Abbs, J. (1976). Labial-mandibular coordination in the production of speech: Implications for the operation of motor equivalence. *Phonetica, 44,* 199–221.

Hunker, C., & Abbs, J. (1984). Physiological analyses of parkinsonian tremors in the orofacial system. In M. McNeil, J. Rosenbek, & A. Aronson (Eds.), *The dysarthrias: Physiology, acoustics, perception, management.* San Diego: College-Hill Press.

Hunker, C., Abbs, J., & Barlow, S. (1982). The relationship between parkinsonian rigidity and hypokinesia in the orofacial system: A quantitative analysis. *Neurology, 32,* 755–761.

Hunker, C., Bless, D., & Weismer, G. (1981). *Respiratory inductive plethysmography: A clinical technique for assessing respiratory function for speech.* Paper presented at the Annual Convention of the American Speech-Language-Hearing Association, Los Angeles, CA.

Kent, R., & Netsell, R. (1975). A case study of an ataxic dysarthric: Cineradiographic and spectrographic observations. *Journal of Speech and Hearing Disorders. 40,* 115–134.

Kent, R., Netsell, R., & Abbs, J. (1979). Acoustic characteristics of dysarthria associated with cerebellar disease. *Journal of Speech and Hearing Research, 22,* 627–648.

Kent, R., & Rosenbek, J. (1982). Prosodic disturbance and neurologic lesion. *Brain and Language, 15,* 259–291.

Kornhuber, H. (1977). A reconsideration of the cortical and subcortical mechanisms involved in speech and aphasia. In J. Desmedt (Ed.), Language and hemisperic specialization in man: Cerebral ERP's. *Progress in Clinical Neurophysiology, 3,* 28–35.

Kuypers, H. (1958). Corticobulbar connections to the pons and lower brainstem in man: An anatomical study. *Brain, 81,* 364–388.

Lane, H., & Tranel, B. (1971). The Lombard sign and the role of hearing in speech. *Journal of Speech and Hearing Research, 14,* 677–709.

Larson, C., & Pfingst, B. (1982). Neuroanatomic basis of hearing and speech. In N. Lass, L. McReynolds, J. Northern, & D. Yoder (Eds.), *Speech, language, and hearing*. Philadelphia: W.B. Saunders.

Leanderson, R., Meyerson, B., & Persson, A. (1972). Lip muscle function in parkinsonian dysarthria. *Acta Otolaryngologica, 74,* 271–278.

Lehiste, I. (1965). Some acoustic characteristics of dysarthric speech. *Bibliotheca Phonetica, Fasc. 2.* Basel: S. Karger.

Lewis, D. (1981). The physiology of motor units in mammalian skeletal muscle. In A. Towe & E. Luschei (Eds.), *Handbook of behavioral neurobiology: Volume 5, Motor Coordination*. New York: Plenum Press.

Lindblom, B., Lubker, J., & Gay, T. (1979). Formant frequencies of some fixed-mandible vowels and a model of speech motor programming by predictive simulation. *Journal of Phonetics, 7,* 147–161.

Lindblom, B., & Sundberg, J. (1971). Acoustical consequences of lip, tongue and jaw movements. *Journal of the Acoustical Society of America, 50,* 1166–1179.

Ludlow, C., & Bassich, C. (1984). Relationships between perceptual ratings and acoustic measures of hypokinetic speech. In M. McNeil, J. Rosenbek, & A. Aronson, (Eds.), *The dysarthrias: Physiology, acoustics, perception, management.* San Diego: College Hill Press.

MacNeilage, P. (1970). Motor control of serial ordering of speech. *Psychological Reviews, 77,* 182–196.

MacNeilage, P., & DeClerk, J. (1969). On the motor control of coarticulation in CVC syllables. *Journal of the Acoustical Society of America, 45,* 1217–1233.

McClean, M. (1984). Recruitment thresholds of lower-lip motor units with changes in movement direction. *Journal of Speech and Hearing Research, 27,* 6–12.

McClean, M., Beukelman, D., & Yorkston, K. Speech-muscle visuomotor tracking in dysarthric and nonimpaired speakers. *Journal of Speech and Hearing Research, 30,* 276–282.

McClean, M., Goldsmith, H., & Cerf, A. (1984). Lower lip EMG and displacement during bilabial dysfluencies in adult stutterers. *Journal of Speech and Hearing Research, 27,* 342–349.

McClean, M., & Sapir, S. (1980). Surface EMG recording of platysma single-motor units during speech. *Journal of Phonetics, 8,* 169–173.

Minifie, F. (1973). Speech acoustics. In F. Minifie, T. Hixon, & F. Williams (Eds.), *Normal aspects of speech, hearing, and language.* Englewood Cliffs, NJ: Prentice-Hall.

Mortimer, J., & Webster, D. (1978). Relationships between quantitative measures of rigidity and tremor and the electromyographic responses to load perturbations in unselected normal subjects and Parkinson patients. In J. Desmedt (Ed.), *Progress in clinical neurophysiology* Vol. 4. Basel: Karger.

Muller, E., & Brown, S. (1980). Variations in the supraglottal air pressure waveform and their articulatory interpretation. In N. Lass (Ed.), *Speech and language: Advances in basic research and practice.* New York: Academic Press.

Muller, E., Milenkovic, P., & MacLeod, G. (1984). Perioral tissue mechanics during speech production. In C. DeLisi & J. Eisenfeld (Eds.), *Proceedings of the second IMAC international symposium on biomedical systems modeling*. New York: Elsevier North Holland.

Neilson, P., & O'Dwyer, N. (1984). Reproducibility and variability of speech muscle activity in athetoid dysarthria of cerebral palsy. *Journal of Speech and Hearing Research, 27,* 502–517.

Netsell, R. (1969). Evaluation of velopharyngeal function in dysarthria. *Journal of Speech and Hearing Disorders, 34,* 113–122.

Netsell, R. (1973). Speech physiology. In F. Minifie, T. Hixon & F. Williams (Eds.), *Normal aspects of speech, hearing, and language.* Englewood Cliffs, NJ: Prentice Hall.

Netsell, R. (1982). Speech motor control and selected neurologic disorders. In S. Grillner, B. Lindblom, J. Lubker, & A. Persson (Eds.), *Speech motor control.* Oxford: Pergammon Pres.

Netsell, R. (1983). Speech motor control: Theoretical issues with clinical impact. In W. Berry (Ed.), *Clinical dysarthria*. Austin, TX: PRO-ED.

Netsell, R., Daniel, B., & Celesia, G. (1975). Acceleration and weakness in parkinsonian dysarthria. *Journal of Speech and Hearing Disorders, 40,* 170–178.

Nestell, R., & Hixon, T. (1978). A noninvasive method for clinically estimating subglottal air pressure. *Journal of Speech and Hearing Disorders, 43,* 326–330.

Ohman, S. (1967). Peripheral motor commands in labial articulation. *Speech Transmission Laboratory—Quarterly Progress & Status Report*, Royal Institute of Technology, Stockholm, 4, 30–63.

Paillard, J. (1983). Introductory lecture: The functional labelling of neural codes. In J. Massion, J. Paillard, W. Schultz, & M. Wiesendanger (Eds.), *Neural coding of motor performance* (pp. 1–19). Berlin: Springer-Verlag.

Penfield, W., & Roberts, L. (1966). *Speech and brain mechanisms*. New York: Atheneum.

Porter, R. (1983). Neuronal activities in primary motor area and premotor regions. In J. Massion, J. Paillard, W. Schultz, & M. Wiesendanger (Eds.), *Neural coding of motor performance* (pp. 23–29). Berlin: Springer-Verlag.

Putnam, A., & Hixon, T. (1984). Respiratory kinematics in speakers with motor neuron disease. In M. McNeil, J. Rosenbek, & A. Aronson (Eds.), *The dysarthrias: Physiology, acoustics, perception, management.* San Diego: College-Hill Press.

Rosenbek, J., & LaPointe, L. (1985). The dysarthrias: Description, diagnosis and treatment. In D. Johns (Ed.), *Clinical management of neurogenic communication disorders*. Boston: Little, Brown and Company.

Rubow, R. (1984). Role of feedback, reinforcement, and compliance on training and transfer in biofeedback-based rehabilitation of motor speech disorders. In M. McNeil, J. Rosenbek, & A. Aronson (Eds.), *The dysarthrias: Physiology, acoustics, perception, management*. San Diego: College Hill Press.

Sapir, S., McClean, M., & Larson, C. (1983). Human laryngeal responses to auditory stimulation. *Journal of the Acoustical Society of America, 73,* 1070–1073.

Schmidt, E., & Thomas, J. (1981). Motor unit recruitment order: Modification under volitional control. In J. Desmedt (Ed.), *Progress in clinical neurophysiology* (Vol. 9). Basel: Karger.

Schwarting, S., Schroder, M., Stennert, E., & Goebel, H. (1982). Enzyme histochemical and histographic data on normal human facial muscles. *Otorhinolaryngology, 44,* 51–59.

Sessle, B., & Wiesendanger, M. (1982). Structural and functional definition of the motor cortex in the monkey (macaca fascicularis). *Journal of Physiology, 323,* 245–265.

Smith, A., & Luschei, E. (1983). Assessment of oral-motor reflexes in stutterers and normal speakers: Preliminary observations. *Journal of Speech and Hearing Research, 26,* 322–328.

Stein, R., & Lee, R. (1981). Tremor and clonus. In V. Brooks (Ed.), *Handbook of physiology* (Vol. 2). Bethesda, MD: American Physiological Society.

Stiles, R. (1976). Frequency and displacement amplitude relations for normal hand tremor. *Journal of Applied Physiology, 40,* 44–54.

Tatton, W., Beddingham, W., Verrier, M., & Blair, R. (1984). Characteristic alterations in the response to imposed wrist displacement in Parkinsonian rigidity and dystonia musculorum deformans. *The Canadian Journal of Neurological Sciences, 11,* 281–287.

Thach, W. (1980). The cerebellum. In V. Mountcastle (Ed.), *Medical physiology.* St. Louis: C.V. Mosby Co.

Warren, D. (1982). Aerodynamics of speech. In N. Lass, L. McReynolds, J. Northern, & D. Yoder. *Speech, language, and hearing.* Philadelphia: W.B. Saunders.

Warren, D. (1986). Compensatory speech behaviors in individuals with cleft palate: A regulation/control phenomenon? *Cleft Palate Journal, 23,* 251–260.

Weismer, G. (1984a). Acoustic descriptions of dysarthric speech: Perceptual correlates and physiological inferences. *Seminars in Speech and Language, 5,* 293–314.

Weismer, G. (1984b). Articulatory characteristics of parkinsonian dysarthria: Segmental and phrase-level timing, spirantization, and glottal-supraglottal coordination. In M. McNeil, J. Rosenbek, & A. Aronson (Eds.), *The dysarthrias: Physiology, acoustics, perception, management.* San Diego: College-Hill Press.

Wiesendanger, M. (1981). The pyramidal tract: Its structure and function. In A. Towe & E. Luschei (Eds.), *Handbook of behavioral neurobiology: Vol. 5. Motor coordination.* New York: Plenum Press.

Woodbury, J.W., Gordon, A., & Conrad, J. (1965). Muscle. In T. Ruch, H. Patton, J.W. Woodbury, & A. Towe (Eds.), *Neurophysiology.* Philadelphia: W.B. Saunders.

Woolsey, C. (1958). Organization of somatic sensory and motor areas of the cerebral cortex. In H. Harlow & C. Woolsey (Eds.), *Biological and biochemical bases of behavior.* Madison, WI: The University of Wisconsin Press.

Yorkston, K., Beukelman, D., Minifie, F., & Sapir, S. (1984). Assessment of stress patterning. In M. McNeil, J. Rosenbek, & A. Aronson (Eds.), *The dysarthrias: Physiology, acoustics, perception, management.* San Diego: College Hill Press.

Yumoto, E., Sasaki, Y., & Okamura, H. (1984). Harmonics-to-noise ratio and psychophysical measurement of the degree of hoarseness. *Journal of Speech & Hearing Research, 27,* 2–5.

CHAPTER 3

Differential Diagnosis

Clinical issues: As she entered my office, I recognized her as the new medical student on the neurology service. She had just completed a morning outpatient clinic. A new patient seen by her team exhibited a complex pattern of symptoms including a "speaking problem." Her assignment was to write a student work-up summary and propose a list of diagnoses to be ruled out. Her questions centered around the characteristics of neurogenic communication disorders. They included:

- *How do you distinguish between a language disorder and a speech disorder?*
- *What is the difference between apraxia and dysarthria?*
- *What factors help you to distinguish among the various types of dysarthria?*

Speech/language clinicians are frequently called upon to provide a differential diagnosis among communication disorders. At times, the differentiation involves distinguishing motor speech from language-based neurogenic communication problems. At other times, the differentiation involves distinguishing between the two motor speech disorders—dysarthria and apraxia of speech. Still other times, it involves distinguishing among the various dysarthrias. The area of differential diagnosis is particularly important because of the implications such diagnoses carry for the identification of underlying neuropathologies. Neurogenic communication disorders with varying etiology, symptomology, and management have been described by Johns and his colleagues (1985). The definitions in Table 3-1, which Wertz (1985) adopted from Darley (1969), will pertain throughout this discussion.

TABLE 3-1.
Definitions of Five Neurogenic Communication Disorders

APHASIA: Impairment, due to brain damage, of the capacity to interpret and formulate language symbols; a multimodal loss or reduction in decoding conventional meaningful linguistic elements (morphemes and larger syntactc units); disproportionate to impairment of other intellectual functions; not attributable to dementia, sensory loss, or motor dysfunction; manifested in reduced availability of vocabulary, reduced efficiency in applying syntactic rules, reduced auditory retention span, and impaired efficiency in input and output channel selection.

LANGUAGE OF CONFUSION: Impairment of language accompanying neurologic conditions; often traumatically induced; characterized by reduced recognition and understanding of and responsiveness to the environment, faulty memory, unclear thinking, and disorientation in time and space. Structured language events are usually normal and responses utilize correct syntax; open-ended language situations elicit irrelevance, confabulation.

LANGUAGE OF GENERALIZED INTELLECTUAL IMPAIRMENT: Deterioration of performance on more difficult language tasks requiring better retention, closer attention, and powers of abstraction and generalization; degree of language impairment roughly proportionate to deterioration of other mental functions.

APRAXIA OF SPEECH: An articulatory disorder resulting from impairment, as a result of brain damage, of the capacity to program the positioning of speech muscles and the sequencing of muscle movements for the volitional production of phonemes. No significant weakness, slowness, or incoordination of these muscles in reflex and automatic acts. Prosodic alterations may be associated with articulatory problem, perhaps in compensation for it.

DYSARTHRIAS: A group of speech disorders resulting from disturbances in muscular control—weakness, slowness, or incoordination—of the speech mechanism due to damage to the central or peripheral nervous system or both. The term encompasses coexisting neurogenic disorders of several or all the basic processes of speech: respiration, phonation, resonance, articulation, and prosody.

Based on work of Darley, F.L. (1969). *Aphasia: Input and output disturbances in speech and language processing.* Paper presented in dual session on aphasia to the American Speech and Hearing Association, Chicago, IL.

Cited in Wertz, R.T. (1985). Neuropathologies of speech and language: An introduction to patient management. In D.F. Johns (Ed.), *Clinical management of neurogenic communicative disorders.* Boston: Little, Brown & Company.

A word of caution is warranted before beginning this discussion. Differential diagnosis of neurogenic communication disorders is at times complicated by the co-occurrence of disorders. Mild dysarthria may accompany aphasia, especially in the period immediately following a stroke. Apraxia and dysarthria may also coexist. Wertz, Rosenbek, and Deal (1970, cited in Wertz, 1985) reported a study in which they documented the presence of coexsisting disorders in a retrospective study of 176 apraxic individuals. They found that apraxia of speech occurred with dysarthria in eight percent of the sample and that apraxia of speech occurred with both dysarthria and aphasia in 14 percent of the sample. Mixed dysarthrias or coexistance of two or more types of dysarthria are also common in the clinical setting. The discussion that follows will be based on differential diagnostic categories uncomplicated by coexistance of one or more different types of dysarthric or different neurogenic communication disorders.

MOTOR SPEECH DISORDERS VERSUS LANGUAGE DISORDERS

Dysarthria Versus Aphasia

Aphasia is a specific language disorder involving deficits that cross all language modalities, including listening, speaking, reading, and writing. Unlike dysarthric individuals, aphasic speakers have difficulty handling any type of symbolic information. Critical to the distinction between aphasia and dysarthria is the fact that aphasia is characterized by deficits in understanding of both verbal and written language. In dysarthria, auditory comprehension and reading skills are preserved. The word-finding difficulties or the inability to retrieve a desired word that characterize aphasia are typically not present in dysarthria. Site of lesion and etiology also distinguish aphasia from dysarthria. Lesions that produce aphasia are restricted to the cortical language areas and related subcortical connections, which for most speakers are located in the left hemisphere. Lesions that produce dysarthria many occur at a variety of sites in either or both the peripheral or central nervous systems. Most typical etiologies for aphasia are left cerebrovascular accident (CVA), tumors, or trauma. Some types of aphasia are characterized by articulatory breakdowns. These breakdowns are particularly frequent in fluent aphasia and are thought to be a problem of phoneme selection rather than production. Errors are usually produced effortlessly and are often not recognized by the speaker.

Dysarthria Versus Dementia

Dementia has been associated with what Wertz (1985) calls "the language of generalized intellectual impairment." Individuals suffering from dementia exhibit language problems, but, unlike the pattern of deficits seen in aphasia, the language problems are roughly equivalent to deficits seen in other areas of intellectual functioning, including memory, reasoning, judgment, orientation, etc. Bayles (1984) states that language impairments can be observed in all stages of dementia even though these deficits may be subtle in the early stages. On the other hand, dysarthria is observed only in a subgroup of dementias associated with movement disorders. These include parkinsonism, Huntington's chorea, and progressive supranuclear palsy, among others.

Dysarthria Versus Language of Confusion

According to Darley's (1969) definition, language of confusion is often traumatically induced. Frequent characteristics include unclear thinking, faulty memory, and irrevelant responses. Confused language may frequently coexist with dysarthria, especially in cases of traumatical head injury. Here, locus of damage may occur in areas important to the control and regulation of movement, for example, upper motoneuron involvement or brain stem contusions (Groher, 1983). It is clear that dysarthria may co-occur with traumatic head injury and language of confusion when frank motor control problems are among the consequences of the injury. However, others suggest dysarthrias after closed head injury may also be associated with "failure to monitor articulation" and at times may be difficult to distinguish from the consequences of cognitive deficits (Hagen, Malkmus, & Burditt, 1979). Although the literature is not conclusive (see Chapter 5 for a more complete review), dysarthria associated with closed head injury may frequently resolve in the first year post-onset. For example, all 14 of the patients followed by Groher (1977) exhibited dysarthria early in their recovery, and six of the nine individuals with pseudobulbar dysarthria resolved completely by six months post-onset.

APRAXIA OF SPEECH VERSUS THE DYSARTHRIAS

Both apraxia of speech and dysarthria are considered motor speech disorders. Apraxia of speech is a deficit of motor programming involving speech production tasks but not automatic or involuntary tasks such as chewing. Dysarthria, on the other hand, is a disorder of motor production involving abnormalities in movement rates, precision, coordination, and strength. In dysarthria, the motor control problems are present regardless of tasks or context. As shown in Chapter 2, speech is regulated at a number of sites in the central and peripheral nervous system. Although the scientific community does not yet understand completely how an activity as complex as speech is executed, movements are not programmed individually.

Perceptually, apraxia of speech has been described as the "combination of slow rate, variable phonemic errors, and disturbed prosody. . ." (Johns & Darley, 1970, p. 581). At first glance, these characteristics appear to be quite similiar to those of dysarthria. However, the experienced observer is able to rely on a few salient differences to make a differential diagnosis in the clinical setting. The following section contains an overview of the characteristics that distinguish apraxia from dysarthria, including site of lesion, description of speech characteristics, pattern and type of articulatory errors, and movement deficits.

Site of Lesion

Although dysarthria may result from lesions at a number of different sites in either the central or peripheral nervous system, apraxia of speech, like aphasia, is associated with unilateral left hemisphere lesion. Similiar site of lesion and etiology help to explain the frequent co-occurrence of apraxia and aphasia. Reports estimate that apraxia occurs in isolation from aphasia, dysarthria, or both only 13 percent of the time, whereas apraxia coexists with aphasia in 65 percent of the population, with dysarthria in eight percent, and with both aphasia and dysarthria in 14 percent (Wertz et al., 1970; cited in Wertz, 1985).

Although the third frontal convolution (Broca's area) is usually involved in apraxia, localizing the lesion responsible for apraxia of speech and associating those lesions with clinical behaviors is not completely understood (see Rosenbek, Kent, & LaPointe, 1984, for a review of this problem). For example, Marquardt and Sussman (1984) found that a number of correlations between volume of lesions and clinical measures of severity were nonsignficant and Kertesz (1984) presented 10 cases with verbal apraxia as the result of subcortical lesions.

Speech Characteristics

At times, the clinician can appreciate the differences between apraxia and dysarthria by listening to and watching the speakers and their attempts to cope with the disorder. Darley (1984) described the behavior of an apraxic speaker in the following way:

> He appears uncertain as to how to position his articulators. He visibly gropes for correct articulation points but, failing to attain them, is frequently off target. More often than not he recognizes his error and tries to correct it, sometimes seeming to struggle effortfully to do so, even using his fingers to try to position his articulators. He may make several trials to produce the correct sound; he may succeed or he may in his successive trials mistakenly assume several different articulatory postures. Parts of his sentences may be fluent and well articulated; these islands of fluent speech make it clear that his problem is not due to inadequacy of innervation of any specific muscle groups. (p. 291)

This description implies that some features of apraxia may be the direct result of the underlying pathology and other features may be the result of speakers' attempts to compensate for the deficits. Thus, slow rate and prosodic abnormalities may be an effort to compensate for a more primary articulatory impairment (Darley, 1969, 1982; Rosenbek et al., 1984).

Articulatory Error Patterns

Articulatory errors of both apraxic and dysarthric speakers have been examined in an effort to distinguish these disorders. Unfortunately for the clinician who is attempting to make a differential diagnosis, examination of the results of traditional, perceptually based articulation inventories often do not provide a clear differential diagnosis. The research efforts of Johns and Darley (1970) illustrate this point. They compared the articulatory performance of three groups of patients: a group of 10 patients with apraxia of speech, a group of 10 patients with dysarthria (six with spastic, two with flaccid, and two with mixed dysarthria), and a group of 10 normal subjects. All speakers performed a variety of speech production tasks under a number of stimulus conditions. Their results suggested that dysarthria and apraxia of speech are similiar in some ways. Not only are articulatory errors present in both, but the error patterns appear to be similiar. They presented a list of 30 phonemes and blends rank-ordered according to difficulty (number of errors produced) in each speaker group. We have plotted these two rank orders against one another in Figure 3-1, which suggests correspondence between the two groups, that is, the most difficult sounds for dysarthric individuals are also the most difficult for an apraxic individual to produce and those that are produced most accurately for one group also tend to be produced most accurately by the other. Although number and pattern of error do not distinguish apraxia from dysarthria, Johns and Darley (1970) state:

> The two groups could be distinguished, however, by the types of articulatory errors they made and the consistency of their errors. Whereas the dysarthric subjects erred more by distortion and substitution (general simplification), the apraxic subjects erred more by substitution and repetition—their substitutions being often unrelated and frequently additive (such as substitution of a consonant cluster for a consonant singleton). Dysarthric errors were highly consistent, apraxic errors highly variable. (p. 582)

Movement Patterns

Because of the growing appreciation of the motor component of apraxia of speech, a number of investigators have begun to examine the movements associated with apraxic production errors. Itoh and Sasanuma (1984) reviewed a series of studies in which they observed the articulatory movements of normal, fluent aphasic, and apraxic speakers using fiberscopic observations of velar movements, x-ray microbeam observation of the lip, velum, and tongue, and voice onset time. They found evidence of deficits in temporal organization of articulatory movements of different structures. For example, in a speaker considered to have "pure" apraxia, they found that mistiming among the movements of the lip, velum, and tongue dorsum resulted in the

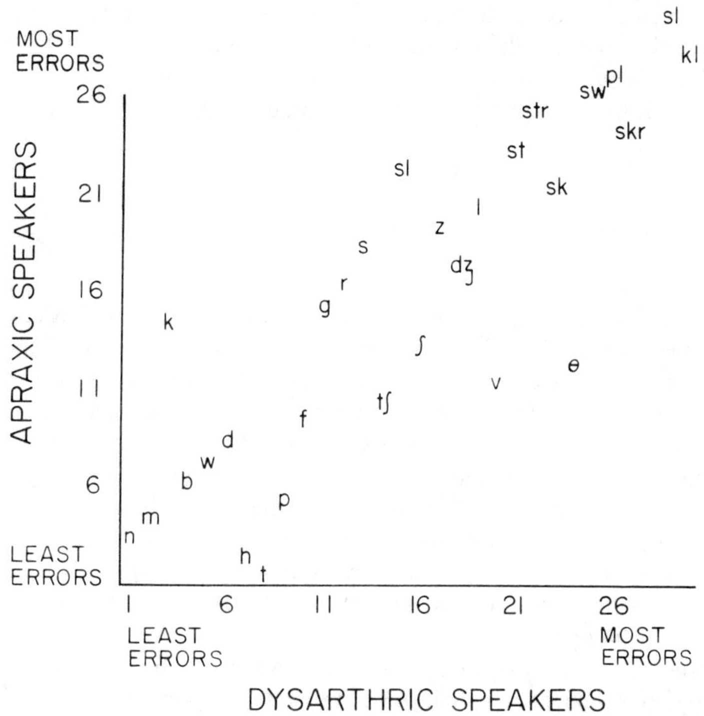

Figure 3-1. A comparison of the rank ordering of difficulty of phonemes for dysarthric and apraxic speakers. (Adapted from data presented in Johns & Darley, 1970.)

perception of a /d/ rather than the target sound /n/. Thus, what judges considered to be a substitution was the result of a slight mistiming of movements. This work supports the notion that apraxia is a motor planning or production problem rather than a problem of phoneme selection.

Fromm, Abbs, McNeil, and Rosenbek (1982) obtained physiological measures of a number of apraxic productions that were judged to be in error. They concluded that the errors were not fluent substitutions, nor were the movement abnormalities similar to those seen in flaccid, ataxic, or spastic dysarthric subjects. Ninety-five percent of all substitutions and addition errors were produced with one or more of the following abnormalities:

1. antagonistic muscle co-contraction
2. continuous, undifferentiated EMG activity
3. muscle activity shutdown
4. movement without voice
5. movement dyscoordination
6. addition
7. groping

Advancements in our understanding of the movement pattern in dysarthric and apraxic speech will not only allow us to better distinguish the two disorders but will also provide a better understanding of the relationship between faulty movements and perceptual judgment of articulatory productions.

Differential Diagnosis in the Clinical Setting

The ability to differentiate apraxia of speech from dysarthria is important for the practicing clinician because the two disorders are both assessed and treated differently. When evaluating the apraxic speaker, it is important to do an in-depth assessment of language skills in order to identify whether or not aphasia is present. When evaluating the dysarthric speaker, however, it is important to do an in-depth assessment of the components of speech production including respiration, phonation, velopharyngeal function, and oral articulation. Treatment for apraxia has been described (Shewan, 1980) as "burning in" the motor program. This involves extensive drill work with appropriately selected material, with focus on achieving target sounds. Treatment of dysarthria at times may be different, focusing instead on improving specific aspects of the physiological support for speech.

Although the two motor speech disorders share a number of characteristics (neurogenic basis, language skills in "pure" apraxia are intact, presence of articulatory errors, reduced speaking rate, reduced prosody, and awareness of errors), the two disorders are sufficiently different to make clinical diagnosis relatively straightforward. Differences between automatic movements and movements during speech are primary distinguishing features. In apraxia, automatic movements are intact; in dysarthria, they are not. Highly consistent articulatory errors are characteristic of dysarthria, whereas inconsistent errors are a hallmark of apraxia. Finally, with most dysarthrias, all speech components are involved. These features coupled with information regarding site of lesion and etiology form the basis for clinical differential diagnosis between the two motor speech disorders.

DIFFERENTIAL DIAGNOSIS AMONG THE DYSARTHRIAS

The Mayo Clinic Studies

Differential diagnosis among the dysarthrias is an area that perhaps has received more systematic attention than any other aspect of the disorder. Diagnosis from the Mayo perspective is based on the simple notion that one type of dysarthria sounds different from others. Darley, Aronson, and Brown provided the following perceptually based descriptions of the dysarthrias:

PSEUDOBULBAR PALSY (Spastic dysarthria) typically makes speech slow and labored, the articulation being rather consistently imprecise, especially on more complicated groups of consonant sounds. Pitch is low and monotonous. Voice quality is harsh and often strained or strangled-sounding. There may be considerable hypernasality, but usually no nasal emission is audible. Associated nonspeech signs are increase of deep tendon reflexes, appearance of the sucking reflex, increased jaw jerk, sluggish tongue movements, and activity of accessory respiratory musculature.

BULBAR PALSY (flaccid dysarthria) produces hypernasality with associated nasal emission of air during speech as its most prominent speech symptom. Inhalation is often audible and exhalation is often breathy, air wastage being manifested also in shortness of phrases. Articulation is often imprecise on either or both of two bases: (1) consonants may be weak through failure to impound sufficient intraoral breath pressure because of velopharyngeal incompetence; (2) immobility of tongue and lips because impairment of the hypoglossal and facial nerves prevents normal production of vowels and consonants. Associated nonspeech signs are fasciculation and atrophy of the tongue, reduced rate of alternating motion of tongue and lips, poor elevation of the soft palate and nasal alar contraction and grimacing as the patient tries to compensate for velopharyngeal incompetence.

AMYOTROPHIC LATERAL SCLEROSIS (combined spastic and flaccid dysarthria) has a developing effect on speech. In an earlier stage either spastic or flaccid speech and nonspeech signs predominate; in an advanced stage both sets of features described above are present. Slow rate, low pitch, hoarse and strained-strangled quality, highly defective articulation, marked hypernasality, and nasal emission combine to make the speaker struggle to produce short, scarcely intelligible phrases, his enormous effort seemingly inadequate amid a great weakness.

CEREBELLAR DISORDERS (ataxic dysarthrias) usually produce one of two patterns of speech deviation, the two seldom appearing concurrently: (1) intermittent disintegration of articulation, together with dysrhythmia and irregularities of pitch and loudness in performing tests of oral diadochokinetic rate; and (2) altered prosody, involving prolongation of sounds, equalization of syllabic stress (by undue stress on usually unstressed words and syllables), and prolongation of intervals between syllables and words. Speech proceeds at an artificially even, measured pace.

PARKINSONISM (hypokinetic dysarthria) reduces vocal emphasis, peaks and valleys of pitch and variations of loudness being flattened out monotonously. Short rushes of speech are separated by illogically placed pauses, the rate being variable, often accelerated. Consonant articulation in contextual speech and syllable repetition is blurred as muscles fail to go through their complete excursion. Difficulty in initiating articulation is shown by repetition of initial sounds and inappropriate silences. The voice is often breathy, and the loudness is reduced sometimes almost to inaudibility.

DYSTONIA (hyperkinetic dysarthria), through involuntary bodily and facial movements, unpredictably causes voice stoppages, disintegration of articulation, excessive variations of loudness, and distortion of vowels. Perhaps in anticipation of these interruptions, normal prosody is altered by slowing of rate, reduction in variations of pitch and loudness, prolongation of inter-word intervals, and interposition of inappropriate silences.

> CHOREOATHETOSIS (hyperkinetic dysarthria) causes involuntary movements that alter the normal breathing cycle and result in sudden exhalatory gusts of breath, bursts of loudness, elevations of pitch, and disintegration of articulation. The overall loudness level may be increased. Anticipated breakdowns are managed by varying the rate, introducing and prolonging pauses, and equalizing stress on all syllables and words. (1968, pp. 841–844)

For additional information, readers are referred to Chapter 4, Chapter 5, and Chapter 6, which outline medical management, the natural course, and speech characteristics of a number of disorders that frequently result in dysarthria.

In a series of studies carried out at the Mayo Clinic in the late 1960s, Darley, Aronson, Brown (1969a, b, 1975) examined the perceptual features of the speech of groups of dysarthric individuals. We will review this work in detail not only because it has become a classic work, but also because the results of these studies, and closely related work that followed them, are still used today as the basis of clinical differential diagnosis among the dysarthrias. In the Mayo Clinic studies, all speakers were unequivocally diagnosed as representing one of seven neurologic categories, including pseudobulbar palsy (N = 30), bulbar palsy (N = 30), amyotrophic lateral sclerosis (N = 30), cerebellar lesions (N = 30), parkinsonism (N = 32), dystonia (N = 30), and choreoathetosis (N = 30). Thirty-second speech samples taken for the most part from reading of the "Grandfather Passage" were judged on a seven-point equal-appearing interval scale for 38 speech dimensions. These dimensions appear in Table 3-2 grouped under the following categories: pitch characteristics, loudness, vocal quality, respiration, prosody, articulation, and general impression dimensions.

Following the perceptual ratings of the various speech dimensions, a listing of the most deviant features (those dimensions with a scaled score of 2.0 or more) was obtained for each of the disorder groups. For example, in the bulbar palsy group, four dimensions had a mean scaled score of two or higher. They were hypernasality, imprecise consonants, breathy voice (continuous), and monopitch. See Table 3-3 for a listing of the most deviant speech dimensions for each of the diagnostic groups. A review of this table suggests many similiarities among`the lists. In fact, four dimensions (monopitch, monoloudness, harsh voice, and imprecise consonants) received mean scale scores of 1.5 or above in all of the neurologic groups and three dimensions (phrases short, reduced stress, and vowels distorted) received such a score in five of the seven groups.

Although these similiarities are important for understanding the nature of the dysarthrias, such similiarities are not useful when attempting to make a differential diagnosis among the dysarthrias, as just the opposite type of information is needed. One would wish to identify the deviant dimensions that occur in only one or two of the dysarthria groups. According to the results

TABLE 3-2.
Speech Dimensions Used in the Mayo Clinic Studies

Pitch Characteristics

Pitch level—Pitch of voice sound consistently too low or too high for individual's age and sex.

Pitch breaks—Pitch of voice shows sudden and uncontrolled variation (falsetto breaks).

Monopitch—Voice is characterized by a monopitch or monotone. Voice lacks normal pitch and inflectional changes. It tends to stay at one pitch level.

Voice tremor—Voice shows shakiness or tremulousness.

Loudness

Monoloudness—Voice shows monotony of loudness, lacking normal variations in loudness.

Excess loudness variation—Voice shows sudden, uncontrolled alternations in loudness, sometimes becoming too loud, sometimes too weak.

Loudness decay—There is progressive diminution or decay of loudness.

Alternating loudness—There are alternating changes in loudness.

Loudness (overall)—Voice is insufficiently or excessively loud.

Voice Quality

Harsh voice—Voice is harsh, rough, and raspy.

Hoarse (wet) voice—There is "liquid sounding" hoarseness.

Breathy voice (continuous)—Continuously breathy, weak, and thin.

Breathy voice (transient)—Breathiness is transient, periodic, intermittent.

Strained-strangled voice—Voice (phonation) sounds strained or strangled (an apparently effortful squeezing of voice through glottis).

Voice stoppages—There are sudden stoppages of voiced air stream (as if some obstacle along vocal tract momentarily impedes flow of air).

Hypernasality—Voice sounds excessively nasal. Excessive amount of air is resonated by nasal cavities.

Hyponasality—Voice is denasal.

Nasal emission—There is nasal emission of air stream.

Respiration

Forced inspiration-expiration—Speech is interrupted by sudden, forced inspiration and expiration sighs.

Audible inspiration—Audible, breathy inspiration.

Grunt at end of expiration—Grunt occurs at end of expiration.

(*continued*)

TABLE 3-2 *(continued)*

Prosody

Rate—Rate of actual speech is abnormally slow or rapid.

Phrases short—Phrases are short (possibly due to fact that inspiration occur more often than normal). Speaker may sound as if he has run out of air. He may produce a gasp at the end of a phrase.

Increase of rate in segments—Rate increases progressively within given segments of connected speech.

Increase of rate overall—Rate increases progressively from beginning to end of sample.

Reduced stress—Speech shows reduction of proper stress or emphasis patterns.

Variable rate—Rate alternately changes from slow to fast.

Intervals prolonged—Prolongation of interword or intersyllable intervals.

Inappropriate silences—There are inappropriate silent intervals.

Short rushes of speech—There are short rushes of speech separated by pauses.

Excess and equal stress—Excess stress on usually unstressed parts of speech, e.g., (1) monosyllablic words, and (2) unstressed syllables of polysyllabic words.

Articulation

Imprecise consonants—Consonant sounds lack precision. They show slurring, inadequate sharpness, distortions, and lack of crispness. There is clumsiness in going from one consonant sound to another.

Phonemes prolonged—There are prolongations of phonemes.

Phonemes repeated—There are repetitions of phonemes.

Irregular articulatory breakdown—Intermittent nonsystematic breakdown in accuracy of articulation.

Vowels distorted—Vowel sounds are distorted throughout their total duration.

Overall

Intelligibility (overall)—Rating of overall intelligibility or understandability of speech.

Bizarreness (overall)—Rating of degree to which overall speech calls attention to itself because of unusual, peculiar, or bizarre characteristics.

From Darley, F.L., Aronson, A.E., & Brown, J.R. (1969a). Differential Diagnostic patterns of dysarthria. *Journal of Speech & Hearing Research, 12,* 246–269; and (1969b). Clusters of deviant speech dimensions in the dysarthrias. *Journal of Speech & Hearing Research, 12,* 462–496.

TABLE 3-3.
Speech Dimensions Judged to Be the Most Deviant with a Mean Scaled-Score of 2.0 or Higher for Each of the Diagnostic Groups (mean scaled socre is in parentheses)

Pseudobulbar Palsy
- Imprecise Consonants (3.98)
- Monopitch (3.72)
- Reduced Stress (3.32)
- Harsh Voice (3.23)
- Monoloudness (2.98)
- Low Pitch (2.82)
- Slow Rate (2.66)
- Hypernasality (2.64)
- Strained-Strangled Voice (2.49)
- Phrases Short (2.41)

Bulbar Palsy
- Hypernasality (3.61)
- Imprecise Consonants (2.91)
- Breathy Voice (Continuous) (2.28)
- Monopitch (2.09)

Amyotrophic Lateral Sclerosis
- Imprecise Consonants (4.39)
- Hypernasality (3.14)
- Harsh Voice (3.00)
- Slow Rate (2.89)
- Monopitch (2.77)
- Phrases (2.69)
- Vowels Distorted (2.60)
- Low Pitch (2.59)
- Monoloudness (2.51)
- Excess and Equal Stress (2.33)
- Intervals Prolonged (2.21)

Cerebellar Lesions
- Imprecise Consonants (3.19)
- Excess and Equal Stress (2.69)
- Irregular Articulatory Breakdowns (2.59)
- Vowels Distorted (2.14)
- Harsh Voice (2.10)

Parkinsonism
- Monopitch (4.64)
- Reduced Stress (4.46)
- Monoloudness (4.26)
- Imprecise Consonants (3.59)
- Inappropriate Silences (2.40)
- Short Rushes (2.22)
- Harsh Voice (2.08)
- Breathy Voice (Continuous) (2.04)

(*continued*)

TABLE 3-3 *(continued)*

Dystonia
- Imprecise Consonants (3.82)
- Vowels Distorted (2.41)
- Harsh Voice (2.40)
- Irregular Articulatory Breakdown (2.28)
- Strained-Strangled Voice (2.14)
- Monopitch (2.14)
- Monoloudness (2.01)

Chorea
- Imprecise Consonants (2.93)
- Intervals Prolonged (2.56)
- Variable Rates (2.29)
- Monopitch (2.23)
- Harsh Voice (2.20)
- Inappropriate Silences (2.17)
- Vowels distorted (2.13)
- Excess Loudness Variations (2.04)

From Darley, F.L., Aronson, A.E., & Brown, J.R. (1969a). Differential diagnostic patterns of dysarthria. *Journal of Speech & Hearing Research, 12,* 246–269.

of the Mayo Clinic studies, such single deviant dimensions occur only rarely. Only the following single dimensions appear to be helpful in making a differential diagnosis. Three dimensions, pitch breaks in pseudobulbar palsy, voice stoppages in dystonia, and short rushes of speech in parkinsonism, received mean scale scores of 1.5 or above in only one neurological group. In addition, four dimensions, excess loudness variations in choreoathetosis and dystonia, nasal emission and audible inspiration in bulbar palsy and amyotrophic lateral sclerosis, and variable rate in choreathetosis and parkinsonism received such a scale score in two neurologic groups. Thus, single speech dimensions are only of limited value when making differential diagnoses.

Clusters of Speech Dimensions in Differential Diagnosis

Spurred by the finding that single speech dimensions are not helpful in differential diagnosis, Darley and colleagues (1969b) further examined the data in order to identify clusters rather than single deviant speech dimensions. These clusters are made up of groups of deviant dimensions that tend to cooccur. It was suggested that the co-occurrence or clustering of deviant dimensions reflects the underlying pathophysiology. For example, in flaccid dysarthria both the speech dimensions of nasal emission and imprecise consonants correlate with short phrases. With the dimension of hypernasality, this correlation approaches significance. Thus, the cluster containing hypernasality, nasal emission, imprecise consonants, and short phrases is assumed to be the result of air wastage through the velopharyngeal port. Applying this correlational method to each of the neurologic groups, eight unique clusters of three or more deviant speech dimensions were found. Unique combinations of these clusters characterized each of the neurological groups. The clusters include:

Cluster 1—Articulatory Inaccuracy, consisting of Imprecise Consonants, Irregular Articulatory Breakdown, and Vowels Distorted. This cluster is articulatory in nature and may be the result of breakdown of coordinate activity such as seen in ataxia or as the result of adventitious involuntary movements of dystonia or chorea.

Cluster 2—Prosodic Excess, consisting of Slow Rate (of speech), Excess and Equal Stress, Phonemes Prolonged, Intervals Prolonged, and Inappropriate Silences. Slowness of repetitive movements is thought to be the chief neuromuscular defect responsible for this cluster.

Cluster 3—Prosodic Insufficiency, consisting of Monopitch, Monoloudness, Reduced Stress, and Phrases Short. Restricted range of movement is the probable underlying neuromuscular defect responsible for this cluster.

Cluster 4—Articulatory–Resonatory Incompetence, consisting of Imprecise Consonants, Vowels Distorted, and Hypernasality. It is thought to result from a combination of impaired force of contraction and reduced range of movement.

Cluster 5—Phonatory Stenosis, consisting of Low Pitch, Harsh Voice, Strained-Strangled Voice, Pitch Breaks, and Voice Stoppages as well as Excess Loudness Variation, Slow Rate, and Phrases Short (which may be compensatory features). This cluster may represent the physiologic narrowing of the laryngeal outlet.

Cluster 6—Phonatory Incompetence, consisting of Breathy Voice, Audible Inspiration, and Phrases Short. This cluster is thought to be the result of a reduction in the force of contraction.

Cluster 7—Resonatory Incompetence, consisting of Hyperasality, Nasal Emission, Imprecise Consonants, and Phrases Short. Like Cluster 6, it may result from reduction in force of muscular contraction and failure to close the velopharyngeal port.

Cluster 8—Phonatory–Prosodic Insufficiency, consisting of Monopitch, Monoloudness, and Harsh Voice. Hypotonia is thought to be responsible for this cluster.

In summary, results of the Mayo Clinic study found that each of the seven neurological disorders could be characterized by a unique set of clusters of deviant speech dimensions and that no two disorders had the same set of clusters. Thus, differential diagnosis can be based on clusters of related dimensions rather than on single features. A listing of clusters characteristic of each of the neurological disorders appears in Table 3-4. For a more complete description of the speech characteristics of various disorders, see Chapters 4, 5, & 6.

TABLE 3-4.
The Clusters Characterizing Each of the Dysarthrias Studied in the Mayo Clinic Research

Pseudobulbar Palsy
Prosodic Excess
Prosodic Insufficiency
Articulatory-Resonatory Incompetence
Phonatory Stenosis
Bulbar Palsy
Phonatory Incompetence
Resonatory Incompetence
Phonatory-Prosodic Insufficiency
Amyotrophic Lateral Sclerosis
Prosodic Excess
Prosodic Insufficiency
Articulatory-Resonatory Incompentence
Phonatory Stenosis
Phonatory Incompetence
Resonatory Incompetence
Cerebellar Lesions
Ariculatory Inaccuracy
Prosodic Excess
Phonatory-Prosodic Insufficiency
Parkinsonism
Prosodic Excess
Prosodic Insufficiency
Phonatory Stenosis
Dystonia
Articulatory Inaccuracy
Prosodic Excess
Prosodic Insufficiency
Phonatory Stenosis
Chorea
Articulatory Inaccuracy
Prosodic Excess
Prosodic Insufficiency
Articulatory-Resonatory Incompetence
Phonatory Stenosis
Resonatory Incompetence

Further Applications of the Mayo Study Techniques

The original Mayo Clinic studies perceptually examined only seven neurological disorders. However, similiar perceptual rating techniques have been applied to a number of other neurological disorders since the early 1970s.

Multiple Sclerosis

Darley, Brown, & Goldstein (1972) reported the results of a perceptual study of the speech characteristics of 168 individuals with multiple sclerosis. Their conclusions indicated that dysarthria was not a universally characteristic symptom in multiple sclerosis. Over 50 percent of the speakers were judged to be normal when overall speech adequacy was rated. The most prominent speech deviations were impaired control of loudness (reported in 77 percent of the speakers), harsh voice quality (reported in 72 percent of the speakers), and defective articulation (reported in 46 percent of the speakers). Impaired use of vocal variability for emphasis, impaired pitch control, hypernasality, inappropriate pitch level, and breathiness were observed also.

Wilson's Disease

Berry and his colleagues (Berry, Aronson, Darley, & Goldstein, 1974; Berry, Darley, Aronson, & Goldstein, 1974) reported the results of a perceptual study of the speech characteristics of twenty individuals with Wilson's disease. Results indicate that the dysarthria associated with Wilson's disease is mixed with ataxic, hypokinetic, and spastic components. Results of a factor analysis indicated that the following clusters of deviant speech dimensions were present: prosodic insufficiency, phonatory stenosis, prosodic excess, and articulatory-resonatory inadequacy.

Motor Neuron Disease

Carrow, Rivera, Mauldin, and Shamblin (1974) reported the results of a perceptual study of speech characteristics in 79 individuals with motor neuron disease. Etiologies included amyotrophic lateral sclerosis (both with and without pseudobulbar symptomatology), progressive muscular atrophy, primary lateral sclerosis, and bulbar palsy. For the group as a whole, the following deviant speech dimensions were common (parentheses include the percentage of the group with that characteristic):

Harshness (80%)
Hypernasality (75%)
Breathiness (65%)
Voice Tremor (63%)
Imprecise Consonants (58%)

For the two groups of individuals with amyotrophic lateral sclerosis, results indicated that those with pseudobulbar signs were judged to have more severe speech disorders than those without such signs. Strained-strangled voice and slow rate were the two deviant speech dimensions that were particularly severe in individuals with pseudobulbar signs.

Shy-Drager Syndrome

Linebaugh (1979) reported the results of a perceptual study of the speech characteristics of 80 individuals with Shy-Drager syndrome. Forty-four percent were found to exhibit dysarthria. Three distinct forms of mixed dysarthria were present, including: a mixed hypokinetic-ataxic dysarthria, a mixed ataxic-spastic dysarthria, and a mixed spastic-ataxic-hypokinetic dysarthria.

Friedreich's Ataxia

Joanette and Dudley (1980) reported the results of a perceptual study of the speech symptomatology of individuals with Friedreich's ataxia. Their results confirmed the presence of three clusters related to ataxic dysarthria, including articulatory imprecision, prosodic excess, and phonatory-prosodic insufficiency. A subgroup of these individuals also exhibited a cluster of characteristics labeled as "phonatory stenosis." This cluster included the deviant speech dimensions of harshness and pitch breaks.

At this time, differential diagnosis in the clinical setting relies primarily on perceptual ratings and clusters of characteristics generated from them. There is considerable research focusing on the physiological aspects of the various dysarthrias. However, this work has not yet been integrated into routine clinical practice to the extent that perceptual observations have.

REFERENCES

Bayles, K.A. (1984). Language and Dementia. In A.L. Holland (Ed.), *Language disorders in adults: Recent advances*. Austin, TX: PRO-ED.

Berry, W.R., Aronson, A.E., Darley, F.L., & Goldstein, N.P. (1974). Effects of penicillamine therapy and low-copper diet on dysarthria in Wilson's disease (hepatolenticular degenerative). *Mayo Clinic Proceedings, 49,* 405–408.

Berry, W.R., Darley, F.L., Aronson, A.E., & Goldstein, N.P. (1974). Dysarthria in Wilson's disease. *Journal of Speech & Hearing Research, 17,* 169–183.

Carrow, E., Rivera, V., Mauldin, M., & Shamblin, L. (1974). Deviant speech characteristics in motor neuron disease. *Archives of Otolaryngeal, 100,* 212–218.

Darley, F.L. (1969). Aphasia: *Input and output disturbances in speech and language processing*. Paper presented in dual session on aphasia to the American Speech and Hearing Associaton, Chicago, IL.

Darley, F.L. (1982). *Aphasia*. New York: Saunders.

Darley, F.L. (1984). Apraxia of speech: A neurogenic articulation disorder. In H. Winitz (Ed.), *Treating articulation disorders: For clinicians by clinicians*. Austin, TX: PRO-ED.

Darley, F.L., Aronson, A.E., & Brown, J.R. (1968). Motor speech signs in neurologic disease. *Medical Clinics of North America, 52,* 835–844.

Darley, F.L., Aronson, A.E., & Brown, J.R. (1969a). Differential diagnostic patterns of dysarthria. *Journal of Speech & Hearing Research, 12,* 246–269.

Darley, F.L., Aronson, A.E., & Brown, J.R. (1969b). Clusters of deviant speech dimensions in the dysarthrias. *Journal of Speech & Hearing Research, 12,* 462–496.

Darley, F.L., Aronson, A.E., & Brown, J.R. (1975). *Motor speech disorders*. Philadelphia: Saunders.

Darley, F.L., Brown, J.R., & Goldstein, N.P. (1972). Dysarthria in multiple sclerosis. *Journal of Speech & Hearing Research, 15,* 229–245.

Fromm, D., Abbs, J.H., McNeil, M.R., & Rosenbek, J.C. (1982). Simultaneous perceptual-physiological method for studying apraxia of speech. In R.H. Brookshire (Ed.), *Clinical aphasiology: Conference proceedings*. Minneapolis: BRK Publishers.

Groher, M. (1977). Language and memory disorders following closed head trauma. *Journal of Speech & Hearing Research, 20,* 212.

Groher, M. (1983). Communication Disorders. In M. Rosenthal, E.R. Griffith, M.R. Bond, & J.D. Miller (Eds.), *Rehabilitation of the head injured adult*. Philadelphia: F.A. Davis Company.

Hagen, C., Malkmus, D. & Burditt, G. (1979). *Intervention strategies for language disorders secondary to head trauma*. Short Course presented at the annual convention of the American Speech-Language-Hearing Association, Atlanta, GA.

Itoh, M. & Sasanuma, S. (1984). Articulatory movements in apraxia of speech. In J.C. Rosenbek, M.R. McNeil, & A.E. Aronson (Eds.), *Apraxia of speech: Physiology, acoustics, linguistics, management*. San Diego: College-Hill Press.

Joanette, Y. & Dudley, J.G. (1980). Dysarthria symptomatology of Friedreich's ataxia. *Brain & Language, 10,* 39–50.

Johns, D.F. (Ed.). (1985). *Clinical management of neurogenic communication disorders*. Boston: Little, Brown.

Johns, D.F. & Darley, F.L. (1970). Phoneme variability in apraxia of speech. *Journal of Speech & Hearing Research, 13,* 556–583.

Kertesz, A. (1984). Subcortical lesions and verbal apraxia. In J.C. Rosenbek, M.R. McNeil, & A.E. Aronson (Eds.), *Apraxia of speech*. San Diego: College-Hill Press.

Linebaugh, C. (1979). The dysarthrias of Shy-Drager syndrome. *Journal of Speech & Hearing Disorders, 44,* 55–60.

Marquardt, T.P. & Sussman, H. (1984). The elusive lesion—apraxia of speech link in Broca's aphasia. In J.C. Rosenbek, M.R. McNeil, & A.E. Aronson (Eds.), *Apraxia of speech: Physiology, acoustics, linguistics, management*. San Diego: College-Hill Press.

Rosenbek, J.C., Kent, R.D., & LaPointe, L.L. (1984). Apraxia of speech: An overview of some perspectives. In J.C. Rosenbek, M.R. McNeil, & A.E. Aronson (Eds.), *Apraxia of speech: Physiology, acoustics, linguistics, management*. San Diego: College-Hill Press.

Shewan, C.M. (1980). Verbal apraxia and its treatment. *Human Communication, 5,* 3.

Wertz, R.T. (1985). Neuropathologies of speech and language: An introduction to patient management. In D.F. Johns (Ed.), *Clinical management of neurogenic communication disorders*. Boston: Little, Brown & Company.

Wertz, R.T., Rosenbek, J.C., & Deal, J.L. (1970). *A review of 228 cases of apraxia of speech: Classification, etilogy, and localization*. Paper presented to the American Speech & Hearing Association, New York.

CHAPTER 4

Congenital Dysarthrias

Individuals with dysarthria frequently have serious underlying neurological disease and syndromes. Therefore, speech/language pathology services are often delivered in conjunction with other medically related services. To provide a resource guide for speech/language pathologists, each of the following chapters contains a review of medical issues related to those neurological conditions that are frequently associated with dysarthria, including a description of the disorder, differential diagnosis, natural course, and medical management. A summary of research describing the speech characteristics related to selected neurological conditions is included to assist the reader in integration of the speech consequences and characteristics of the neurological disorder. Reference to the speech symptoms will be made throughout the book during discussions of specific assessment and intervention procedures. References are provided so that the interested reader can pursue the study of specific disorders in-depth.

This chapter reviews those dysarthrias that are congenital, Chapter 5 contains a review of disorders with an adult onset and a nonprogressive course, and Chapter 6 contains a review of the degenerative dysarthrias. This organizational approach was adopted because the age of onset and natural course of the disorders has such a strong impact on management. For example, although we will focus exclusively on the speech aspects of cerebral palsy, the onset of the disorder before language has developed has important implications. Thus, the need to attend to the issue of language development becomes critical in this population when it is not in disorders that have their onset in adulthood.

CEREBRAL PALSY

Medical Aspects

Description and Diagnosis

Cerebral palsy can be defined as a nonprogressive motor disorder that stems from an insult to the cerebral level of the central nervous system during the prenatal or perinatal period. It is important to realize, however, that even though cerebral palsy stems from a static lesion of the nervous system, the manifestations and complications of the disorder will change with the growth of the child into adolescence and adulthood. Although the incidence of cerebral palsy is between 2 and 2.5/1000 with a prevalence of about 400,000 school-aged children, figures for adults are difficult to obtain (Erenberg, 1984; Lord, 1984). The population most at risk are low birth weight infants who comprise only six percent of all live births but nearly 30 percent of all cerebral palsy cases (Kudrgavcev, Schoenberg, Kurland, & Groover, 1983). Specific factors associated with the presence of cerebral palsy are hypoxia, periventricular hemorrhage, mechanical birth trauma, intrauterine infection, and kernicterus; however, in almost 50 percent of the cases, there are no identified perinatal complications (Erenberg, 1984).

The diagnosis of cerebral palsy rests primarily on clinical information and observation of the child's development over time. The hallmarks of cerebral palsy are the persistence of primitive reflexes in the child and delays in developmental milestones. For instance, the Moro or startle reflex, which commonly becomes more difficult to elicit after two to three months of age in an unimpaired child, may last indefinitely in an individual with cerebral palsy. There is also a failure of more mature postural mechanisms (such as the equilibrium response to occur. The infant may display poor feeding ability, unexplained irritability, disordered sleep patterns, and as she or he grows, may have poor balance and an early hand preference (before one year). Diagnostic studies such as computerized tomography and electroencephalography (EEG) are not always correlated with the clinical picture. The most useful studies are thyroid function studies to eliminate hypothyroidism and urine metabolic studies to eliminate a congenital degenerative disease (Erenberg, 1984).

Major Classifications

There are four overall classes of cerebral palsy, with the spastic variety accounting for the vast majority of cases (75 percent). Within the spastic category are the subclasses of hemiparesis (30 percent), diparesis (25 percent), and quadriparesis (20 percent). Other classes include athetoid (5 percent), dystonic athetoid or ataxic (10 percent), and a mixed variety (10 percent) (Erenberg, 1984).

Hemiplegia is often undiagnosed at birth and is usually brought to the physician's attention when the infant fails to match peer development at three to nine months. It usually involves the arm to a greater extent than the leg and may also occur with a sensory deficit. Mental retardation is less common in this form than with quadriplegia or diplegia. Quadriplegia again is more severe in the upper extremities. Diplegia (also called Little's disease) involves limbs bilaterally, more commonly the legs and is most closely associated with a low birth weight.

Ataxic or dystonic cerebral palsy is associated with hypotonia at birth and may therefore be diagnosed late. The athetoid condition also may not be fully apparent for a year or two after birth, with initial hypotonia and gradual onset of involuntary athetoid and choreic movements. This particular diagnosis commonly does not involve mental retardation (Brett, 1983).

Associated Problems

Some limitation in intellectual and cognitive functioning occurs in 50 to 70 percent of persons with cerebral palsy; the hemiplegic and athetoid types are less likely to be associated with mental retardation than the others. Behavioral problems, perhaps linked with intellectual deficits, are less frequently seen, including hyperactivity, decreased attention span, or emotional lability. Depression may occur, especially in adolescents coping with body image issues. Various ocular abnormalities such as refractive errors, visual field defects, and extraocular muscle imbalances may interfere with learning and movement abilities. Deafness may occur in up to seven percent of the cases, particularly in the athetoid type of cerebral palsy. Seizure disorders may be present in 30 percent or more; EEG results do not generally correlate well with intellectual function, however. Speech/language impairments are common in the classes associated with bulbar dysfunction and involuntary movement. Orthopedic complications occur in response to chronic muscle imbalances and involuntary movement. Scoliosis, hip dislocations, and muscle/tendon contractures are examples that frequently require correction; uncorrected, these can lead to osteoarthritis, seating problems, pressure sores, and additional problems with secondary scoliosis. Dental needs in addition to those normally exhibited by the growing child may also result from chronic involuntary movements (Erenberg, 1984; Lord, 1984).

Natural Course

As was mentioned previously, although the definition of cerebral palsy contains the term *nonprogressive*, the manifestations of this primarily motor disorder will change as the body changes through growth. Periods of rapid growth, such as infancy and adolescence, may bring an exacerbation of symptoms and a regression of functional status until new skills are acquired and a new level of neuromuscular equilibrium is attained. Over time, new complications of spasticity and dystonia may become evident as the orthopedic disorders mentioned earlier occur in response to overuse and postural abnormalities. However, the basic level of intellectual functioning and neurological dysfunction should remain relatively unchanged.

Virtually 100 percent of hemiplegic children will walk in time; the functional use of the hemiplegic arm, however, depends largely on the degree of sensory deficit present. Current figures indicate that about 50 percent are employable as adults. Most diplegic children can walk during childhood; however, it is not uncommon to see them revert to the use of a wheelchair during adolescence because of the increased efficiency of mobility provided. Diplegic children tend to integrate well into the mainstream classroom situation and about one-third will later be employed. The outlook for quadriplegia is less optimistic. In mild cases, ambulation and at least some level of independence in self-care is possible; in one-quarter of the cases of quadriplegia, total care is needed to sustain life (Lord, 1984).

Therapy and Other Management Issues

The family outlook and support system is crucial to successfully habilitating the child and adult with cerebral palsy. Therefore, families should be included early in educational efforts, to alert them to expected developmental crises and achievements, and they should be urged to participate in peer support groups for encouragement and practical advice on the care of the disabled child. Physical therapy, in the form of early intervention programs, is a controversial but common ingredient in the management of cerebral palsy. The child and family are encouraged, via various techniques, to facilitate normal patterns of sensation and movement and to inhibit abnormal reflexes and postures. As these are often applied in groups, opportunities for fostering socialization are maximized. Early and aggressive orthopedic surgery is called for to prevent childhood hip dislocation with its resultant problems and to correct fixed deformities, aid in restoring muscle balance, improve postural stability, and maximize function (Bleck, 1984; Erenberg, 1984). Training in functional activities as well as environmental adaptation to achieve the optimal level of independence in self-care activities is mandatory to allow development of the child's sense of mastery and achievement. In the area of adaptive equipment, motorized mobility devices have been prescribed for increasingly younger children, allowing access to the community and enhancing the child's ability to explore the environment.

Specific therapies to control spasticity and involuntary movement have been relatively unsuccessful. Neuromuscular biofeedback has had some limited success in the areas of head control and the treatment of certain gait abnormalities. Surgery for the treatment of spasticity, including cerebellar stimulation implants, has had no beneficial effects (Erenberg, 1984). Although systemic medications are used to treat spasticity, none have been found to be ideal. Diazepam (Valium) is sometimes effective, but has the adverse effect of drowsiness and may be detrimental to learning abilities. Dantrolene sodium (Dantrium), another antispasticity drug, may cause muscle weakness, drowsiness, nausea, and significant hepatitis in 0.2 percent of patients. Baclofen (Lioresal), although generally more benign, may still cause drowsiness and gastrointestinal side effects. Most of the anticonvulsants (including diphenytoin, phenobarbital, carbamazepine) as well can cause central nervous system (CNS) effects such as drowsiness and ataxia; some reports suggest that learning potential may be adversely affected.

For young children, two areas should additionally be addressed. The first, nutrition, may suffer from the preserved primitive bite and tongue thrust reflexes; instruction should be given to parents or caretakers in order to overcome these obstacles to adequate nutrition. The second area, educational needs, should also be considered early; as it is difficult for these children to use their bodies effectively to explore the world, it is important that ways to achieve these aims be considered. Adequate communication and seating to provide social contact for these children is crucial to educational and personal development. For adults, attention should be given to employment potential and training, independent living situations, and a program for regular exercise and maintenance.

Speech Characteristics

Occurrence of Dysarthria

Although the reported incidence of speech disorders associated with cerebral palsy varies, a review shows that speech disorders are a common sequela of this neurological disorder. On the low end of the range, Wolfe (1950) indicated that 31 to 59 percent of individuals with cerebral palsy show some degree of dysarthria. On the other end of the range, Achilles (1955) reported 88 percent of 151 speakers with cerebral palsy exhibited disordered articulation. As with other types of dysarthria, the motor speech problems of individuals with cerebral palsy are not limited to disorders of oral articulation.

Speech Components

RESPIRATORY FUNCTION. In early studies that investigated the speech characteristics of individuals with cerebral palsy, Blumberg (1955) and Achilles (1955) reported that athetoid individuals have poorer respiratory control than do spastic individuals. In a series of studies that examined the respiratory function of speakers with cerebral palsy, Hardy (1964) reported that the breathing rates of spastic children demonstrated significantly reduced respiratory reserve and, therefore, reduced vital capacities. He also reported that the respiratory patterns of children with cerebral palsy were less flexible than those of normal children. This reduction in flexibility may result from a number of different factors, including muscular weakness and excessive involuntary oppositions of antagonistic muscles. Hardy (1983) expanded these observations by writing that the spastic subgroup demonstrated reduced ability to expire below their resting respiratory levels due to the involvement of their abdominal muscles.

A reduction in vital capacity is not necessarily associated with inadequate respiratory support for speech. Hardy (1961) indicated that the absolute volume of air capacity does not determine whether or not speakers with cerebral palsy have severe dysarthria. Rather, he observed that children with cerebral palsy utilized more air volume per syllable than normal speakers. Together with a reduced vital capacity, the inefficient valving of the breath stream results in respiratory support for speech that is often inadequate. For example, 16 of 41 children were found to have problems with velopharyngeal closure. In addition to velopharyngeal dysfunction, laryngeal and oral articulation dysfunction may contribute to insufficient intraoral air pressure.

LARYNGEAL FUNCTION. A number of authors have reported that laryngeal dysfunction is a common characteristic of speakers with cerebral palsy. For example, Rutherford (1944) and Leith (1954) concluded that athetoid individuals demonstrate a monotonous pitch level. Clement and Twitchell (1959) described the voice of athetoid speakers as low in pitch with weak intensity, exhibiting a forced, throaty voice quality. Berry and Eisenson (1956) noted the whispered, hoarse phonation of speakers with cerebral palsy. Ingram and Barn (1961) reported inspiratory voice, periodic involuntary abduction of the vocal folds, and involuntary dysphonia. McDonald and Chance (1964) wrote that adductor spasm of laryngeal muscles in cerebral palsy may prevent the initiation of voicing or interrupted phonation during speech. Although the informal observations of phonatory performance of cerebral-palsied speakers have been reported, little instrumental research has been completed in this area.

VELOPHARYNGEAL FUNCTION. Although velopharyngeal dysfunction in many speakers with cerebral palsy has been reported clinically, careful study of this speech component in this population has been quite limited. Hardy (1961) and Carr (1959) studied athetoid speakers using cinefluorography. They reported velopharyngeal function to be inconsistent and uncoordinated. Hardy found that 39 percent of his cerebral-palsied speakers demonstrated problems with velopharyngeal closure. Netsell (1969) studied isolated vowel positions of six children with cerebral palsy and dysarthria, and reported larger oral openings without palatal lifts and smaller oral openings when the palatal lift was in position. It was hypothesized that the speakers attempted to radiate more sound orally in the presence of velopharyngeal incompetence. Kent and Netsell (1978) studied articulatory abnormality in athetoid cerebral palsy and concluded that all five of their subjects demonstrated some difficulty in achieving velopharyngeal closure, as they exhibited instability of velar position.

ORAL ARTICULATION. Of all the speech components, oral articulation has received the most systematic study. Irwin (1955) observed the articulatory performance of 128 speakers with spastic cerebral palsy, 86 speakers with athetoid cerebral palsy, and 52 speakers with tension athetosis. No strong statistical differences between the three subgroups were reported. However, a significant increase in the mastery of speech sounds was observed with increasing age. Byrne (1959) found that speech elements involving the movement of the tongue tip were the most frequently misarticulated by children with cerebral palsy. Both Byrne (1959) and Irwin (1955) reported that cerebral-palsied children misarticulated voiceless sounds more frequently than the voiced cognates. Hixon and Hardy (1964) investigated the relationship among speech defectiveness, rates of repetition of consonant-vowel syllables, and rates of repetitive nonspeech movements. They concluded that restrictions of motility in the posterior portion of the tongue may exert important influences on the production of speech in spastic and athetoid speakers. In addition, speech movements of the articulators can be used to accomplish an adequate evaluation of restricted mobility of speech articulators in cerebral-palsied children. Byrne (1959) reported no consonant or vowel articulation differences for spastic as compared to athetoid cerebral-palsied children.

The articulatory performance of adult speakers with cerebral palsy has also been studied. Kent and Netsell (1978) studied the articulatory movements of five athetoid cerebral-palsied speakers using cinefluorography. Their findings supplemented their earlier work (Kent, Netsell, & Bauer, 1975), in that large ranges of jaw movements, inappropriate tongue positioning, and abnormalities in the timing and range of velopharyngeal movements were observed. In addition, articulatory transition times were prolonged. Platt, Andrews, Young, and Quinn (1980) and Platt, Andrews, and Howie (1980) indicated that adults with spastic cerebral palsy did not differ from speakers with athetoid cerebral palsy in articulatory error pattern and that differences between severely and less severely disabled individuals were of degree rather than quality. In addition, they reported that both groups of cerebral-palsied speakers demonstrated imprecision of fricative and affricate manners of articulation, and inability to achieve the extreme positions in the articulatory space. Their subjects demonstrated a predominance of within-manner errors. Errors that cross manner of articulation boundaries were uncommon. Devoicing of voiced consonants was frequently observed. More errors occurred in word-final as compared to word-initial positions.

Overall Adequacy

The overall performance of subgroups of speakers with cerebral palsy has also been investigated. Shapiro (1960) and Hedges (1955) reported that there is little indication that listeners can distinguish spastic and athetoid speakers. However, Platt and colleagues (1980) reported that speech of spastic cerebral-palsied speakers was more intelligible and less articulatorily impaired than speakers with athetoid cerebral palsy.

Several attempts have been made to relate selected speech characteristics of overall speech intelligibility. Andrews, Platt, and Young (1977) found that specific features contribute to the intelligibility problem of adults with athetoid and spastic dysarthria, including reduced vowel target space, poor anterior lingual place accuracy for consonants, and reduced articulatory precision for fricative and affricate consonants. Subsequently, these authors suggest that both groups of cerebral-palsied speakers exhibited word-final consonant errors, devoicing of voiced consonants, and extensive within-manner errors. In a recent study, Ansel (1985) and Ansel and Kent (1986) sought to identify the specific acoustic features that would predict speech intelligibility in groups of adult cerebral-palsied male speakers. These researchers concluded that the acoustic factors of vowel duration and F1 and F2 formant location and noise duration were major predictors of speech intelligibility scores. Thus, the physiological parameters of temporal control and tongue position appear to influence speech intelligibility. Obviously, the relationship between specific speech parameters and speech intelligibility is very complex. However, because improvement in speech intelligibility is such a central focus of nearly all dysarthria intervention programs, further research in this area would be extremely beneficial.

MOEBIUS SYNDROME

Medical Aspects

Description and Clinical Characteristics

Moebius syndrome is a rare congenital bilateral facial and abducent paralysis affecting cranial nerves VI and VII. A number of additional characteristics are also described in some cases, including involvement of other cranial nerves, musculoskeletal deformities, reduced muscle mass in the extremities, ocular ptosis, and ear deformities (Merz & Wojtowicz, 1967). Occurrence of the disorder is sporadic with the male to female ratio being equal (Gorlin, Pindborg, and Cohen, 1976). A suggestion of familial incidence occurs in a small number of reports.

The pathology of the disorder is unclear. Meyerson and Foushee (1978) have briefly reviewed some speculations, including theories suggesting either nuclear or nerve agenesis or underlying muscular deficits. Pitner, Edwards, and McCormick (1965) have suggested that there may be two variants of the disorder, one myopathic and the other neuropathic.

Medical Management

A variety of surgical intervention strategies have been reported for maxillary or mandibular deformities, limb anomalies, eye muscles and platysma and temporalis muscle transplants (Edgerton, Tuerck, & Fisher, 1975; Federman & Stoopack, 1975; Gutman, Sharon, & Laufer, 1973; Sogg, 1961).

Speech Characteristics

In describing the speech/language and hearing problems in a group of 22 children with Moebius syndrome, Meyerson and Foushee (1978) reported flaccid dysarthria in 20 cases. They characterized the dysarthric features as limited strength, range, and speed of movement of the articulators, and inaccurate consonant production. The dysarthria ranged in severity from mild distortion of phonemes requiring bilabial closure or lingual elevation to unintelligible speech. Small mouth opening and micrognathia contributed to a "muffled" quality in some of the subjects. Two of the subjects were characterized as being velopharyngeally incompetent. Fourteen of the 22 subjects also reported feeding problems. Other problems occurring in this population were cleft palate, hearing loss, mental retardation, and delayed language development.

Kahane (1979) reported physiological and acoustic measures of speech production of an eight year old male. Articulatory characteristics were summarized as follows:

1. Absence of bilabials resulted from paralysis of orbicularis oris superioris.
2. Lingua-alveolar sounds were produced as lingua-dentals.
3. Lingua-velar sounds were often produced pharyngeally with the tongue resting on the floor of the mouth and with slight thrusting of the apex.
4. Sibilant and fricative sounds were generally interdentalized and were not accompanied by clinically notable amounts of nasal emission.
5. Vowel productions were distorted largely by imprecise placement of the tongue during speech.

REFERENCES

Andrews, G., Platt, L.J., & Young, M. (1977). Factors affecting intelligibility of cerebral palsied speech to the average listener. *Folia Phoniatrica*, *29*, 292–301.

Ansel, B. (1985). *Acoustic predictors of speech intelligibility in cerebral palsied-dysarthric adults.* Unpublished doctoral dissertation, University of Wisconsin, Madison.

Ansel, B., & Kent, R. (1986). Predictors of speech intelligibility in cerebral palsied-dysarthric adults. Paper presented at the third Biennial Clinical Dysarthria Conference, Tucson, AZ.

Achilles, R. (1955). Communication anomalies of individuals with cerebral palsy: I Analysis of communication processes in 151 cases of cerebral palsy. *Cerebral Palsy Review, 16*, 15–24.

Berry, M., & Eisenson, J. (1956). *Speech disorders.* New York: Appleton-Century-Crofts.

Bleck, E.E. (1984). Where have all the CP children gone? The needs of adults. *Developmental Medicine & Child Neurology, 26*, 674–676.

Blumberg, M. (1955). Respiration and speech in the cerebral palsied child. *American Journal of Disabled Children, 89*, 48–53.

Brett, E.M. (Ed.). (1983). *Pediatric Neurology.* Edinburgh: Churchill Livingston.

Byrne, M. (1959). Speech and language development of athetoid and spastic children. *Journal of Speech & Hearing Disorders, 24*, 231–240.

Carr, K. (1959). *A study of velopharyngeal movement patterns in cerebral palsied speakers.* Unpublished master's thesis, University of Iowa.

Clement, M., & Twitchell, T. (1959). Dysarthria in cerebral palsy. *Journal of Speech & Hearing Disorders, 4*, 118–122.

Edgerton, M. T., Tuerck, D.B., & Fisher, J.C. (1975). Surgical treatment of Moebius syndrome by platysma and temporalis muscle tranfers. *Plastic and reconstructive surgery*, 305–311.

Erenberg, G. (1984). Cerebral Palsy. *Postgraduate Medicine, 75*(7), 87–93.

Federman, R., & Stoopack, J.C. (1975). Moebius syndrome. *Journal of Oral Surgery, 33*, 676–678.

Gorlin, R.J., Pindborg, J.J., & Cohen, M.M. (1976). *Syndromes of the face and neck* (2nd ed.). New York: McGraw-Hill.

Gutman, D., Sharon, A., & Laufer, D. (1973). Moebius syndrome: Surgical management of a case. *British Journal of Oral Surgery, 11*, 20–24.

Hardy, J. (1961). Intraoral breath pressure in cerebral palsy. *Journal of Speech & Hearing Disorders, 26*, 310–319.

Hardy, J. (1964). Lung function of athetoid and spastic quadriplegic children. *Developmental & Child Neurology, 6*, 378–388.

Hardy, J. (1983). *Cerebral Palsy.* Englewood Cliffs, NJ: Prentice-Hall.

Hedges, T. (1955). *The relationship between speech understandability and the diadochokinetic rates of certain speech musculatures among individuals with cerebral palsy.* Unpublished doctoral dissertation, Ohio State University.

Hixon, T., & Hardy, J. (1964). Restricted motility of speech articulators in cerebral palsy. *Journal of Speech & Hearing Research, 29*, 293–306.

Ingram, T., & Barn J. (1961). A description and classification of common speech disorders associated with cerebral palsy. *Cerebral Palsy Bulletin, 2*, 254–277.

Irwin, J. (1955). Phonetic equipment of spastic and athetoid children. *Journal of Speech & Hearing Disorders, 20*, 54–67.

Kahane, J. (1979). Pathophysiological effects of Moebius syndrome on speech and hearing. *Archives of Otolaryngology, 105*, 29–34.

Kent, R. & Netsell, R. (1978). Articulatory abnormalities in athetoid cerebral palsy. *Journal of Speech & Hearing Disorders, 43*, 353–373.

Kent, R., Netsell, R., & Bauer, L. (1975). Cineradiographic assessment of articulatory motility in the dysarthrias. *Journal of Speech & Hearing Disorders*, *40*, 467–480.

Kudrgavcev, T., Schoenberg, B.S., Kurland, C.T., Groover, R.V. (1983). Cerebral palsy—Trends in incidence and changes in concurrent neonatal mortality: Rochester, MN, 1950-1976. *Neurology*, *33*, 1433–1438.

Leith, W. (1954). A comparison of judged speech characteristics of athetoid and spastics. Unpublished master's thesis, Purdue University.

Lord, J. (1984). Cerebral Palsy: A clinical approach. *Archives of Physical Medicine & Rehabilitation*, *65*, 542–548.

McDonald, E., & Chance, B. (1964). *Cerebral Palsy*. Englewood Cliffs, NJ: Prentice-Hall.

Merz, M., & Wojtowicz, S. (1967). The Moebius syndrome. *American Journal of Ophthalmology*, *63*, 837–840.

Meyerson, M., & Foushee, D. (1978). Speech, language and hearing in Moebius syndrome. *Developmental Medical and Child Neurology*, *20*, 357–365.

Netsell, R. (1969). Changes in oropharyngeal cavity size of dysarthric children. *Journal of Speech & Hearing Research*, *12*, 646–649.

Pitner, S. Edwards, J., & McCormick, W. (1965). Observations of the pathology of the Moebius syndrome. *Journal of Neurology, Neurosurgery and Psychiatry*, *28*, 362–373.

Platt, L., Andrews, G., Young M., & Quinn, P. (1980). Dysarthria of adult cerebral palsy: I. Intelligibility and articulatory impairment. *Journal of Speech & Hearing Research*, *23*, 28–40.

Platt, L., Andrews, G., & Howie, F.M. (1980). Dysarthria of adult cerebral palsy: II. Phonemic analysis of articulation errors. *Journal of Speech & Hearing Research*, *23*, 41–55.

Rutherford, B. (1944). A comparative study of loudness, pitch rate, rhythm, and quality of speech of children handicapped by cerebral palsy. *Journal of Speech & Hearing Disorders*, *9*, 262–271.

Shapiro, J. (1960). *An investigation of the ability of auditors to assess athetoid and spastic cerebral palsy by listening to speech samples*. Unpublished masters's thesis, Syracuse University.

Sogg, R.L. (1961). Congenital facial diplegia syndrome of Moebius. *Archives of Neurology*, *65*, 16–19.

Wolfe, W. (1950). A comprehensive evaluation of fifty cases of cerebral palsy. *Journal of Speech & Hearing Disorder*, *15*, 234–251.

CHAPTER 5

Adult-Onset, Nonprogressive Dysarthrias

There are a group of dysarthrias whose onset occurs in adulthood. The typical course of these disorders involves a sudden onset, followed by a period of neurologic recovery and later stabilization. Etiologies of these dysarthrias include stroke and traumatic brain injury. Type and characteristics of the speech problems vary considerably and are dependent on the site and extent of the neurological damage.

STROKE

Medical Aspects

Population

Stroke is responsible for almost 10 percent of deaths in the United States; each year there are 500,000 new cases. Most strokes occur in people over age 55; the average age is 70. Seventy to 80 percent survive their first episode and the 10-year survival rate is about 50 percent. The medical risk factors include arterial hypertension (for both ischemic and hemorrhagic types), diabetes mellitus, hyperlipidemia, oral contraceptives use in women over the age of 35 who smoke, and cardiac disease. Other factors implicated in association with stroke are obesity, cigarette smoking, and life stresses. Any patient with a history of transient neurological deficits and the previously listed factors is at extremely high risk for developing a stroke (Goldstein, Bolis, Fiesci, Gorini & Millikan, 1979; Meyer & Shaw, 1982).

There are two types of stroke, ischemic and hemorrhagic. Ischemic strokes result from (1) a sudden blockage, due to atherosclerosis, of a major blood vessel supplying the brain (the internal carotid arteries, vertebrobasilar artery, or their branches), (2) a blood or air embolus that lodges in a vessel, causing complete occlusion, or (3) a microinfarct or "lacune," which results from the effects of chronic hypertension. Hemorrhagic infarcts are caused by (1) subarachnoid hemorrhage due to a congenital defect or hypertension, (2) intracerebral hemorrhage, or (3) arteriovenous malformations (Meyer & Shaw, 1982).

Certain syndromes are quite common or distinctive. Middle cerebral artery syndrome and anterior cerebral artery syndrome result from unilateral carotid artery disease, involving stenosis of the artery, ulceration, or occlusion of an atheromatous plaque. Middle cerebral artery syndrome is manifested by contralateral hemiplegia and hemisensory defect, aphasia if the lesion is on the dominant side, visual/perceptual deficits if the lesion is on the nondominant side, and apractagnosia. Anterior cerebral artery syndrome, however, is identified by paralysis of the contralateral leg with sensory loss and occasional bowel and bladder incontinence. Vertebrobasilar artery syndromes may be caused by trauma, atherosclerosis, or arthritic compression of the vessels. Posterior inferior cerebellar artery syndrome (PICA, Wallenburg's, or lateral medullary syndrome) involves vertigo, dysphagia, ataxia, nausea and vomiting, and homolateral loss of facial sensation with contralateral sensory loss over the body. Basilar artery or pontine infarcts can result in coma or *locked in syndrome* with quadriplegia but intact intellectual functioning. Thalamic syndrome, though rare, is distinctive for its unilateral sensory loss with intense continuous pain (Toole, 1984).

Diagnosis

The history of onset and the clinical appearance of the patient can be helpful in both localizing the lesion and in determining the etiology. Thrombotic or atherosclerotic strokes tend to be stepwise in progression, whereas embolic strokes tend to occur suddenly and completely; hemorrhage often is associated with severe headache and nausea. Beyond this, computerized tomography (CT scan) is commonly used to differentiate between the two types of stroke. An ischemic infarct is seen as a hypodense area against normal brain tissue; hemorrhage is seen as a hyperdense area that enhances when contrast material is injected. If CT scanning is not available, a nuclear brain scan or blood flow study may be done to grossly identify the location of the lesion. Recently, magnetic resonance imaging has also been used to visualize the brain anatomy after cerebral damage.

Some tests may be used to identify the cause of the stroke or to evaluate the patient for possible surgical treatment of the cause, rather than strictly for diagnosis of the presence or absence of stroke. Echocardiography is useful in embolic stroke to localize the source of the embolus, often the left ventricle of the heart. Cerebral angiography may be utilized to better identify the anatomy of an arteriovenous malformation in a hemorrhagic stroke.

Ultrasound studies of the carotid arteries can be used to determine if there is a surgically correctable obstruction. Electroencephalography (EEG) is used to distinguish seizure activity from possible recurrence or enlargement of a stroke (Meyer & Shaw, 1982).

Natural Course

As mentioned before, a stroke may be heralded by a transient loss of neurological function, called a transient ischemic attack (TIA) or reversible ischemic neurologic defect (RIND). Fifteen to 40 percent of these patients will have a cerebral infarct within five years (Goldstein, Bolin, Fieschi, Gorini, & Millikan, 1979). After a stroke, there will generally be a period of hypotonicity for 4 to 48 hours with depressed deep tendon reflexes, a lack of voluntary movement, and possible urinary retention. Following this, there is a return of muscle tone and the onset of spasticity. If movement is to return to an extremity, some indication will be seen in the first 48 hours. Most motor recovery takes place within the first three to six weeks; upper extremity function may continue to improve over the first six months, especially in those patients most severely affected at the outset. The return of language function may continue at a slow rate for an even longer time. Motor return usually occurs in a proximal to distal sequence; gross patterns of flexion or extension will precede any isolated voluntary function (Kaplan & Cerullo, 1986). Incontinence after the first few days is not common and, if present, may indicate an abnormality in the genitourinary tract (Brocklehurst, Andrews, Richards, & Laycoch, 1983). Positive prognostic indicators include strong family support, preservation of visuoperceptual abilities, early return of voluntary movement, and good trunk control. Negative factors include prolonged coma, incontinence past the first 48 hours, the presence of unilateral neglect, and profound aphasia.

The long-term prognosis for recurrence of stroke varies according to the type of lesion. Patients who have atherosclerotic infarcts are certainly at higher risk for repeated espisodes of stroke, especially if they also have hypertension or diabetes mellitus. It is difficult to identify clearly what percentage will go on to recurrence as "silent strokes," or TIAs may confuse the picture. In about 80 percent of strokes with embolic origins, a second episode will occur if the patient is untreated; up to 20 percent of these may occur within 10 days of the initial episode. Patients with hemorrhagic strokes also have a varied outcome. Those with an intracerebral hemorrhage have little chance of rebleeding from the same site. However, among patients with untreated aneurysms, almost half will rebleed and 78 percent of these recurrences are fatal (Adams & Victor, 1985; Gordon, Drenth, Jarvis, Johnson, & Wright, 1978; Henley, Pettit, Todd-Pakropek, & Tupper, 1985).

Certain complications occur frequently enough after a cerebrovascular accident to merit comment. Spasticity with resulting joint contractures is not uncommon; the upper extremity is usually carried in an adducted, internally rotated, and flexed position while the lower limb is extended and externally rotated. Clonus associated with leg spasticity may interfere with independent ambulation and may require bracing or other intervention.

Shoulder subluxation, or a downward displacement of the humeral head in the glenoid fossa, as a result of muscle imbalance or flaccidity may cause pain or traction on the brachial plexus; it may eventually improve with the onset of spasticity. Shoulder-hand syndrome is yet another disorder of the upper extremity with no definitely proven cause. This syndrome is thought to be a manifestation of sympathetic overactivity and is characterized by a painful upper limb with swelling, temperature changes, and contractures of the finger joint. Frozen shoulder may be the end result of all the previously mentioned disorders and consists of a significant decrease in the range of motion at the shoulder because of capsular and soft tissue tightness. It may be quite painful and a significant impediment to independence in activities of daily living. Depression may be significant and is probably more common than generally acknowledged; evidence of vegetative symptoms such as a loss of appetite, disturbed sleep patterns, and anhedonia may indicate the need for antidepressant medication.

Medical Treatment

The most effective treatment for stroke is prevention. Since hypertension and cardiac disease are the most strongly linked precursors of cerebrovascular disease, good control of these disorders will be the most effective means of prevention. Other factors such as smoking, diet, and stress are not as directly associated with cerebrovascular disease but should also be addressed (Meyer & Shaw, 1982).

Transient ischemic attacks should be treated aggressively because of the high percentage of persons who go on to complete a stroke. Standard medical treatment consists of the use of antiplatelet drugs such as aspirin, dipyridamole (Persantine), and more recently, vasodilator drugs. If the patient with TIAs has evidence of significant narrowing of the carotid arteries and his or her transient symptoms are reflective of ischemia in cortical areas supplied by branches of the carotid arteries, then surgical endarterectomy of the carotid arteries may be done.

For those patients who are first seen by medical personnel with an *evolving stroke* (whose symptoms are continuing to worsen), treatment with an anticoagulant (Heparin) might be instituted to halt further thrombosis. If a stroke is thought to be embolic and the patient has an identifiable source of such emboli, then he or she may receive long-term oral anticoagulation (Coumadin). A controversial surgical procedure designed to improve blood flow to the ischemic area, called an EC-IC bypass (external carotid–internal carotid), is being performed in some institutions, but is not routine (Toole, 1984).

Although many patients with completed strokes are treated with antiplatelet drugs to prevent recurrences, there is no treatment that can reverse the neurological deficits. However, function can be considerably improved by providing the patient with physical and cognitive retraining. Physical therapy can be utilized to improve the patients' independence with mobility skills (transfer skills, wheelchair usage, and ambulation). Some physical therapists use neuromuscular facilitation programs to encourage resumption of normal movement patterns and muscle tone. Excessive spasticity can be treated with a number of drugs, including diazepam (Valium), baclofen (Lioresal), and dantrolene sodium (Dantrium). The major side effects of all these drugs include central nervous system sedation and possible weakness of nonparetic muscles. Dantrolene sodium may have hepatotoxic effects as well, and the patient must have periodic blood testing. Other treatments such as nerve blocks and motor point blocks may be directed at specific muscle groups that are interfering with independence. The patient may require lower extremity bracing to provide ankle and knee stability as well as other assistive devices. Occupational therapists can provide instruction in performing basic and advanced levels of daily living activities, evaluate the need for environmental adaptation and equipment, and retrain the patient in perceptual and fine motor skills. Recreation therapists may offer the patient some insight into new or old leisure skills that are available to them despite neurological deficits. Resocialization and community reintegration is also an important component of rehabilitation. Other medications that might be commonly used after stroke would include urologic agents (e.g., Probanthine or Ditropan to help in controlling hyperactive bladders—primary side effects including confusion, urinary retention, and dry mouth), antidepressants (Elavil, nortriptyline—side effects may include hypotension, dry mouth, arrhythmias), and anti-inflammatory agents (Motrin, aspirin, Indocin, Naprosyn, Feldene—side effects usually include gastrointestinal upset).

Speech Characteristics

The communication disorders of aphasia and apraxia of speech are much more commonly associated with stroke than is dysarthria, and the prevalence of dysarthria following stroke is not well documented. The characteristics of the dysarthria depend on the area of the resulting lesion in the central nervous system.

Unilateral Cortical Lesions

A unilateral lesion of the corticobulbar fibers may produce a contralateral weakness of the articulators. Transient, mild dysarthria may result from this weakness. Typically, articulation is the most severely affected, and phonation may be minimally affected. Speech symptoms associated with velopharyngeal dysfunction and respiratory dysfunction are extremely uncommon in unilateral stroke. With severe, acute hemiplegia, articulation may be imprecise, but this disorder is usually resolved in a few days (Darley, Aronson, & Brown, 1975).

Bilateral Cortical Lesions

Bilateral lesions of the corticobulbar fibers are necessary to produce permanent dysarthria secondary to stroke. The resulting dysarthria shows primarily characteristics of spastic dysarthria. This motor disorder is commonly referred to as *pseudobulbar palsy.* This condition is commonly caused by bilateral stroke, but may result from infantile cerebral palsy, severe brain injuries, multiple sclerosis, progressive degeneration of the brain, encephalitis, and extensive brain tumors (Darley, et al., 1975).

Studies of the performance of speech mechanism subsystems of subjects with spastic dysarthria due to bilateral stroke are limited. Darley, Aronson, and Brown, (1969a, 1969b) made no direct measures of respiratory function for the pseudobulbar group. However, they perceptually observed "short breath groups." This characteristic might have resulted from laryngeal dysfunction.

Phonatory disorders are commonly observed in speakers with pseudobulbar palsy. Kammermeier (1969) observed that pitch variability was reduced for pseudobulbar as compared to normal speakers. Darley, and colleagues (1969a, 1969b) reported harsh voice quality in 29 of 30 speakers in this group. Strained-strangled voice quality was observed in 20 of 30 pseudobulbar speakers. In addition, pitch breaks, breathiness of voice, shortness of phrases, and slow rate of speech were also reported. Twenty-nine of the 30 subjects demonstrated monotony of pitch, and 27 of 30 exhibited monotony of loudness. In an instrumental study of laryngeal aerodynamic resistance, Smitheran and Hixon (1981) presented the case of an individual with multiple bilateral strokes and a marked strained-strangled voice quality. Measures of laryngeal resistance for this speaker were 85 percent higher than the average resistance of normal male speakers.

The articulatory/resonance disorders of pseudobulbar dysarthria included imprecise consonants for all subjects. Hypernasality was perceived in 20 of 30 subjects. Twenty-five of the 30 subjects exhibited slowed speaking rate (Darley et al., 1975).

Lesions in the Area of Vertebrobasilar Circulation

The vertebral arteries and the basilar artery and their branch supply blood to a number of areas, including the upper cervical spinal cord, the cerebellum, the medulla oblongata, the pons, and most of the remaining mesencephalon. Infarcts in these areas are less common than cortical infarcts, accounting for 15 percent of all cerebrovascular accidents (CVAs). The speech characteristics associated with dysarthria or stroke vary, depending on the site of lesion.

Brainstem strokes may result in a flaccid paralysis of the speech muscles. The two major muscular abnormalities are weakness and hyptonia. These abnormalities are seen in all movements of affected muscles including those movements that are reflexive, automatic, or voluntary in origin. Darley and colleagues (1975) summarize the perceptual speech characteristics of a group of 30 individuals with bulbar palsy as follows:

> the combination of auditory characteristics that best distinguishes flaccid dysarthria from other types consists of marked hypernasality often coupled with nasal emission of air, continuous breathiness during phonation, and audible inspiration (stridor on inhalation). (p. 127)

Fisher (1978) presented case studies of three stroke patients who showed weakness and pyramidal signs on one side combined with cerebellar-like ataxia on the same side. Pathologic study in each case showed an infarct in the basis pontis at the level of the junction of the upper one third and lower two thirds on the side opposite the neurologic deficit. Two of these three individuals demonstrated slight dysarthria.

Grunwell and Huskins (1979) described a woman who experienced a large post fossa cerebellar hematoma caused by bleeding from an angioma. Due to severe ataxia, she was wheelchair-bound and demonstrated an ataxic dysarthria. Her speech was slow, but characterized by "excessive rhythmicity." Monoloudness and monopitch were present along with articulatory imprecision. Frequent errors of voicing, aspiration, and nasality were observed.

TRAUMATIC BRAIN INJURY

Medical Aspects

Epidemiology

Injuries to the head resulting in either temporary or permanent brain damage are extremely common. However, the actual number of head injures is difficult to estimate for at least two reasons. First, head injuries frequently go unreported. Second, no consistent definition of such an injury has been used across studies. For example, diagnoses such as facial lacerations, skull fractures, or brain contusions may all be reported as head injury. For purposes of this text, the discussion will be restricted to traumatic brain injury. Based on emergency room records, the incidence of traumatic brain injury is 200/100,000 population with about 400,000 patients admitted to the hospital each year in the United States. Traumatic brain injury is responsible for 25 percent of all deaths due to trauma; of all men who have died of traumatic brain injury, only 34 percent lived long enough to be admitted to the hospital (Grossman & Gildenberg, 1982). The incidence for children is similar, with a morbidity rate of 10/100,000 children per year (Shapiro, 1983).

The occurrence of brain injury is two to three times higher in men than in women for all ages. However, the greatest difference in incidence between the sexes occurs in the group between 15 to 24. Another high-risk group is the elderly over age 75. Road accidents (including motorcycle, bicycle, other vehicles, and pedestrians) account for the majority of traumatic brain injuries. Among children, falls constitute another major cause for head injuries. Both chronic and acute types of brain injuries can be attributed to some sports (Jennett & Teasdale, 1981; Rosenthal, Griffith, Bond, & Miller, 1983). Although some advances have been made in modifying sports equipment and practices and in mandating the use of safety equipment on motor vehicles, recent trends to repeal such safety and speed laws may impact the future statistics regarding traumatic brain injury.

Classification of Brain Injuries

The major categories of brain injuries are penetrating and closed. Penetrating injuries include bullet or knife wounds, or other sharp instruments seen in pediatric cases, such as pencils and knitting needles. On the whole, penetrating injuries are less frequent in the civilian population than in the military and will often manifest more focal neurological findings than the closed head injury. The biomechanics of closed head injury are important in understanding the resultant neuropathology. With a blow to the head or a simple fall, a compression injury may result in a local indentation of the skull, with the lesion appearing directly below the site of impact (the *coup* lesion). With acceleration injuries, a number of different mechanisms may occur singly or in combination. A simple linear translation motion of the brain substance may occur and result in lesions distal or opposite to the site of impact (the *contrecoup* lesion). This occurs frequently in children whose bony skulls are immature and more yielding to pressure than the adult bony skull. When a rotational force occurs, shear strains are applied to the brain substance, resulting in more diffuse injury. Any combination of these forces may occur with multiple sites and types of injuries (Shapiro, 1983).

The actual pathological findings may include a skull fracture, found frequently in fatal injuries. However, the presence of a skull fracture by itself does not indicate a significant traumatic brain injury. Brain lesions may be focal, for example, in extradural or subdural hematomas or intracerebral contusions. These contusions are frequently found on the undersurface of the temporal and frontal lobes and at the anterior poles of the temporal lobe, regardless of the actual site of impact. This is probably due to the bony structure of the skull. Diffuse white matter lesions may also occur, especially in the corpus callosum and the superior cerebellar peduncles (Grossman & Gildenberg, 1982; Jennett & Teasdale, 1981).

A further distinction can be made between the primary impact damage and secondary damage due to the brain's response to injury. This might include such reactions as edema, cerebral hypoxia, and cerebral ischemia. Elevated intracranial pressure has been shown to affect regional cerebral blood flow. It is felt that many of the focal residua of traumatic brain injury may be due to infarcts produced by elevated intracranial pressure.

Another type of injury that falls under the general category of closed head injury is the minor head injury or cerebral concussion. This is characterized by a brief loss of consciousness, followed by evidently complete recovery without any focal neurological signs. Although pathological studies in humans are few (because few patients die in conjunction with minor head injury), it appears from animal studies that there are changes in the functioning of the neuronal mitochondria and altered permeability of the blood-brain barrier (Bakay & Glasauer, 1980).

In chronic traumatic brain injury or post-traumatic dementia ("Boxer's Brain"), lesions are often found in deep central structures of the brain such as the thalamus and basal ganglia. These lesions result in a parkinsonian-type neurological picture, as well as dementia.

Acute Management

Severe brain injuries are frequently associated with major damage to other body systems, so that immediate concerns are maintenance of adequate respiration and circulation. A clinical assessment tool used throughout the world is the Glasgow Coma Scale devised by Teasdale and Jennett (1976). This scale attempts to quantify levels of consciousness by assigning scores to eye movements, motor responses, and verbal responses based on the best performance of the patient. (See Table 5-1.) Glasgow Coma Scale scores of eight or less are considered indicative of severe brain injury; scores of twelve or better define minor injury.

Many centers rely heavily on intracranial pressure monitoring devices to assist in planning therapies and surgeries. Computerized tomography (CT) scans and magnetic resonance imaging (MRI) are the most widely used methods of localizing lesions within the brain and have contributed, in conjunction with monitoring, to direct surgical interventions. Cerebral angiography may be performed if there is any suspicion of the presence of a vascular abnormality. Regional cerebral blood flow studies done with radioactive tracer are most helpful in monitoring the secondary effects of edema and ischemia. Electroencephalography is no longer routinely performed as an initial diagnostic tool, but may be used in places where CT or MRI scanning is not available, or in later diagnosis of seizure disorders.

Medical treatments used acutely might include hyperventilation of the patient to decrease the carbon dioxide content of the blood, the administration of osmotic diuretics to reduce blood volumes, and the administration of barbiturates to reduce oxygen demand. The use of steriods, although used widely at one time, have not been shown to be beneficial in reducing morbidity (Grossman & Gildenberg, 1982). Hypothermia has also been used in

TABLE 5-1.
The Glasgow Coma Scale.

Eye Opening	4	Spontaneous
	3	To command
	2	To pain
	1	Nil
Best Motor Response	6	Obeys commands
	5	Localizes pain (purposeful)
	4	Flexor withdrawal (semipurposeful)
	3	Abnormal flexor (decorticate)
	2	Extensor (decerebrate)
	1	Nil
Verbal Commands	5	Oriented
	4	Disoriented
	3	Words
	2	Sounds
	1	Nil pain
	Total possible 15	

an attempt to decrease general metabolic demands; none of these methods has been clearly more effective than others (Jennett & Teasdale, 1981).

Course of Recovery

In general, rapid recovery after traumatic brain injury probably occurs on a biochemical basis; restoration of neurotransmitter function, oxygenation, and perfusion to brain tissue may also play a part (Jennett & Teasdale, 1981; Rosenthal, Griffith, Bond, & Miller, 1983). Recovery occurring over hours to days indicates that the neural system is likely to be still intact, although damaged. Restoration of function may be seen even after months or perhaps years; the reason for this recovery is poorly understood. It has been explained on the basis of redundant neural pathways or by the adaptation of alternative areas of the brain with previously unused potential.

In severely brain-injured individuals, roving eye movement and spontaneous eye-opening are usually the first functions to appear; they may appear deceptively purposeful even in unresponsive patients. The motor response is the best indicator of recovery in these patients and usually occurs in the sequence listed in the Glasgow Coma Scale. Improving motor abilities may be accommpanied by emerging movement disorders such as tremors or dystonic movements. These movement disorders generally improve over time. The verbal response also improves along the same scale: initially, the person may be noisy and disinhibited; this is usually followed by a period of confusion, disorientation, and possible delusional or hallucinatory behavior. Verbal ability may be difficult to evaluate in critically injured persons who may be intubated or otherwise unable to produce audible speech. Early talking after traumatic brain injury may be deceptive; it has been estimated that 38 percent of those admitted to the hospital who later died of their head injuries talked at some stage (Bakay & Glasauer, 1980).

The end of coma is usually marked by the patient's ability to follow one-stage commands and to communicate in some manner with others. However, post-traumatic amnesia (the length of time from the point of injury to return of continuous memory) may persist beyond the end of coma by weeks. The end of post-traumatic amnesia correlates closely with complete orientation; the patient will often describe this event as "waking up." At this time, other, more subtle, behavior abnormalities may manifest themselves and will be discussed in more detail later in this chapter.

Three states of reduced wakefulness may be seen after severe brain injury and may not follow the normal course of recovery. The *locked-in syndrome* may be seen when there has been complete disruption of motor pathways through the ventral pons; the person is awake and sentient, but is also quadriplegic and mute. When the rostral brain stem is affected, a state known as akinetic mutism or *coma vigil* may be seen. In this case, the neurologic status may fluctuate, but eye movements may occur. The last of these syndromes is the *persistent vegetative state.* In this state, there is essentially no cortical function. However, because the brain stem is intact, numerous reflexes may occur. Respiration is maintained spontaneously, chewing and teeth grinding may occur. The patient may display a palmar grasp reflex. Roving eye movements are frequently present and patients will react to painful stimuli with eye opening and reflex movements of the limbs. Patients may continue, with good nursing and medical care, to live for years in this state. One study demonstrated that, of the patients with a firm diagnosis of persistent vegetative state at one month, only seven percent ever reached the level of moderate disability. This improvement was always apparent by three months after injury. After three months, 10 percent of those diagnosed with persistent vegetative state showed some improvement, but all remained severely disabled and totally dependent (Rosenthal, et al., 1983).

The course of individuals admitted to the hospital with a minor head injury (or post-concussional syndrome) is somewhat variable. Many are discharged without any neurological abnormalities by examination or patient's report. Frequently, however, within three months, complaints of persistent headache, memory difficulties, and difficulty in completing work or household chores are reported. Other symptoms include dizziness, poor concentration, fatigue, and irritability (Grossman & Gildenberg, 1982; Jennett & Teasdale, 1981).

Physical and Neurological Complications and Sequelae

The patient with traumatic brain injury acquired in a vehicular accident is likely to have other injuries in such areas as the thoracic, abdominal, and skeletal systems. Of particular consequence to future communication abilities are craniofacial fracture and cervical spine fractures/dislocations. Long-term musculoskeletal problems may include the formation of heterotopic bone in limbs where spasticity and paresis occur, especially at the hip, shoulder, and elbow. Untreated, this may significantly decrease functional range of motion at the involved joint and compromise seating, mobility, and hand use. Treatment consists of the administration of disodium etidronate (Didronel) and surgical resection of the abnormal bone (Garland & Rhoades, 1978).

Permanent neurological sequelae and complications are usually the most physically disabling impairments outside the cognitive or behavioral realms. Cranial nerve deficits are observed in about 32 percent of persons with severe head injures (Jennett & Teasdale, 1981). Anosmia is frequently not diagnosed until after discharge from the hospital and is common even in mild injuries. Visual pathways can be assessed grossly by the use of optokinetic drums or strips, as well as with visual evoked responses. Visual field testing will require some cooperation on the part of the patient. Oculomotor muscle dysfunction may result from both intracranial damage and from orbital fractures causing entrapment. The facial nerve is second only to the olfactory nerve in frequency of involvement. Signs of recovery should be present within eight weeks of injury if recovery is to occur; nerve conduction and eletromyographic studies may assist in assessing prognosis. Vestibular dysfunction may be the basis for dizziness or vertigo in some patients. Clinically, oculovestibular and caloric testing are helpful; electronystagmograms can also be obtained at a later stage. Auditory loss may be more frequent than is presently known; of those tested, greater than 50 percent are abnormal, especially with high frequency losses. Brainstem auditory evoked responses may be obtained from even comatose patients to indicate intactness of the auditory pathways. Tinnitus is often present without any objective eighth nerve findings on auditory or vestibular testing (Jennett & Teasdale, 1981; Rosenthal et al., 1983).

Disorders of movement are also quite common in the traumatically brain-injured population. Hemiparesis is present in 49 percent of the severely brain injured. The other most frequently encountered disorders include spasticity, bradykinesia, ataxia, tremors, rigidity, and apraxia. Sensory impairment may occur from decreased cortical function such as deficits in graphesthesia, stereognosis, two-point discrimination, simultaneous tactile discrimination, and deep pain. Disorders of peripheral nerve function, especially at the brachial plexus in motorcycle injuries, may result in local paralysis or causalgias (Jennett & Teasdale, 1981; Rosenthal et al., 1983).

Epileptic seizures occur frequently in the first week following traumatic brain-injury. Among all brain-injured patients admitted to the hospital, five percent will develop a seizure disorder after the first week (later or post-traumatic epilepsy). Only 18 to 25 percent of those with early seizures will have a permanent disorder. Factors that increase the chance of developing late epilepsy include brain penetration, subdural hematomas, and hygromas. Greater than 50 percent of those patients who develop later epilepsy do so in the first year; however, there is a significant risk of having a first seizure up to four years post-injury (Jennett & Teasdale, 1981; Rosenthal et al., 1983).

Endocrinologic disorders resulting from pituitary and hypothalamic lesions are not uncommon after brain injury. Diabetes insipidus, with polyuria and polydipsia and fluid wasting, is usually transient and is treated with increased fluid intake and use of vasopressin. Hyperphagia is more uncommon and is not presently treatable. Hypopituitarism is rare and can be adequately controlled with hormone replacement (Roberts, 1979).

Many sequelae directly involving the brain may be seen after brain injury. The most common of these are infection and hydrocephalus. Meningitis usually involves a fracture or direct penetration of the brain substance. Fractures involving the nasal sinuses are especially correlated with later infection. Post-traumatic hydrocephalus may result from:

1. reaction to blood in the vectricles causing adhesions to form
2. resorption of necrotic brain tissue (hydrocephalus ex vacuo)
3. decreased reabsorption of cerebrospinal fluid (normal pressure hydrocephalus) (Rosenthal et al., 1983).

Cognitive and Behavioral Sequelae

The cognitive impairment that remains after severe or even mild brain injury may frequently persist despite the resolution of motor or sensory deficits. Cognitive and behavioral deficits have a greater impact on the resumption of normal occupation than do neurologic sequelae. The areas most affected appear to be initiative and activity level, attention and concentration, memory, language and thinking, problem-solving, and judgment. Persons often demonstrate decreased drive and stamina as well as a slowness of movement or reaction after traumatic brain injury. Studies have indicated that even in patients with good recovery, significant reductions in attention and concentration, rapid processing of information, and endurance in problem solving exist (Stuss, Ely, Hugenholz, Richard, LaRochelle, & Poirier, 1985). Memory in all areas can be affected, but especially in complex new learning situations. The recovery of memory and learning is much slower than other functions; however, the meaning of this in relation to everyday activities is unknown. Brain-injured individuals frequently display impaired understanding of propriety and situations requiring safety precautions. These individuals may be at risk for further accidents because of these deficits.

The behavior of the brain-injured individual may be attributable to the premorbid personality, organic damage sustained during the injury, and the reaction to the injury itself. Frontal lobe lesions are manifested by decreased drive, apathy, lethargy, social disinhibition, poor judgment, inappropriate sexual and aggressive behavior, and dull affect. Some patients, on the other hand, display an inappropriate euphoria with emotional lability and a tendency to underestimate their disabilities. Children will often display a syndrome of irritability, restlessness, and aggressive behavior. Brain-injured individuals are not immune to reactive or affective syndromes seen in all people after a devastating illness or accident, such as anger, frustration, or depression. This may be reflected in the behavior of family and friends who are adjusting to the change in role demanded of them in response to their family member's new persona and physical disabilities.

Treatment Options

Treatment modalities for the moderately or severely brain-injured patient span virtually the entire spectrum of medical, surgical, behavioral, and cognitive tools presently available. Neurosurgery would commonly be done in response to a worsening or nonresolving mass effect causing compression of neural structures acutely or subacutely. Chronically, a patient may require a cerebrospinal fluid shunting procedure to reduce hydrocephalus or a cranioplasty to replace missing bone mass. Numerous orthopedic procedures may be necessary to deal with the long-term effects of spasticity and hemiparesis, including such procedures as tendon lengthening, muscle tendon transfers, or resection of heterotopic bone.

The early nutritional status of brain-injured patients is of much concern in light of numerous other injuries, impaired swallowing and cognition, and vigorous posturing that may lead to a catabolic state. Placement of a gastrostomy or a jejunostomy tube for alternative feeding is often necessary; later a feeding and swallowing stimulation program may improve a patient's level of independence. Another early consideration is attention to positioning in bed to avoid joint contractures and to prevent pressure ulcers from occurring.

As most patients with severe head injuries have a significant degree of spasticity, rigidity, and/or hemiparesis, early intervention with physical therapy is important. Strategies to decrease the adverse sequelae of spasticity and rigidity may include the use of antispasticity medications (such as diazepam, baclofen, or dantrolene sodium), inhibitive total contact casting of the extremities or splinting, the use of ice packs, motor point and nerve blocks, and gentle range of motion exercises. Other problems commonly addressed by the therapist are balance training, cardiovascular conditioning, and muscle reeducation. Both occupational and physical therapists will be involved in formulating proper seating and mobility equipment and environmental control units if necessary. There are no ideal remedies for rigidity and tremors, but drugs used in this situation may include levodopa, propanolol, izoniazid, anticholinergic medications (e.g., Congentin, Benadryl), or even anticonvulsants.

These is no firm evidence that perceptual retraining is successful in decreasing perceptual impairments; however, these exercises may enable the patient to maximize use of the residual abilities. Exercises usually include increasing sensory feedback, visual scanning and organizational techniques, and utilizing vestibular and proprioceptive stimulation to heighten the patient's interaction with the environment.

Behavioral manifestations of agitation and irritability are often best managed by manipulation of the environment (adequate rest in a quiet private room, controlled exposure to stimuli, etc.) and the use of behavioral principles to foster desired results (positive reinforcement, clearly measurable expectations, etc.). Medications may be used, but most have a sedative effect as well. Haloperidol (Haldol) is a phenothiazine used in small doses for increased agitation; its major side effects are sedative and movement disorders that may be permanent with chronic usage. Propanolol, also used for control of agitation, is a beta-adrenergic blocking agent long used for controlling heart rate. This drug seems beneficial for brain-injured patients as its sedative effects are minimal. Antidepressants and lithium carbonate may also be used in a selected population. In those patients with primarily frontal lobe symptoms of lethargy and apathy, some success has been obtained with amphetamine and Ritalin therapy (Stern, 1978).

The area of cognitive remediation is a controversial one. Proponents of cognitive retraining feel that alteration of the brain's capacity for relearning or new learning can be fostered by repetition and intensive exposure to subsets of information or processing that have been affected by brain injury. Tasks are designed to improve the executive skills, basic level of orientation, psychomotor skills, visual processing skills, memory functions, and communication skills. It has been difficult to evaluate the success of such programs, as meaningful and functional tests of such skills are, for the most part, lacking. However, attention to these areas may at the very least allow the patient and his or her family to address these deficits and construct acceptable methods of dealing with them on a daily basis.

Skills of daily living should also be addressed. Together with self-care issues, these may include safety consciousness, monetary understanding, driving, social skills, and other abilities necessary for independent living.

Outcome and Prognosis

Many measures of outcome have been created and implemented for brain-injured individuals in order to evaluate rehabilitative techniques and to assist medical professionals in better determining prognosis and appropriate timing of intervention. Two premorbid factors have a bearing on overall recovery from traumatic brain injury—psychosocial status and age. Patients of more stable socioeconomic status are more likely to return to work after traumatic brain injury. Individuals who are white-collar workers are also more likely to return to work (Gilchrist & Wilkinson, 1976; Roberts, 1979). With respect to age, the younger the patient, the more likely he or she is to survive the injury. Morbidity increases with increasing age. This may be due to the medical consequences accompanying severe brain injury rather than to the injury itself (Rosenthal et al., 1983).

The type of injury will also have an effect on survival and recovery. The presence of coma after injury is a negative prognostic factor, particularly when one looks at the duration and depth of coma, as measured by the Glasgow Coma Scale. The motor response is the most powerful predictor of outcome. The presence of an intracranial intradural hematoma requiring surgical evacuation is associated with increased mortality and morbidity (Rosenthal et al., 1983). Post-traumatic amnesia can be used in combination with other descriptors of coma to predict outcome; severe disability generally does not occur unless post-traumatic amnesia is greater than 14 days. In fact, 83 percent of patients with post-traumatic amnesia of less than 14 days will make a good recovery (defined by Jennett & Bond [1975] as being able to resume normal vocational and social activities, although often in the context of persisting minor physical or mental deficits). The presence of a skull fracture has no significant effect on outcome.

Although there may be individual exceptions, the statistics on overall outcome indicate that the major part of recovery is accomplished by three to six months after injury. Of those who have a good recovery by 12 months, about two-thirds have done so by three months and fully 90 percent by six months (Rosenthal et al., 1983). Of all patients with severe brain injury, about half are dead within six months. Between 12 and 26 percent will achieve a good recovery. The rest will be significantly disabled and about half will remain dependent on others for activities of daily living. The outcome after severe brain injury has been reported by Jennett and Teasdale (1981) as follows:

Dead at six months	50%
Persistent vegetative state	2–5%
Severe disability	7–14%
Moderate disability	15–19%
Good recovery	12–26%

The situation for children is quite different. However, what may initially appear to be a good outcome for a child may still represent a loss because mental and physical development may not reach their true potential. Children under age 15 are rarely in a vegetative state or severely disabled (totally dependent for all activities of daily living, but conscious). Ninety percent or more are moderately disabled or better at three years after their injuries. In fact, independent ambulation can be expected in 70 to 80 percent of children in a coma for up to three months. However, cognitive impairment commonly persists despite physical recovery and, as noted, may be even more disabling to children who must accomplish so much new learning (Shapiro, 1983).

Speech Characteristics

Occurrence of Dysarthria

The dysarthric characteristics associated with traumatic brain injury have been addressed by only a few research groups and, as yet, are poorly described. Rusk, Block, and Lowman (1969) found that approximately one third of a group of 96 head trauma patients evidenced dysarthria in their acute illness. A follow-up study by the same authors between five and 15 years later revealed that of the original 30 patients, the dysarthria of approximately half of the patients had improved significantly and half had not changed. Thompsen (1983) observed that in the closed-head-injured population, individuals with dysarthria showed little or no improvement up to 15 years post-injury.

Sarno, Buonagura, and Levita (1986) tested a group of 125 closed head injury subjects on a battery of language tests. Their results indicated that 29 percent exhibited classical aphasia; 34 percent exhibited dysarthria and subclinical aphasia; and 36 percent exhibited subclinical aphasia. These authors defined subclinical aphasia as "linguistic processing deficits on testing in the absence of clinical manifestations of linguistic impairment." The dysarthrias observed ranged in severity from "mild articulatory imprecision of consonant sound to completely unintelligible speech." The finding that dysarthric subjects also exhibited subclinical aphasia was unexpected. The authors state, "The severity of such linguistic impairment is all the more dramatic because such deficits generally are not expected to be present in patients with dysarthria."

Characteristics of Dysarthria

There appear to be no research studies that focus primarily on describing the dysarthric characteristics of the closed-head-injured population. However, there is growing evidence from a series of intervention studies of the diversity of characteristics that depend upon the locus and severity of the brain injury. Predominantly ataxic dysarthria has been reported in some closed-head-injured patients by Simmons (1983), Yorkston and Beukelman (1981a), Yorkston, Beukelman, Minifie, and Sapir (1984). Predominantly flaccid dysarthria was reported for a head-injured man by Netsell and Daniel (1979). Yorkston and Beukelman (1981b) described individuals with closed head injury who exhibited mixed flaccid-spastic and mixed spastic-ataxic dysarthria. To date, there have been no articles reporting the incidence of the various types of dysarthria in the closed-head-injured population.

Mutism After Brain Injury

A number of syndromes whose features include speechlessness after arousal from coma have been described. *Persistent vegetative state* (Jennett & Plum, 1972) is a term that refers to individuals who exhibit no cognitive interaction with their environment, as reflected by failure to follow commands and total inability to communicate. *Locked-in syndrome* (Bauer, Gerstenbrand, & Rumpl, 1979; Plum & Poser, 1980) is a term used to describe patients with relatively preserved language comprehension. Many of these individuals may communicate by eye blinking or vertical eye movement. The occurrence of mutism in a series of 350 head-injured patients was reported by Levin, Madison, Bailey, Meyers, Eisenberg, and Guinto (1983). They reported that three percent were mute after recovery of consciousness, despite the fact that these individuals communicated through nonspeech channels. Their findings led them to suggest:

> two types of mutism may be distinguished after head injury. Interruption of speech following a left focal basal ganglia lesion is typically associated with more rapid recovery of consciousness and has a better prognosis for linguistic outcome, whereas mutism produced by severe diffuse brain injury is more likely to lead to residual linguistic disorder. (p. 606)

Von Cramon (1981) reported the course of recovery of speech in 11 individuals who had suffered from acute traumatic midbrain syndrome. During the initial stage, mutism was characterized by the "complete loss of voluntary control of the laryngeal muscles." These individuals were unable to cough or clear their throats voluntarily, but were able to do so reflexively. During the second stage of mutism, nonverbal utterances occurred that often signaled emotions such as pain, disgust, or affirmation. The final stage of mutism occurs when the individual produces verbalization in response to a stimulus, but not spontaneously. Speech is usually accompanied by a whisper or breathy phonation during this phase.

Sapir and Aronson (1985) reported the cases of two closed-head-injured individuals with aphonia in the presence of intact cough and swallowing abilities and only mildly impaired articulation. They argue against paralysis of the vocal folds and suggest that the aphonia may be due to a frontal lobe-limbic system disturbance. They state:

> One explanation is that the aphonia was a consequence of an affective disorder secondary to damage or disturbance of the limbic system and its neocortical and subcortical, especially reticular and thalamic, connections. . . . These neural systems allegedly do not participate in motor coordination nor in the execution of phonatory gestures, but seem to function as a drive-controlling mechanism that determines, by its activity, the readiness to phonate as well as the intensity of phonation. . . . (pp. 292–293)

In this chapter, the medical aspects and speech characteristics of nonprogressive, adult-onset dysarthrias has been presented. In the following chapter, a group of adult-onset dysarthrias with a progressive course will be reviewed.

REFERENCES

Adams, R.D., & Victor, M. (1985). *Principles of neurology.* New York: McGraw-Hill.

Bakay, L., & Gasauer, F.E. (1980). *Head Injury.* Boston: Little, Brown & Co.

Bauer, G., Gerstenbrand, F., & Rumpl, E. (1979). Varieties of locked-in syndrome. *Journal of Neurology, 221,* 77–91.

Brochlehurst, J.C., Andrews, K., Richards, B., & Laycoch, P.J. (1983). Incidence and correlates of incontinence in stroke patients. *Journal of the American Geriatrics Society, 33*(8), 540.

Darley, F., Aronson, A., & Brown, J. (1969a). Differential diagnostic patterns of dysarthria. *Journal of Speech & Hearing Research, 12,* 462–496.

Darley, F., Aronson, A., & Brown, J. (1969b). Clusters of deviant speech dimensions in the dysarthrias. *Journal of Speech & Hearing Research, 12,* 462–496.

Darley, F., Aronson, A., & Brown, J. (1975). *Motor Speech Disorders.* Philadelphia: W.B. Saunders.

Fisher, C. (1978). Ataxic Hemiparesis. *Archives of Neurology, 35,* 126–128.

Garland, D.E. & Rhoades, M.E. (1978). Orthopedic management of brain-injured adults, Part II. *Clinical Orthopedics and Related Research, 131,* 111.

Gilchrist, E., & Wilkinson, M. (1976). Some factors determining prognosis in young people with severe head injuries. *Archives of Neurology, 36,* 355.

Goldstein, Bolis, L., Fieschi, C., Gorini, S., & Millikan, C.H. (Eds.). (1979). *Cerebrovascular Disorders and Strokes: Advances in Neurology,* (Vol. 25). New York: Raven Press.

Gordon, E.E., Drenth, V., Jarvis, L., Johnson, J., & Wright, V. (1978). Neurophysiologic syndromes in stroke as predictors of outcome. *Archives of Physical Medicine & Rehabilitation, 59,* 399.

Grossman, R.G., & Gildenberg, P.L. (1982). *Head Injury: Basic and Clinical Concepts.* New York: Raven Press.

Grunwell, P., & Huskins, S. (1979). Intelligibility in acquired dysarthria—a neurophonetic approach: Three studies. *Journal of Communication Disorders, 12,* 9–22.

Henley, S.H., Pettit, S., Todd-Pakropek, A., & Tupper, A. (1985). How goes home? Prediction factors in stroke recovery. *Journal of Neurology, Neurosurgery & Psychiatry, 1985, 48,* 1.

Jennett, W.B., & Bond, M. (1975). Assessment of outcome after severe brain damage. A practical scale. *Lancet, 1,* 480.

Jennett, W.B., & Plum, F. (1972). The persistent vegetative state: A syndrome in search of a name. *Lancet, 1,* 734.

Jennett, W.B., & Teasdale, G. (1981). *Management of Head Injuries.* Philadelphia: FA Davis.

Kammermeier, M. (1969). *A comparison of phonatory phenomena among groups of neurologically impaired speakers.* Unpublished doctoral dissertation, University of Minnesota.

Kaplan, P.E., & Cerullo, L.J. (1986). *Stroke Rehabilitation.* Boston: Butterworths.

Levin, H.S., Madison, C.F., Bailey, C.B., Meyers, C.A., Eisenberg, H.M., & Guinto, F.C. (1983). Mutism after closed head injury. *Archives of Neurology, 40,* 601–606.

Meyer, J.S., & Shaw, T. (Eds.). (1982). *Diagnosis and management of strokes and TIAs,* Menlo Park: Addison-Wesley Publishing Co.

Netsell, R., & Daniel, B. (1979). Dysarthria in adults: Physiologic approach to rehabilitation. *Archives of Physical Medicine & Rehabilitation*, *60*, 502–508.

Plum, F., & Poser, J.B. (1980). *Diagnosis of Stupor and Coma* (3rd ed.). Philadelphia: FA Davis.

Roberts, A.H. (1979). *Severe Accidental Head Injury: An Assessment of Long-term Prognosis*. London: The Macmillan Press.

Rosenthal, M., Griffith, E.R., Bond, M.R., & Miller, J.D. (1983). *Rehabilitation of the Head Injured Adult*. Philadelphia: FA Davis.

Rusk, H., Block, J., & Lowmann, E. (1969). Rehabilitation of the brain injured patient: A report of 157 cases with long term follow-up of 118. In E. Walker, W. Caveness, & M. Critchley (Eds.), *The late effects of head injury*. Springfield: Charles C. Thomas.

Sapir, S., & Aronson, A.E. (1985). Aphonia after closed head injury: Aetiologic considerations. *British Journal of Disorders of Communication*, *20*, 289–296.

Sarno, M. T., Buonaguro, A., & Levita, E. (1986). Characteristics of verbal impairment in closed head injured patients. *Archives of Physical Medicine & Rehabilitation*, *67*, 400–405.

Shapiro, K. (1983). *Pediatric Head Trauma*. Mount Kisco, NY: Futura Publishing Co.

Simmons, N. (1983). Acoustic analysis of ataxic dysarthria: An approach to monitoring treatment. In W. Berry (Ed.), *Clinical Dysarthria*. Austin, TX: PRO-ED.

Smitheran, J., & Hixon, T. (1981). A clinical method of estimating laryngeal airway resistance during vowel production. *Journal of Speech and Hearing Disorders*, *46*, 138–146.

Stern, J.M. (1978). Cranio-cerebral injured patients. *Scand. Journal of Rehabilitation Medicine*, *10*, 7.

Stuss, D.T., Ely, P., Hugenholtz, H., Richard, M.T., LaRochelle, S., Poirier, C.A., & Bell, I. (1985). Subtle neuropsychological deficits in patients with good recovery after closed head injury. *Neurosurgery*, *17*, 41.

Teasdale, G., & Jennett, B. (1976). Assessment and prognosis of coma after head injury. *Acta Neurochir (Wien)*, *34*, 45.

Thompsen, V. (1983). Standardized methods of assessing and predicting outcome. In M. Rosenthal, E. Griffith, M. Bond, & J.D. Miller (Eds.), *Rehabilitation of the head injured adult*. Philadelphia: F.A. Davis.

Toole, J.F.(Ed.). (1984). *Cerebrovascular Disorders* (3rd ed.). New York: Raven Press.

Von Cramon, D. (1981). Traumatic mutism and the subsequent reorganization of speech functions. *Neuropsychologia*, *19*, 801–805.

Yorkston, K.M., & Beukelman, D.R. (1981a). *Assessment of intelligibility of dysarthria speech*. Austin, TX: PRO-ED.

Yorkston, K.M., & Beukelman, D.R. (1981b). Ataxic dysarthria: Treatment sequences based on intelligibility and prosodic considerations. *Journal of Speech & Hearing Disorders*, *46*, 398–404.

Yorkston, K.M., Beukelman, D.R., Minifie, F.D., & Sapir, S. (1984). Assessment of stress patterning in dysarthric speakers. In M.McNeil, A. Aronson, & J. Rosenbek, (Eds.), *The dysarthrias: Physiology, acoustics, perception, management*. San Diego: College-Hill Press.

CHAPTER 6

The Degenerative Dysarthrias

This chapter contains a review of the medical aspects, speech characteristics, and management of a diverse group of dysarthrias with a degenerative natural course. Onset of these disorders occurs after childhood, and in most cases, the disorders are insidious, with signs and symptoms appearing gradually. Many progressive neuromotor disorders result in dysarthria, however, we will not review them all here. Rather, we have selected those disorders that occur frequently in a clinical caseload of speech/language pathologists together with those disorders that are uncommon but whose speech characteristics have been studied carefully and are reported in the literature.

The chapter begins with reviews of those disorders referred to by neurologists as *movement disorders*. Movement disorders can be divided into two general clinical types: the akinetic-rigid syndrome of parkinsonism and those conditions characterized by abnormal involuntary movements known as the dyskinesias. The five categories of dyskinesia are tremor, chorea, myclonus, tic, and dystonia. In the following sections, each of these categories will be reviewed briefly. Included among the dyskinesias reviewed here are dystonia, Huntington's disease, and Wilson's disease. Amyotrophic lateral sclerosis (a motoneuron disease), Friedreich's ataxia (a spinocerebellar disorder), multiple sclerosis (a disease of the white matter), and myasthenia gravis (an autoimmune disorder characterized by abnormal fatiguability and weakness of skeletal muscles) are reviewed.

PARKINSON'S DISEASE

Medical Aspects

Parkinsonism is a general syndrome that encompasses the symptoms of "rest" tremor, rigidity, paucity of movement, and impaired postural reflexes, and is due to the loss of dopaminergic neurons in the basal ganglia (especially the substantia nigra) and brainstem. It can be divided into three subgroups depending upon its etiology and associated signs and symptoms:

1. Idiopathic or primary Parkinson's disease (also known as paralysis agitans), which will be the focus of this discussion
2. Secondary parkinsonism, which includes a number of disorders with extrapyramidal features and that have an identifiable causal agent, some of which would include toxins (1-methyl-4-phenyl-1,23,3,6-tetrahydropyridine or MPTP), infections (Von Economo's encephalitis), drugs (neuroleptics), repeated trauma or multiple strokes
3. Heterogeneous system degenerations such as progressive supranuclear palsy, striatonigral degeneration, Shy-Drager syndrome, or orolivopontocerebellar degeneration (Marttila, 1983)

The remainder of the discussion will focus on idiopathic Parkinson's disease. In order to diagnose Parkinson's disease, at least two of the classic signs mentioned previously must be present. However, since most of the secondary and degenerative types of parkinsonism also have these symptoms (particularly rigidity and bradykinesia), a search must be made for signs and symptoms that are not typically seen. Some of these signs would be pyramidal tract signs (exaggerated reflexes, extensor plantar responses), intention tremor, ataxia or other evidence of cerebellar dysfunction, or profound early dementia (Marttila, 1983).

The diagnosis of Parkinson's disease is made on clinical grounds. In the patient who does not show the classic signs of tremor, rigidity, and akinesia, computerized tomography (CT scans) may be helpful in the differential diagnosis.

Population Characteristics

The average annual incidence of parkinsonism (excluding drug-induced cases) is 18.2 per 100,000. The prevalence in white populations is estimated to be between 66 and 187 per 100,000. There is no significant difference between males and females. The incidence increases sharply above the age of 64 and the peak of incidence is between 75 and 84 years of age. There has been a trend toward increased age at the time of diagnosis; in 1967, the mean age at onset was 55.3 years (Hoehn, & Yahr, 1967; Rajput, Offord, Beard, & Kurland, 1984).

Causes

There are three areas presently being investigated as possible etiologies: genetic, age-related, and environmental. There have been two familial subgroups identified with variants of parkinsonism. The first, with autosomal dominant transmission, has tremor as the predominant sign with a strong family history of benign tremor. The second autosomal recessive form shows symptoms of akinesia and rigidity. However, twin studies have not shown any genetic transmission of typical idiopathic Parkinson's disease.

It has been argued by some that Parkinson's disease is an accelerated form of normal aging with a loss of substantia nigra neurons. Again, however, twin studies do not support this. Another argument against the aging theory is that the "parkinsonian" traits of normal elderly people do not respond to treatment with levodopa.

The third possibility, that of an environmental toxin, has received some support by the development of a severe form of parkinsonism in a number of drug abusers. A derivative of meperidine, MPTP, has been shown to cause a severe loss of dopaminergic substantia nigra neurons. Although the pathology found after the use of this drug is not identical to that of Parkinson's disease (which includes other regions of the brain), it is the best model available. Other studies have suggested common exposures among patients from similar geographic areas that may trigger eventual cell death (Lang & Blair, 1984).

Natural Course

Parkinson's disease typically has an insidious onset; in retrospect, patients recall increasing difficulties with "stiffness" and "muscle aches" that they had attributed to the normal course of aging. The problem that initiates the first visit to a physician is most commonly tremor. The tremor of Parkinson's disease is of the distal extremities and occurs at rest (the pill-rolling phenomenon). Patients who initially show symptoms of tremor apparently have a slower progression of the disease, at least in the first 10 years (Hoehn & Yahr, 1967).

Early in the disease, the patient might notice increasing difficulty in repetitive or alternating movements such as walking. When a joint is passively moved through its range, a "catch" can be felt; this phenomenon is known as *cogwheeling*. This rigidity affects all striated muscles, causing difficulties in respiration, facial expression, swallowing, mastication, and speech. Progression of rigidity can lead to flexion contractures of the fingers, elbows, cervical spine, hips, and knees with ensuing loss of mobility.

Bradykinesia (or akinesia, in its most extreme form) is a slowness or decrease in spontaneous movements. Often the earliest manifestation of this is a decrease in the frequency of eye blinking (normal range 14 to 17 per minute). Paucity of facial movement leads to a mask-like appearance. With progression of the disease, the patient may not be able to perform simple volitional acts (called *freezing*) such as initiating ambulation or arising from a chair; these episodes can often be overcome by diverting the patient's attention from the desired act or by an emotional response. Loss of postural reflexes, shuffling gait, retropulsion (the tendency to fall backwards), and festination (progressive rapidity of forward movement with a loss of control) all severely affect safe ambulation.

Controversy exists as to whether dementia is a feature of Parkinson's disease. In some patients, specific memory deficits are present on testing, and patients may complain of slowness in problem solving. However, objective testing of these patients is difficult because of the extreme slowness of motor responses, poor handwriting, and dysarthria. Agreement certainly exists that if dementia is prominent and occurs before major motoric disability, a diagnosis other than Parkinson's disease should be considered, for example, Alzheimer's disease or progressive supranuclear palsy (Morris, 1982).

Prior to treatment with levodopa, over one-quarter of patients were dead or severely disabled within five years of their diagnosis; eighty percent were in this category after 10 to 14 years of observation, nearly three times that of the normal population (Hoehn & Yahr, 1967). It was initially thought that treatment with levodopa decreased the mortality to only 1.3 to 1.9 times higher than normal; recent studies question whether these apparent improvements were due to methodological inadequacies of these studies (Marttila, 1983; Rajput et al., 1984).

Medical Management

The major method of treatment is pharmacological; the discovery that levodopa could cross the blood-brain barrier and be metabolized to dopamine in the brain revolutionized the treatment of Parkinson's disease. Essentially, all symptoms of parkinsonism respond to levodopa; rigidity and bradykinesia, however, respond more promptly and fully than tremor. There are many fluctuations in the clinical response to levodopa, even within the individual (known as the *on-off* response), probably due to differences in absorption and dopamine receptor responsivity. Levodopa is usually combined with a dopamine decarboxylase inhibitor (carbidopa), which decreases the inactivation of levodopa in the peripheral tissues and decreases the dosage required (Bianchine, 1976). Unfortunately, in recent years it has become apparent that there are a number of therapeutic problems with levodopa usage, including the failure to respond, the loss of response with prolonged treatment, the occurrence of involuntary movements with long-standing therapy, and the previously mentioned fluctuations in response (Lang & Blair, 1984). Drug holidays (a few days of complete withdrawal from all drugs while the patient is hospitalized) are sometimes effective in temporarily allowing a decrease in dosage. The other drugs used in treatment are the anticholinergics (primarily for tremor), the dopamine agonist-ergot derivatives (such as bromocriptine, pergolide, & lisuride), and amantadine hydrochloride.

Neurosurgery is used far less frequently since the advent of levodopa; however, stereotactic thalamotomy is more effective than levodopa in alleviating the tremor of Parkinson's disease, and is usually considered for the patient with an incapacitating tremor that is unresponsive to other forms of therapy (Kelly & Gillingham, 1980).

Physical therapy does not contribute to halting the progression of the disease; however, it can be very useful in preventing secondary complications due to rigidity and imbalance. Patients and their families should be trained in the use of walkerettes or wheelchairs, if necessary. Range of motion exercises can prevent unnecessary contractures that would further hinder mobility and care of the patient. Proper positioning in bed and while working can ameliorate the cervical flexion which can affect vision and mobility. Occupational therapists can assist the family in evaluating the home for safety and can prolong the independence of the patient through the use of assistive devices for dressing and eating. The speech/language pathologist can not only address the question of dysarthria but can evaluate and correct swallowing difficulties, thereby decreasing the risk of aspiration and subsequent pneumonia.

Speech Characteristics

Extensive research has been focused on the description of the speech patterns of individuals with Parkinson's disease. The prevalence of speech disorder in the parkinsonian population is high. Logemann, Fisher, Boshes, and Blonsky (1978) studied 200 parkinsonian speakers and reported that 89 percent of their sample exhibited laryngeally related problems and 45 percent demonstrated articulatory problems. Of the 65 parkinsonian patients studied by Buck and Cooper (1956), 37 percent had normal speech or were mildly involved, 22 percent had a moderate degree of speech involvement, and 29 percent had severely impaired speech.

Perhaps the most complete overview of parkinsonian speech characteristics comes from the work of Darley, Aronson, and Brown (1969a, 1969b, 1975). They recorded the speech of 32 individuals with Parkinson's disease and rated the speech samples on the 38 dimensions listed in Chapter 3. They concluded:

> reduced variability in pitch and loudness, reduced loudness level overall, and decreased use of all vocal parameters for achieving stress and emphasis. Markedly imprecise articulation is generated at variable rates in short bursts of speech punctuated by illogical pauses and often by inappropriate silences. Voice quality is sometimes harsh, sometimes breathy. (p. 195)

Speech Components

RESPIRATORY FUNCTION. With few exceptions, researchers have supported the conclusion that for parkinsonian speakers, respiratory function is reduced as compared to normal speakers. De la Torre, Mier, and Boshes (1960) observed reduced vital capacities in the 17 parkinsonian males that they studied. Two-thirds of the group demonstrated vital capacities that fell below 40 percent of predicted vital capacity for their age and sex. Irregular breathing patterns observed in the group were attributed to disruption in the normal agonist-antagonist synergy of the respiratory muscles. Ewanowski (1964) studied 12 parkinsonian subjects and a matched number of normal subjects and found no differences between quiet respiratory patterns of the two groups.

Several investigators instructed their subjects to sustain phonation as a measure of respiratory support. Canter (1965a) and Boshes (1966) reported that their parkinsonian subjects were reduced in their ability to sustain phonation. However, Ewanowski (1964) and Kreul (1972) reported similar ability to sustain phonation between the parkinsonian and normal subjects. The differences in these results are probably related to the severity of the parkinsonism in the various groups of subjects.

The pattern of respiratory support for speech has also been investigated. Kim (1968) employed an ink-recording respirometer with a face-mask. He reported that all of his patients but one showed a varied degree of ability to alter automatic respiratory rhythms to speak or voluntarily hold their breath. Both Kim and Hunker, Bless, and Weismer (1981) reported that dysarthric speakers with Parkinson's disease may have "inflexible" respiratory patterns for speech. In part, this inflexibility may be reflected in reduction of lung volume excursions or restricted use of chest wall part combinations to achieve lung volume displacements.

LARYNGEAL FUNCTION. Impairment of laryngeal subsystem performance for speech has been measured in numerous studies that consistently reported an important reduction in laryngeal function for patients with Parkinson's disease. Several studies have shown that parkinsonian subjects produce average fundamental frequency levels that are higher than normal speakers (Canter, 1965a, b; Kammermeier, 1969; Ludlow & Bassich, 1983). A reduction in pitch variability was reported by Grewel (1957). Ludlow and Bassich concluded that pitch variability was restricted, in that the downward pitch inflection at the ends of sentences or parts of sentences is lacking.

Although persons who routinely listen to parkinsonian speakers often complain that they do not speak loudly enough, the research reports are contradictory. Canter (1963) analyzed the speech of 17 speakers with Parkinson's disease and found that they did not differ from normal speakers in mean peak sound-pressure levels. Also, the two groups did not differ on range of peak sound-pressure levels. Ludlow and Bassich (1983) reported that mean intensity in sentences was significantly reduced for parkinsonian speakers. In addition, the literature would suggest that reduced loudness variability is common. Darley and colleagues (1975) reported that voice was frequently deviant in parkinsonian speakers. Perhaps one contribution to the vocal pattern is the tendency of parkinsonian speakers to be unable voluntarily to produce speech at very low intensity levels (Canter, 1965a). Ludlow and Bassich (1983) reported that the maximum range of intensity for parkinsonian speakers on a loudness imitation task was reduced. As a group, parkinsonian speakers also show extensive disorders of vocal quality. Darley and colleagues reported harsh voice quality and breathy voice (continuous) ranked sixth and seventh, respectively, as deviant speech dimensions for this population.

VELOPHARYNGEAL FUNCTION. A review of research reveals that although hypernasality is sometimes observed in parkinsonian speakers, nasal emission is not. Mueller (1971) reported no measured nasal emission during speech in any of the 10 parkinsonian speakers he studied. Darley and colleagues (1975) reported that only 8 of their 32 subjects demonstrated hypernasality to a minor degree (mean severity value of 1.16 on a 7-point scale). No subject was judged to display nasal emission during speech.

ORAL ARTICULATION. Canter (1965b) reported that the primary articulatory characteristics of parkinsonism result from inadequate articulatory valving during production of plosives and breakdowns in the coordination of laryngeal and oral activity. Logemann and Fisher (1981) reported that manner errors were most characteristic of parkinsonism dysarthria. Spirantization of stops (the tendency of stops to be fricated) is characteristic of these patterns. Caligiuri (1985), Hirose, Kiritani, and Sawashima (1982), Hirose, Kiritani, Ushijima, Yoshioka, and Sawashima (1981), Hunker, Abbs, and Barlow (1982), and Leanderson, Persson, and Ohman (1970) suggest that persons with Parkinson's disease have reduced articulatory displacements as compared to normal speakers and incoordination of agonist and antagonist muscle groups. Caligiuri (1985) noted that at normal speaking rates, rigid parkinsonian speakers exhibited significantly lower lip displacement amplitudes than nonrigid parkinsonian speakers.

Weismer (1984) reported that parkinsonian subjects had longer vowel durations than both the geriatric and young adult subjects. The shortest closure durations were produced by parkinsonian subjects for initial voiceless stops, whereas the longest durations were produced by geriatric subjects. For fricative durations, parkinsonian speakers had shorter durations than both the geriatric and young adult subjects. In summarizing his research, Weismer wrote:

> The data presented here suggest that parkinsonian subjects have segmental and phrase-level durations which are slightly shorter than the corresponding durations of the appropriate control group, and that frequent spirantization is a typical feature of parkinsonian dysarthria. Several characteristics of parkinsonian dysarthria, such as the continuation of vocal fold vibration into voiceless stop closures and somewhat inflated inter- and intrasubject variabilities seem to be characteristic of geriatric speech and not unique to the neurogenic disorder. The only characteristic of parkinsonian dysarthria that might be considered an exaggerated aging effect is the shortened voiceless interval . . . (pp. 125–126)

Overall Aspects of Speech

There is considerable variation in speaking rate among parkinsonian speakers. Canter (1969b) reported median speaking rate during oral reading for his subjects at 172.6 as compared to 177.6 words per minute (wpm) for normal subjects. However, the performance range for his subjects was 69.6 to 249.6 wpm. Kreul (1972) reported that his parkinsonian subjects read aloud at a mean rate of 142.5 wpm, and Boshes' (1966) subjects read with a range from 50 to 70 wpm. Kammermeier (1969) reported a mean oral reading rate of 127 wpm (range 110 to 152). Netsell, Daniel, and Celesia (1975) studied the "rushes of speech" that were demonstrated by one parkinsonian speaker. Eleven of their 22 subjects demonstrated short rushes of speech. They observed:

> The reciprocal of these periods in the later syllables corresponds to rates in excess of 13 per second. Considering that the upper limit for voluntary control of such repetition rates is fewer than 10 per second, the 13 per second rate is interpreted as evidence that the subject is in some neuromuscular mode over which he (the speaker) has no immediate control. (pp. 172–173)

During the rushes of speech, the researchers report that lip contacts were not made during the production of /p/, thus supporting the conclusion that the speech articulators failed to reach the necessary position for production of a particular speech sound before beginning the movement to the following sound (articulatory undershoot).

Several clinical researchers not only suggest that there is variability among parkinsonian speakers, but also that variability may be seen from task to task within a speaker. Weismer (1984) is speaking of intelligibility differences from situation to situation when he states:

> Although the data is derived from connected utterances, the clinical experience of large difference in intelligibility of parkinsonian speech in the clinical setting versus "spontaneous" situations is confirmed in our experiment. Most of the parkinsonian subjects in the current experiment were quite intelligible when producing the experimental sentences, but much less intelligible when engaged in spontaneous speech. (p. 127)

Relationship Between Movement and Tremor

Hunker and Abbs (1984) support the hypothesis that a phase relationship exists between the onset of voluntary movement and the resting tremor cycle, and that this phase relationship is responsible for the delays in movement initiation. In other words, some of the delay in initiating movements in patients with tremor at rest comes from "waiting" to get into the correct time of the cycle. The support for this conclusion was the observation that "voluntary movements of symptomatic structures were executed in-phase with the ongoing resting tremor oscillations." Inferiorly and superiorly directed movement trajectories were initiated during the appropriate negative or positive phases of the resting tremor cycle

Effects of Medical Management

Several authors have written about the effects of surgical and pharmacological treatment on the speech performance of dysarthric speakers. Sarno (1968) reported that the long-term gains are poor even though individuals show marked speech improvement during periods of therapy. The carryover effects of speech therapy appear to be poor with these speakers, although exceptions do occur.

Buck and Cooper (1956) studied the effect of neurosurgery on the speech of persons with Parkinson's disease. Of the 46 patients who underwent either anterior choroidal artery occlusion or chemopallidectomy, in approximately 50 percent speech impairment remained the same as presurgery or was improved; in the other 50 percent there was a slight decline in speech efficiency following operation. Therefore, the authors concluded that:

> Improvement in speech should not be a prime goal in selecting patients for surgical treatment of parkinsonism. Rather, patients should be selected on a basis of the degree of incapacitation due to rigidity or tremor. (p. 1290)

Samara and colleagues, (1969) studied the brains of 27 deceased parkinsonian patients who had undergone stereotaxic thalamic surgery. The following conclusions were drawn:

1. A lesion strictly confined to the ventrolateral nucleus (VL) of the thalamus may be followed by language and/or speech deficits.
2. No definite relationship existed between postoperative language or speech deficits and partial involvement of thalamic nuclei surrounding the VL nucleus, H fields of Forel, subthalamic nucleus, or red nucleus. Also, mild encroachment on the internal capsule could be tolerated without language or speech deficits, so long as the pyramidal tract remained intact.
3. The size of the lesion was not related to postoperative language or speech deficits.
4. Postoperative language deficits were mild and improved in time, whereas speech disturbances could be either mild, moderate, or severe.
5. When language deficits did occur, they followed surgery on the left dominant hemisphere in most instances. In contradistinction, no definite relationship was found between the side of surgery and speech deficits.
6. Language and speech disturbances are most frequently associated with bilateral rather than unilateral surgery, regardless of the cerebral hemisphere involved in the second operation.

Rigrodsky and Morrison (1970) studied the speech of 21 parkinsonian patients under various conditions of L-dopa therapy. They report:

> Although statistical significance was obtained for only one aspect (the time factor—overall rate of speaking, appropriateness of phrasing and pauses, and rhythm and fluency of speech) of speech in favor of improvement during maximal dosages (4-8 gm daily), there appeared to be a trend in the direction of improved speech during L-dopa therapy. These findings are not nearly as dramatic as the improvement in physical symptoms observed in the same patients. However, the speech changes all occurred within less than one month; greater changes might have been observed had the patients been followed for a longer period with maximal dosages. (p. 150)

PROGRESSIVE SUPRANUCLEAR PALSY

Medical Aspects

Progressive supranuclear palsy is an extrapyramidal syndrome first described by Steele, Richardson, and Olszewki (1964). Symptoms include ophthalmoplegia (mainly of vertical gaze), dystonic rigidity of the neck, pseudobulbar palsy, mild dementia, and spastic dysarthria. The following parkinsonian symptoms have been cited in subsequent reports: akinesia, lack of facial expression, poor postural reflexes, and hypokinetic dysarthria (Behrman, Carroll, Janota, & Matthews, 1969; Blumenthal & Miller, 1969; Hanson & Metter, 1980; Klawans & Ringel, 1971). Neuropathological alterations are found in the following structures (Steele et al., 1964): subthalamic nucleus, red nucleus, substantia nigra, superior colliculus, periaqueductal grey matter, globus pallidus, and dentate nucleus of the cerebellum. The disease has an onset in middle and later life and life expectancy after diagnosis averages five to seven years. This relatively uncommon disease is more frequent in males than females (Steele, 1972).

Diagnosis

Progressive supranuclear palsy can be distinguished from Parkinson's disease in several ways (Cummings & Benson, 1983). In progressive supranuclear palsy, the posture is extended rather than bowed as in Parkinson's disease. In progressive supranuclear palsy, rigidity primarily affects the axial structures, in Parkinson's disease, the limbs are primarily affected. Also, tremor is unusual in progressive supranuclear palsy.

Medical Treatment

Currently, there is no generally effective medical treatment for progressive supranuclear palsy. Although reports vary, most suggest that the remarkable response to levodopa seen in Parkinson's disease does not occur in progressive supranuclear palsy. Cummings and Benson (1983) summarize the literature findings: akinesia improves in some patients treated with levodopa, rigidity and extraocular movements improve in a few patients, and dementia is consistently unaffected.

Speech Characteristics and Intervention

Dysarthria is usually severe in individuals with progressive supranuclear palsy. Individuals may exhibit anarthria or mutism in the later stages (Steele, 1972). To date, few studies of the speech characteristics of a group of individuals with progressive supranuclear palsy have been reported. However, clinical descriptions suggest the occurrence of both spastic and hypokinetic dysarthria and language deficits. Lebrun, Devreax, and Roussea, (1986) report that speech and language symptoms vary considerably from patient to patient.

Hanson and Metter (1980) report the effects of delayed auditory feedback (DAF) intervention with an individual with progressive supranuclear palsy. They report that their patient's speech was characterized "by accelerated speech rate, weak vocal intensity, monopitch, imprecise consonant articulation, and poor speech intelligibility" (p. 269). When the patient spoke under conditions of 100 msec delay, speaking rates were consistently reduced. This reduction in speaking rate was accompanied by an increase in vocal intensity and an increased judged rating of speech intelligibility. Because the effect was not maintained when the DAF unit was not employed, the patient was fitted with a miniature, solid state, battery-powered unit. See Chapter 10 for a more detailed description of DAF application with dysarthric individuals.

DYSTONIA

Medical Aspects

The dystonias are a group of motor disorders characterized by abnormal involuntary movements and postures. The term *dystonia* was coined by Oppenheim, who described patients with sustained posturing and also tonic and clonic spasms of muscles in different parts of the body. These spasms are typically activated with voluntary motor activity. Although dystonia is attributed to disturbances of the extrapyramidal system, the underlying neuropathology and mechanisms have not yet been described (Marsden & Harrison, 1974). Dystonias may be symptomatic of a neurological process such as cerebral anoxia, birth trauma, Wilson's disease, encephalitis, and especially drugs such as phenothiazines and butyrophenones. However, they are often idiopathic or inherited conditions. The severity of dystonia may range from catastrophic to a mild nuisance. There is neither weakness nor wasting of muscle. Sensory, sphincter, and reflex alternations do not occur. In EMG studies of dystonia, several research groups (Herz, 1944a, b; Yanagisawa & Goto, 1971) have observed a tonic, nonreciprocal pattern of activity in agonist and antagonist muscles during any voluntary or postural contraction.

The primary dystonias are slowly progressive disorders that can plateau anywhere in the course of the illness. They begin insidiously and almost always with action dystonia (Fahn, 1984). In contrast, most secondary dystonias begin with dystonia at rest and even with sustained postures. Some secondary dystonias have an obvious sudden beginning, such as on recovery from an acute encephalopathic event. Secondary dystonias may also be associated with metabolic disease (e.g., Wilson's disease, Hallervorden-Spatz disease), and tend to have a more rapidly progressive course than do the primary dystonias. Some secondary dystonias are due to environmental causes, such as head trauma, encephalitis, and exposure to toxins, and tend to have a course that stabilizes and does not progress. Drugs that block the dopamine D2 receptor (antipsychotics and the substituted benzamides, e.g., metoclopramide) can induce two types of dystonia; acute dystonic reaction and delayed persistent dystonia (*tardive dystonia*). Acute dystonic reaction can be reversed readily with administration of anticholinergics or diazepam. Tardive dystonia is not only persistent, but is also frequently unresponsive to therapeutic attempts.

Diagnosis

Marsden, Harrison, and Bundy (1976) report criteria for the diagnosis of idiopathic torsion dystonia:

1. The presence of dystonic movements and postures (but arbitrarily excluding isolated spasmodic torticollis)
2. Normal prenatal history and early development
3. No history of any known precipitating illness or exposure to drugs known to provoke torsion dystonia prior to the onset of the disease
4. No evidence of intellectual, pyramidal, cerebellar, or sensory deficit on clinical examination
5. Failure of laboratory investigations, including copper studies, to demonstrate any cause for the disease

Population

In 72 individuals who were diagnosed as dystonic based on the preceding criteria (Marsden et al., 1976), the age of onset ranged from 1 to 59 years. Approximately 70 percent experienced onset in childhood and 30 percent experienced adult onset. The ratio of females to males was 1.2:1. The duration of the disease was 16 years with a range of 1 to 47 years.

Signs, Symptoms, and Natural Course

The distribution of signs and symptoms in dystonia is usually categorized as generalized (affecting many areas of the body), segmental (limited involvement, e.g., arm and neck, both arms, or neck and trunk but sparing the legs), and focal (signs limited to a single arm or a hand). In the study by Marsden and colleagues, generalized dystonia developed in 85 percent of those with onset at or before age 10, in 60 percent of those with onset between age 11 and 20, and only four percent of those with onset after age 20. Cooper (1969) describes the initial patterns for three groups of patients:

1. Childhood form. Onset occurs at four to six years of age; initial symptom nearly always is flexion inversion of the foot with progression to generalized dystonia within four to six years of onset.
2. Adolescent form. Onset occurs at 8 to 13 years of age; initial symptom is usually in the foot, but sometimes in the arm; the rate of progression is slower than the childhood form.
3. Adult form. Initial symptoms usually start in the arm; this form usually develops into axial (trunk) dystonia with relative sparing of the extremities.

In the childhood form, there appear to be two patterns of inheritance (Eldridge, 1970). The autosomal recessive form begins in early childhood, is progressive over a few years, and is restricted to Jewish patients. The dominant form begins later, usually late in childhood or adolescence, progresses more slowly than the autosomal recessive form, and is not limited to an ethnic group. According to Marsden and colleagues (1976), the "typical" picture of segmental dystonia in adults was onset with dystonic postures and spasms affecting one arm, with subsequent spread to the other arm and neck or the neck alone. Focal dystonia usually involves symptoms in one area of the body, such as the arm (writer's cramp) or the face (cranial dystonia). The syndrome of cranial dystonia, also known as blepharospasm-oromandibular dystonia, Breughel's syndrome, or Meige's syndrome, was described in 1910 by Henry Meige. The primary features of this syndrome are a blepharospasm, a prolonged tonic contraction of the orbicularis oculi muscles, and both fluctuating and sustained contractions of facial, lingual, and mandibular muscle groups (Golper, Nutt, Rau, & Coleman, 1983). Dystonic spasms disappear during sleep and are triggered by initiation of speech or presentation of food or drink to the mouth.

The functional disabilities of the 72 patients in the study by Marsden and colleagues (1976) were assigned according to the criteria of Bundy, Harrison, and Marsden (1975):

Mild Disability

Grade 1: leading a normal life; no symptoms

Grade 2: mild disability; continuing full-time work

Moderate Disability

Grade 3: works with difficulty

Severe Disability

Grade 4: not at work; independent at home

Grade 5: wholly dependent on others

Table 6-1 summarizes the levels of disability of the 72 individuals in the Marsden sample from Marsden and colleagues.

Medical Management

Usually the underlying disorder of dystonia is not treatable, except in some cases of secondary dystonia. Wilson's disease can be treated with D-penicillamine. Drug-induced dystonia requires the elimination of the drug. Some patients with tardive dystonia have improved with anticholinergics (Burke, Fahn, & Gold, 1980). Symptomatic therapy is initiated when no specific therapy is available. Fahn and Jankowic (1984) report that anticholinergics have the highest percentage change of benefit. Some patients will benefit from diazepam, levodopa, or bromocriptine. Surgical approaches are considered when chemical therapies have failed. These may include lesioning peripheral nerves and unilateral or bilateral thalamotomies. Thalamotomy has been effective for contralateral limb dystonia in some patients, but has not been effective for axial dystonia (Fahn & Jankowic, 1984).

Speech Characteristics

Due to varying severity and symptom patterns, not all individuals with dystonia exhibit dysarthria. However, in the dystonias involving the mouth, face, and larynx, a variety of symptoms may be observed. Several researchers

TABLE 6-1.
Levels of Patient Disability

			DISABILITY	
Age at Onset	**Number**	**Mild (%)**	**Moderate (%)**	**Severe (%)**
1–10	34	21	29	50
11–20	14	40	33	27
21–40	7	57	29	14
41–60	9	56	31	13

From Marsden, C., Harrison, M., and Bundy, S. (1976). Natural history of idiopathic torsion dystonia. *Advances in Neurology*, *14*, 177–187.

have studied groups of dystonic speakers. Kammermeier (1969) studied a group of eight dystonic speakers along with groups with pseudobulbar palsy, bulbar palsy, cerebellar lesions, and parkinsonism. He reported that the dystonic patients demonstrated the lowest mean fundamental frequency, were second lowest in the amount of pitch variability, and demonstrated the shortest percentage of phonation time as a portion of total speaking time of any of the five groups. Portnoy (1979) suggested that hypokinetic dysarthria may be an early indicator of tardive dyskinesis.

The Mayo Clinic study (Darley et al., 1969a, b) of 30 dystonic patients showed that in dystonia, phonation, articulation, and prosody were all significantly disturbed. For example, 27 of 30 patients displayed vocal harshness, 17 produced strained-strangled sound during speech, 9 demonstrated excessive loudness, and 11 exhibited voice stoppages. Slow speaking rate was observed in 23 of 30 dystonic speakers, and short phrases were demonstrated in 11 speakers. All 30 dystonic speakers demonstrated imprecise consonants, and 24 displayed disordered vowels and irregular articulatory breakdowns.

In his review of the dystonias, Fahn (1984) described the speech mechanism movements that might be observed in dystonic speakers. The major dystonic feature of laryngeal muscles is an action dystonia of the adductors, causing spastic dysphonia (spasmodic). Lingual dystonia often accompanies other forms of oromandibular dystonias. Occasionally, however, it is an isolated phenomenon. It may be present at rest, with either a sustained protrusion of the tongue or an upward deflection, so that the tongue is curved and touches the hard palate. More often it occurs as an action dystonia. The tongue appears normal when not in use, but abnormal lingual movements appear when the patient begins to speak or bring food to the back of the pharynx for deglutition. Dystonic movements of the jaw indicate that the abnormal movements involve muscles innervated by cranial nerve V, termed *oromandibular dystonia*. The two most common manifestations of the mandibular dystonia are a pulling down or a pulling up of the jaw. The movements are often repetitive, in part because the patient is trying to overcome the involuntary pulling of the muscles. Commonly, lower facial muscles are involved in association with jaw dystonia.

Golper and colleagues (1983) described the perceptual speech characteristics of 10 individuals with focal cranial dystonia. They summarize their findings as follows:

> five subjects displayed abnormal contractions of cranial muscles which were to varying degrees exacerbated by speech initiation. The speech impairment varied depending upon the primary muscle groups affected. Speech intelligibility was decreased as a function of the severity of the dystonia and the location of involvement rather than the number of muscle groups affected. The most noticeable decreases in intelligibility were found in two subjects with severe oromandibular dystonia. Those

> subjects with relatively mild to moderate impairment across several muscle groups maintained remarkably intelligible speech. However, their speech was judged as sounding bizarre. . . . Although there were differences among the dysarthric subjects in loci and degree of dystonia, the prominent speech characteristics were similar to the dystonia patients of Darley et al. (1975). . . (pp. 132–133)

HUNTINGTON'S DISEASE

Medical Aspects

Huntington's disease is a degenerative disorder of the nervous system characterized by a triad of clinical features including chorea, dementia, and a history of familial occurrence. Inheritance is via an autosomal dominant trait with complete penetrance. Thus, half the offspring of an afflicted individual will develop the disease. Males and females are equally likely to have the disease. Average age of onset of symptoms is 35 to 40 years and average course from onset to death is 14 years. Prevalence in the United States is 40 to 70 per one million population (Hogg, Massey, & Schoenberg, 1979).

Natural Course

Personality changes usually occur before the onset of chorea. These alterations include: irritability, untidiness, and loss of interest (Cummings & Benson, 1983). Transient facial grimacing, head nodding, and flexion-extension movements of the fingers may be the first manifestation of the choreic movements. In advanced stages of disease, the speed of movement slows and patients acquire an athetotic or dystonic character.

Diagnosis

The diagnosis of Huntington's disease is made on the basis of clinical findings of choreiform movement disorder and dementia occurring on a familial basis rather than on laboratory findings. Although there are no pathognomonic laboratory findings, diagnosis is supported by demonstrating diminished caudate volume on CT scans. Huntington's disease may be distinguished from other types of chorea, including Sydenham's chorea, a self-limited disease of children usually associated with episodes of inflammatory or infectious processes, and tardive dyskinesis, a movement disorder developed in individuals who are chronically exposed to neuroleptic drugs. The predominate movements in tardive dyskinesia usually involve the mouth and tongue, but hands, legs, trunk, and respiratory muscles may also develop choreoathetosis (Crane, 1968; Maxwell, Massengill, & Nashold, 1970; Portnoy, 1979).

Because of the hereditary nature of Huntington's disease and the fact that age of onset occurs after child-bearing age, attention has focused on the study of "at-risk" individuals in order to identify the incipient signs of the disorder. At present, no test definitively discriminates nonaffected at-risk persons from presymptomatic carrier-victims of the disease (Cummings & Benson, 1983). Medical applications under investigation include use of levodopa, which increases chorea in symptomatic patients. This test, however, has not been completely validated with at-risk individuals (Klawans, Goetz, & Perlik, 1980).

Medical Treatment

No medical treatment changes the course of disease for afflicted individuals. Major tranquilizers and other dopamine antagonists such as tetrabecazine have been used to control the choreiform movements (Swash, Roberts, Zakko, & Heathfield, 1972). Unfortunately, dementia is not improved by drugs that effectively suppress choreiform movements (Cummings & Benson, 1983).

Speech Characteristics

Speech symptoms may range from little or no dysarthria in cases where choreic movements are restricted to the limbs and body, to speech that is so severely impaired that it is unintelligible. Speech may be disrupted by sudden movements of the respiratory muscles, tongue, and face (Wilson & Bruce, 1955). Darley and colleagues (1975) summarize the perceptual characteristics of 30 individuals with hyperkinetic dysarthria of chorea as follows:

> a highly variable pattern of interference with articulation; episodes of hypernasality, harshness, and breathiness; and unplanned variations in loudness. In the speaker's apparent attempt to avoid the inevitable interruptions and to compensate for them, his rate of speech is variably altered, phonemes and intervals between words are prolonged, stress is equalized and inappropriate silences appear. (p. 210)

Speech symptoms are so closely related to the underlying movement disorder that marked improvement in speech symptoms is dependent on modification of the severity of the movement disorders. Ramig (1986) reported the results of a detailed acoustic analysis of phonation in individuals with Huntington's disease. She found abnormalities including low frequency segments (abrupt drops in fundamental frequency of approximately one octave), vocal arrests, and reduced maximal vowel duration. Changes due to behavioral speech intervention have not been reported, although speech may improve coincident with medication management of the choreic movements (Beukelman, 1983)

WILSON'S DISEASE

Medical Aspects

Wilson's disease is a rare, hereditary disorder caused by inadequate processing of the dietary intake of copper. Pathological changes occur in the liver, the brain, and the cornea of the eye as a result of excessive accumulation of copper in the tissue over a period of years. Neurological abnormalities include incoordination, tremor, dysarthria, drooling, dysphagia, and masklike face. Wilson's disease may present as a neurologic syndrome, a psychiatric disturbance, or a hepatic disorder (Cartwright, 1978).

Natural Course

Neurological degeneration begins to appear in adolescence or early adulthood. Darley and colleagues (1975) describe the natural progression of the disorder as follows:

> In later stages they usually exhibit severe ataxia with a bizarre intention tremor involving both upper extremities, marked rigidity of trunk and extremities, or a combination of the two. They also demonstrate marked dysarthria, dysphagia, drooling, and masked expression. If undiagnosed and untreated, the disease is fatal. (p. 243)

Medical Management

Although there is no method for reversing the metabolic deficit, the destructive effects of tissue copper deposition can be prevented by appropriate treatment. The current drug of choice for removing tissue copper and preventing its deposition is a chelating agent, D-penicillamine (Goldstein, Tauxe, McCall, Gross, & Randall, 1969). Although lifelong treatment is necessary, in most cases penicillamine will reverse many of the neurologic manifestations (Cummings & Benson, 1983). Unfortunately, advanced cases may fail to improve.

Speech Characteristics

Dysarthria was recognized as a prominent neurological feature when the disorder was first described by Wilson in 1912. Berry, Darley, Aronson, and Goldstein (1974) reported the results of a study in which they perceptually analyzed the speech of 20 individuals with Wilson's disease. The data suggested the presence of a mixed dysarthria with prominent ataxic, spastic, and hypokinetic features. Further speech samples were obtained at two points of medical treatment for 10 of the 20 individuals. Their findings indicated that a regimen of D-penicillamine and a low copper diet produces a significant remission of dysarthria.

AMYOTROPHIC LATERAL SCLEROSIS

Medical Aspects

Amyotrophic lateral sclerosis (ALS) is a progressive degenerative disease involving the motoneurons of both the brain and spinal cord in adults. Some motoneuron diseases, such as spinal muscular atrophy, involve primarily the lower motoneurons; others, such as primary lateral sclerosis, involve the upper motoneurons. Classical ALS involves both types of motoneurons. Upper motoneuron signs include muscle weakness, increased muscle tone (spasticity), hyperreflexia, extensor plantar reflexes, and pseudobulbar palsy (manifested by hypertonic bulbar muscles, increased perioral reflexes, and exaggerated emotional responses). Lower motoneuron signs include muscle weakness, muscular atrophy, and diminished or absent deep tendon reflexes.

Population Characteristics

The average worldwide incidence of ALS ranges between 0.4 and 1.8 per 100,000 population, and the prevalence rates range between 4 and 6 per 100,000 population (Tandan & Bradley, 1985a). Ninety-five percent of all cases are sporadic. However, there are two familial inherited types of ALS. The familial adult type is based on an autosomal dominant inheritance, whereas with juvenile onset, the inheritance mechanism may be autosomal dominant or recessive (Tandan & Bradley, 1985b). For sporadic ALS in the United States and Europe, the mean age at onset is 56 years with a male to female ratio of 2:1 (Emery & Holloway, 1982). Between 14 and 39 percent of individuals with ALS survive for five years, about 10 percent live up to 10 years, and a few live for 20 years. There appear to be several factors that determine the course and duration of the disease for the individual patient. The prognosis becomes less positive progressively with each of the following symptoms: musculature atrophy, upper motoneuron involvement, respiratory insufficiency, and predominant bulbar (brain stem) symptoms (Tandan & Bradley, 1985a).

Etiology

A long list of possible causative mechanisms have been investigated without any being overwhelmingly convincing (Tandan & Bradley, 1985b; Amico & Antil, 1981). The possibility of genetic factors at least contributing to the development of the full-blown disease seems tempting in view of the fact that familial forms do exist. Other general factors that have been mentioned are the aging phenomenon and the association of ALS with neoplasia. Some degree of loss of motoneuron cells does occur in normal aging; if ALS is a form of "premature aging" it is unclear as to what the mechanism would be. The incidence of malignancy coexisting with ALS is 0.7 to 10 percent above the normal population. However, no humoral or other factor has been identified to explain a causal connection. A viral theory of causation is attractive because of the existence of such viruses as the poliomyelitis virus, which selectively affects anterior horn cells. A slow, virus-type infection is most likely although no viral particles have been identified and tissue transplantation in animals has not resulted in ALS. It is even more likely that the answer may be a combination of viral infection and immune factors; there has been evidence for increased cell-mediated immunity to poliovirus antigens and for the presence of circulating and renal immune complexes. Other suggested mechanisms have included exposure to metals and minerals, endogenous toxins, abnormal nucleic acids or membrane properties, or a defect in neurotransmitters. Patients have mentioned an increased history of trauma or surgery in ALS as opposed to controls; however, no explanation has been forwarded for this observation.

Signs, Symptoms, and Natural Course

The most common presenting symptom is a focal or segmental weakness (63 percent); the most common form is a paraparesis (20 percent), but the weakness may be more focal at outset. About one-third of all patients complain of hand clumsiness, another one-third of leg weakness, which may be manifested as tripping over carpets or on steps. Twenty-two percent show bulbar symptoms (dysarthria in 45 percent, dysphasia in 42 percent, dysphonia in 12 percent, and dyspnea in 6 percent). It is not unusual for patients to complain of muscle pain and cramping or paresthetic-like pains even though ALS is a disease of the motoneuron cells (Adam, 1986; Gubbay, Kahana, Zilber, & Cooper, 1985).

ALS is a progressive disease with a median survival of three years from the time of onset of symptoms (Tandan & Bradley, 1985a). Those showing bulbar symptoms tend to have a more rapid course (median of 2.2 years). There is a subgroup of patients (perhaps up to 25 percent) who have a prolonged course; some have been reported to survive more than 20 years. Increasing weakness of the extremities, inability to swallow without aspiration, and decreased ability to speak ensue. Death is usually on the basis of respiratory failure or infection. Extraocular muscle movements are usually spared as is sphincter control. There have been some reports of dementia (in up to 5 percent) but there is some doubt that this is directly related to the presence of ALS.

Neuropathology

The motoneurons of the brain stem and spinal cord show simple atrophy, shrinkage, and cell loss (Hirano & Iwata, 1979). In individuals with extensive upper motoneuron signs there is a depletion of Betz cells and large pyramidal neurons from the fifth layer of the motor cortex and widespread degeneration of the corticospinal tracts (Hughes, 1982). In sporadic ALS the posterior columns of the spinal cord are uninvolved (Lawyer & Netsky, 1953). In the familial ALS, there is evident involvement of the posterior columns, Clarke's nucleus, and spinocerebellar tracts in at least 50 percent of the cases (Emery & Holloway, 1982). Studies have shown a reduction in the number of large motoneurons in the cervical and lumbar spinal cord (Tohgi, Tsukagnoshi, & Toyokura, 1977). In the peripheral nervous system, several studies have reported a marked reduction in the numbers of large myelinated fibers in the ventral roots (Hanyu, Oguchi, Yanagisawa, & Tsukagnoshi, 1981; Sobue, Matsouka, & Maukai, 1981). Further, data indicate that ALS is predominantly a neuropathy, as evidenced by considerable loss of large myelinated fibers from all levels of the nerve.

Diagnostic Testing

Because of the serious implications associated with the diagnosis of ALS, it is essential to diagnose treatable disorders with symptoms similar to ALS. However, because there is no specific biochemical marker for ALS, definitive diagnosis is difficult early in the disease. Diagnosis is primarily clinical, with supportive evidence from electrophysiological testing. On the electromyogram, evidence of denervation (the presence of fibrillations) and reinnervation (large, polyphasic motor unit action potentials) from two or more extremities outside any peripheral nerve or root distribution is evidence supporting the diagnosis of ALS. Nerve conduction studies are within normal limits. In rapidly progressing cases, repetitive stimulation of a nerve may show a decremental amplitude response of the compound motor action potential, indicating defective neuromuscular transmission. Single fiber electromyography may show increased fiber density and jitter. Serum muscle enzymes (creatine phosphokinase or CPK) may be elevated in some patients, although not to the level expected in an inflammatory muscle disease. The cerebrospinal fluid examination is normal. Myelograms or computerized tomography may be helpful in excluding other possible disease mechanisms such as cervical spondylosis, tumors of the foramen magnum or high cervical spinal cord, or syringomyelia. Other diseases to be excluded include polymyositis, post-polio syndrome, diabetic amyotrophy, or Charcot-Marie-Tooth neuropathy (Amico & Antil, 1981; Tandan & Bradley, 1985a).

Medical Management

There is no known cure for ALS, nor is there a chemical agent that has been shown to significantly change the natural course of the disease. Failed treatments include antiacetylcholinesterase preparations (except temporarily in those cases of rapid progression which show a decremental response to repetitive nerve stimulation), antiviral agents, immunosuppressants and plasmapheresis, and snake neurotoxin. The use of thyrotrophic releasing hormone (TRH) has provided transient improvement in muscle weakness in 50 percent of ALS patients (Brooke, Florence, Heller, Kaiser, Phillips, Gruber, Babcock, & Miller, 1986); however, there have been no demonstrated long-term benefits.

Because of this, the treatment of ALS relies on the alleviation of distressing or disabling symptoms with the ongoing evaluation and intervention of a multi-disciplinary team (Adam, 1986; DeLisa, Mikulic, Miller, & Melnick, 1979). The early management of muscle weakness relies on the prevention of disuse weakness and the strengthening of unaffected muscles (exercise of involved muscles could lead to an accelerated loss of anterior horn cells). The use of energy conservation techniques and work simplification along with adaptive devices is also helpful. Light-weight plastic orthoses may prolong a patient's ability to ambulate. The use of static orthoses and exercise to maintain joint range of motion is important to prevent uncomfortable contractures. For muscle cramping, a trial of quinine or phenytoin (Dilantin) may be warranted; as atrophy progresses, muscle cramping will spontaneously decrease.

Spasticity is not often an overwhelming problem. Most drugs have not been proven effective. The use of stretching exercises, judicious use of local motor point blocks, and perhaps baclofen (Lioresal) may be helpful. Various types of adaptive equipment may address the problem of decreased mobility, including electric mobility devices with various means of control. A decreased ability to perform activities of daily living is expected; again, adaptive equipment for the patient's or caretaker's use may be helpful. Environmental control units can use sensitive switches to allow access to television, lights, and telephone.

A problem peculiar to ALS patients is the maintenance of adequate nutrition. Progressive muscular atrophy will lead to cachexia, predisposing the patient to skin breakdown and continuing loss of protein stores. In addition, dysphagia will lead to decreased ingestion of food without aspiration. Cricopharyngeal myotomy or laryngeal closure and laryngectomy have been used in selected groups of patients. When aspiration is not preventable, alternative feeding methods must be considered. Some possibilities include oral-esophageal tubes, cervical esophagostomy, gastrostomy (surgical or percutaneous), or jejunostomy. Related to swallowing are problems with saliva in ALS patients. Thick, viscous mucus may impede swallowing and must be liquified. Measures include adequate fluid intake, the use of Papase tablets or meat tenderizer, or the use of a mechanical aspirator. On the other hand, sialorrhea is a problem for other patients. Anticholinergic drugs to decrease oral secretions are not a long-term solution; an aspirator or surgery must be considered.

The major area for long-term management for the ALS patient is respiratory care. The issue of artificial ventilation at the time of respiratory failure is one that should be discussed with the patient and his or her family well before it becomes an issue (Tandan & Bradley, 1985a). Home ventilation is a possibility, albeit an expensive and labor-intensive one. Respiratory failure usually accelerates 12 to 15 months prior to death. Pulmonary function tests administered periodically allow some prediction of a time span. Abnormal maximal expiratory pressures are an accurate measure of early involvement. A forced vital capacity of less than fifty percent of predicted indicates an increased likelihood of respiratory failure. In patients with chest wall and diaphragmatic weakness, training of accessory respiration muscles may be a temporary aid. All ALS patients should receive prophylactic influenza and pneumococcus vaccines to prevent pneumonias. If a patient decides against prolongation of life by mechanical ventilation, sedatives and narcotic administration may decrease the anxiety associated with hypoxia; supplemental oxygen supplies may also be helpful.

The incidence of depression in ALS patients is not different from other patients with chronic disease and the suicide rate is not unusually high. However, patients and their families benefit from ongoing counseling regarding issues relating to chronic illness and acceptance of death or grieving; hospice services may also be helpful.

Speech Characteristics

The speech characteristics associated with ALS vary, depending on the course of the disease. For individuals with initial symptoms appearing in areas served by the bulbar (lower cranial) nerves, motor speech and swallowing disorders occur quite precipitously. However, for individuals with initial symptoms in areas served by the spinal nerves, speech symptoms may occur late in the course of the disease. In either case, most persons with ALS are anarthric during the later stages of the disease and require an alternative communication system. Saunders, Walsh, and Smith (1981) reported that 75 percent of their 100 ALS patients were unable to speak at the time of their death.

Type of Dysarthria

The characteristic speech of the individuals with ALS has been classified as a mixed dysarthria by Darley and colleagues (1975). Symptoms associated with both spastic and flaccid dysarthria are often present; however, as the disease progresses the contributions of each type of dysarthria may change. As the individual becomes excessively weak, the symptoms associated with the flaccid dysarthria usually become more apparent. As the disease progresses, the spastic symptoms often cannot be expressed by the excessively weakened neuromuscular system.

Perceptual Characteristics

The most extensive investigation of mixed dysarthria associated with ALS was completed by Darley and colleagues (1975). According to these researchers, the most deviant speech disorders in order of rated severity were imprecise consonants, hypernasality, harsh voice quality, slow rate, monopitch, short phrases, distorted vowels, low pitch, excess and equal stress, prolonged intervals of reduced stress, prolonged phonemes, strained-strangled quality, breathiness, audible inspiration, inappropriate silences, and nasal emission.

Speech Components

A review of the previous list of speech characteristics reveals that, as in most dysarthrias, individuals with ALS demonstrated impairment in all components of the speech mechanism. On a case-by-case basis, the distribution of impairment varies from individual to individual.

RESPIRATORY FUNCTION. Putnam, Hixon, and Stern (1982) studied two individuals with ALS who demonstrated abnormality for speech breathing. These individuals used limited lung volume ranges for speech that may have resulted from reduction in vital capacity. For some individuals with ALS, respiratory impairment becomes so severe that they choose to be ventilated with a respirator.

LARYNGEAL FUNCTION. The phonatory subsystem may reveal a mixed dysarthria. Aronson (1980) writes:

> If spasticity is predominant, hyperadduction of the true and false vocal folds, technically a pseudobulbar dysphonia, will require that the exhaled air be forced through a constricted glottis. Such elevated laryngeal resistance to the exhaled air stream, coupled with a reduced exhalatory force, decreases the volume of voice in addition to producing a strained hoarseness or harshness. . . A greater flaccid (lower motor neuron) component produced adductor vocal-fold weakness. . .extreme breathiness and reduced loudness.

VELOPHARYNGEAL FUNCTION. Velopharyngeal incompetence with resulting hypernasality and nasal emission is commonly associated with ALS. Often the nasal emission is not easily perceived, because of the lack of respiratory support in these individuals. Nevertheless, inadequate closure of the velopharyngeal port decreases the ALS speaker's ability to impound air pressure in the oral cavity for consonant sound production.

ORAL ARTICULATION. The tongue and the lips frequently exhibit excessive weakness. Carrow, Rivera, and Mauldin, et al., (1974) found tongue atrophy to be a prevalent neurological sign in persons with severely reduced speech intelligibility. Dworkin, Aronson, and Mulder (1980) measured tongue protrusion strength on a nonspeech task. Their data showed that healthy males could generate 2,086 grams (range = 1,300 to 3,356 grams), whereas men with ALS averaged 1,129 grams (range = 211 to 1,754 grams).

FRIEDREICH'S ATAXIA

Medical Aspects

Friedreich's ataxia is one of a heterogeneous group of degenerative spinocerebellar disorders. Cummings and Benson (1983) classify the spinocerebellar degenerations into three groups. Those affecting predominantly the spinal cord include Friedreich's ataxia and its variants and hereditary spastic ataxia. Those affecting predominantly the cerebellum include cerebellar cortical degeneration and cerebellar nuclear degeneration (dentatorubral atrophy). Those affecting predominantly the brain stem and cerebellum include olivopontocerebellar atrophy.

The most common type of Friedreich's ataxia is the result of an autosomal recessive trait. Males and females are affected in equal proportion with age of onset between 11 and 12 years. Most patients die within 20 years of the onset of symptoms. The disorder is usually first observed as it affects the lower extremities with gait disturbance. Dysmetria of the upper extremities and dysarthria occur later. A number of abnormalities frequently occur as part of this syndrome, including skeletal deformities (pes cavus, hammer toes, and kyphoscoliosis), loss of vibration and position sense, absent muscle stretch reflexes in the lower extremities, nystagmus, limb weakness, optic atrophy, pigmentary retinal degeneration, vestibular involvement, and myocardial degeneration (Brain & Walton, 1969; Menkes, 1974). A constant feature of the neuropathology of Friedreich's ataxia is the degeneration of the large myelinated sensory fibers, posterior roots, and dorsal root ganglion cells.

Medical Treatment

Currently, there is no medical treatment that changes the progressive course of the disorder. However, supportive measures to maximize mobility and other aspects of daily function are important.

Speech Characteristics

Dysarthria has long been recognized as a symptom of Friedreich's ataxia. In 1877, Charcot described it as a disease in which the tongue became too "thick." In 1964, Heck reported that speech defect is a common finding in Friedreich's ataxia, with an estimated incidence of 63 percent to 93 percent. Brain and Walton (1969) state that the speech of persons with Friedreich's ataxia is invariably dysarthric in the later stages of the disease.

Perceptual Characteristics

Numerous attempts have been made to describe precisely the characteristics of the dysarthria associated with Friedreich's ataxia. In 1937, Zentay classified the dysarthric speech resulting from cerebellar lesions as ataxic speech, adiadokokinesis, explosive-hesitant speech, and scanning speech. By 1958, Alajouanine, Scherer, Sabouraund, and Gremy had studied ataxic dysarthric speech using oscillographic tracings. They reported two patterns: the first showed amplitude variations from one word to another, which they labeled as explosive or scanned speech quality; the second was described as variations disturbing the continuity of phonemes.

In 1980, Joanette and Dudley rated the speech of 22 Friedreich's ataxia patients using 16 of the speech dimensions reported by Darley and colleagues (1975). They concluded that two speech factors were present: a general dysarthria, including reduced intelligibility, monoloudness, prolonged phonemes, inappropriate silences, imprecision consonants, and distorted vowels; and a vocal stenosis type, including harshness, pitch breaks, and pitch level.

Respiratory Function

As early as 1929, Hiller studied the dysarthria of Friedreich's ataxia and concluded that the primary speech problem of patients with cerebellar lesions is one of respiratory control. In 1982, Putnam and colleagues studied the respiratory kinematics techniques described in Chapter 6. They reported that for all three cases, in spite of chest wall disorganization, weakness, or component part deficits, the patients were still able to exchange enough air and move it under enough pressure to produce an acoustic speech signal. However, in all three cases, velopharyngeal incompetence made respiratory efforts and compensations somewhat futile.

MULTIPLE SCLEROSIS

Medical Aspects

Multiple sclerosis (MS) is a disease of the white matter of the central nervous system which is characterized by progressive neurological deficits and, most commonly, a remitting/relapsing course. Although it is a relatively common disease and has been the object of intensive research in recent years, no definite knowledge exists of its etiology or effective therapies.

The macroscopic lesions of MS are multiple plaques that are scattered throughout the nervous system, predominantly in the white matter. These are commonly seen in the periventricular area and tend to be symmetrical (McFarlin & McFarland, 1982). Microscopically, the lesion is shown to cause destruction of the myelin sheath with preservation of the axon, except in very chronic cases. The lesions are generally associated with small veins and venules, surrounded by lymphocytes, plasma cells, and macrophages. In an "acute" plaque, edema is seen in the vicinity of the affected nerve fiber. Resolution of this edema may be an explanation for the early reversal of some neurologic deficits after an exacerbation. The persistent neurologic signs are thought to be due to impaired saltatory conduction along the nerve axon (Hallpike, Adams, & Tourtelotte, 1983).

Research into possible etiologies indicates there may be an environmental agent (e.g., a virus), a deranged immune response, or a combination of the two. Geographic studies indicate that the highest prevalence of the disease is in the higher latitudes in both the northern and southern hemispheres. Migrants from a higher prevalence area to a lower prevalence area and vice versa have a prevalence that is midway between both areas. The critical age of exposure appears to be about 15 years. This may also indicate some genetic predisposition to the disease; certain HLA antigens have been found in MS patients. Because of the similarities between MS and other demyelinating diseases (e.g., postinfectious encephalomyelitis, subacute sclerosing panencephalitis, and progressive multifocal leukoencephalopathy) that are caused by viruses and because of its similar onset to slow viral diseases (e.g., Creutzfeldt-Jakob disease) a search for a viral cause has been made. No viral components have yet been identified; however, new nucleic acid hybridization techniques may prove fruitful in future identification. The presence of lymphocytes and macrophages in MS lesions and of elevated IgG levels in the cerebrospinal fluid have led to the consideration of a malfunctioning immune system. Again, however, there has been no evidence of cross-reactivity between patients; it seems more likely that the immune response is a reaction to an environmental agent (Ellison, Visscher, Graves, & Fahey, 1984).

Population Characteristics

In the northern part of the United States, the prevalence is about one in 1,000 of the population; it is one-third to one-half that in the southern states. About 95 percent of all cases begin between the ages of 10 and 50 years with a median onset age of 27 years. Although it is a disease of younger people, it not unusual to be first diagnosed at 50 to 60 years; in these patients, there are usually signs of chronicity. The female to male ratio is 1.5:1 (Arnason, 1982).

Signs, Symptoms, and Natural Course

Charcot first comprehensively described MS in 1877 with his triad of nystagmus, scanning speech, and intention tremor. The most common symptoms in this population are balance abnormalities (70 percent), impaired sensation (71 percent), paraparesis (62 percent), difficulty with micturition (62 percent), optic neuritis (55 percent), and impotence (5-80 percent) (Hallpike, et al., 1983). Optic neuritis is the acute or subacute loss of central vision with peripheral sparing in one eye; it is the first symptom of MS in 16 to 30 percent of all patients. A young adult with isolated optic neuritis has a 17 to 65 percent risk of developing MS in later life. Other reliable symptoms of MS are intranuclear opthalmoplegia or bilateral ocular paresis, tic douloureux or trigeminal neuralgia in a young adult, Lhermitte's symptom (an electric shock-like sensation down the spine and into the legs), acute transverse myelitis, and a "sensory useless" hand. Fatigue for which no objective explanation can be found is both a common and quite disabling complaint. On physical examination, vibration and position sense are frequently decreased or absent. Intention tremor, ataxia, and hyperreflexia are common (Poser, 1984).

Vision and hearing are commonly ignored in evaluation but cranial nerve dysfunction, scotomas, and decreased visual and auditory acuity are not uncommonly present. Definite evidence of cognitive impairment is present in over half of patients with neuropsychological testing; impaired abstract conceptualization and recent memory are the areas most frequently involved. Signs of bladder dysfunction appear at some time in 50 to 80 percent of all patients. This may include frequency of urination, incontinence, or urinary retention; urinary tract infection and stones can be a source of significant morbidity in this population. Sexual dysfunction can occur in all phases of arousal and performance in males; this is probably present in female patients as well, although studies are nonexistent (Poser, 1984).

The average life expectancy in a young male after onset is 35 years. A number of studies have shown that disability scores calculated five years after onset correlate well with disability at 10 and 15 years; careful evaluation of function, therefore, can be of prognostic value (Hallpike, et al., 1983). Prognosis is worse in males, if the age of onset is greater than 35 years, if a chronic progressive pattern is present at the onset, or if cerebellar symptoms occur at the initial presentation (Poser, 1984).

The clinical course can be divided into the following five classes:

1. Relapsing and remitting—About 70 percent of young patients with MS begin in this category with full recovery from neurologic signs and symptoms after each episode
2. Chronic progressive—This is most commonly present in patients older at the outset
3. Combined relapsing/remitting with chronic progressive—This is the eventual outcome in the majority of patients

4. Benign—About 20 percent of all patients have a normal life span with relatively normal functioning and little or no progression
5. Malignant—Five to ten percent of patients (usually young) show rapid and extensive involvement of cognitive, cerebellar, and pyramidal systems, leading to death (Poser, 1984).

Diagnostic Testing

A plethora of tests exist that are useful in the diagnosis of MS, none of which are sufficient for diagnosis. The hot bath test is probably the oldest; small increases in the body temperatures of MS patients can temporarily worsen existing neurological signs and can precipitate new ones. Although this test is positive in 60 percent of patients, it is not specific to MS. The laboratory examination of cerebrospinal fluid (CSF) reveals the presence of oligoclonal bands of IgG, which are abnormal clusters of immunoglobulins. Myelin basic protein, which is a breakdown product of myelin and may be an indicator of disease activity, also can be found in CSF.

Two imaging techniques are useful in deleting CNS plaques. Computerized tomography (CT) scans can show cerebral atrophy, hypodense areas, or enhanced lesions (clearly correlated with disease activity). Magnetic resonance imaging (MRI) uses a property of atomic nuclei called *spin* to visualize changes in the hydrogen in brain tissue. A strong magnetic field is applied to the area to be studied, causing an alignment of the nuclei of the tissue; when this field is removed, the nuclei "spin," producing a radio frequency signal that matches the secondary spin frequency of the nucleus. These signals can be processed into images similar to those of CT scans. It appears that MRI is more sensitive than CT in demonstrating low density but there is no evidence yet that it is any more useful than an enhanced CT scan in aiding in the diagnosis of MS.

Evoked potentials (EPs), produced by stimulating the peripheral nervous system and recording surface cortical potentials, is the third major modality used for diagnosis. Usually the latency and amplitude of the cerebral potentials are measured and compared to laboratory normals; even more useful is comparing the right-sided potentials to the left and noting differences. Visual evoked potentials, which use rapidly shifting or reversing patterns as a stimulus, can be useful in detecting a subclinical lesion but are not specific enough to be used in following the clinical course. Results can be affected by acuity, level of cooperation, and decreased luminance. Brainstem auditory evoked potentials (BAEPs) are obtained using monaural clicks and may be performed on a sleeping subject. By measuring and comparing interwave latencies it is possible to demonstrate a second lesion when a nonbrainstem locus of dysfunction is present or when clinical observations are equivocal. An audiogram is essential to the interpretation of BAEPs. Somatosensory evoked potentials utilize the stimulation of a peripheral nerve in the upper or lower extremity. Similar measurements are made with respect to latency and amplitude; the normalcy of the peripheral nervous system must be monitored to ensure accuracy of testing. The blink reflex study is used less frequently since the advent of evoked potential testing; it measures the latencies of the ipsilateral and contralateral responses to the stimulation of the supraorbital nerve (Poser, 1984).

Various neuro-ophthalmologic tests are used to measure visual acuity, visual fields, and the ocular fundus when indicated. Neuropsychological testing may be done not only to measure cognitive deficits but also to investigate possible depression. Disorders of bladder function that do not readily respond to treatment may require study of bladder pressure by cystometry or of the sphincter musculature by electromyography; when studied together, simulating function, it is known as urodynamics.

To be used in the diagnosis of multiple sclerosis, neurological deficits should be present in different anatomical locations and should be present for at least 24 hours at separate points in time. Clinical and laboratory criteria have been used to form the following diagnostic classifications: clinically definite MS, laboratory supported definite MS, clinically probable MS, and laboratory supported probable MS (Poser, 1984).

Medical Management

A statement by Dr. Richard Masland at Columbia University quoted in a *New England Journal of Medicine* editorial summarizes the state of therapies for MS:

> There are few areas of scientific inquiry which have spawned more inadequate studies and unwarranted recommendations than that of the therapy of MS. (McFarlin, 1983, p. 215)

The history of the disorder is one of a long and continuing series of false claims of cure for this disease. It is difficult to ascribe a therapeutic effect in many studies because of the differing courses of MS patients and the remitting/relapsing nature of the disease. There are no good markers of disease activity, no pathogenesis is known, and treatments are generally studied in the most advanced group of patients who are least likely to benefit from any therapy (McFarlan, 1983). In view of this, a number of therapies for the disease itself as well as for its complications are reviewed.

Adrenocorticotropic hormone (ACTH) and other corticosteroids can be used in an acute relapse; they are thought to suppress the synthesis of IgG. They are given intravenously or intramuscularly at first and tapered over a three-month period. Some of the adverse effects of steroids include infection, hemorrhage, hypertension, diabetes, electrolyte disturbances, insomnia, irritability, hallucinations, indigestion, and ankle edema (Hallpike, et al., 1983). Other immunosuppressants such as cyclophosphamide and azathioprine have also been administered; one study found a combination of cyclophosphamide and ACTH most effective in precipitating a remission (Hauser, Dawson, Lehrich, Beal, Kevy, Propper, Mills, & Weiner, 1983). Untoward effects can include alopecia, nausea, hematuria, and leukopenia. Another report suggested a positive effect of hyperbaric oxygen on long-term slowly progressive MS (Fischer, Marks, & Reich, 1983). Other treatments have included transfer factor, levamisole, plasmapheresis, and interferon; none have produced a clearly beneficial effect. Diet therapy has enjoyed many rebirths; although many benefits have been claimed, no scientific long-term studies have shown conclusively that diet can affect the disease process. Many of the diets (e.g., the Swank diet) are based on a low-saturated fat consumption and may be beneficial for the overall health of the patient (Scheinberg, 1983).

Most therapy is aimed at controlling the manifestations of the disease and at preventing complications. The care of the MS patient requires the expertise of a wide variety of practitioners: neurologists, physiatrists, physical and occupational therapists, speech therapists, community nursing personnel, vocational counselors, psychologists, and social workers. The education of the patient and his or her family and friends and their active participation in the health care process may be the single most effective treatment.

Drug therapy is used to treat spasticity that interferes with daily functioning. Common drugs include baclofen (adverse effects include drowsiness, mental confusion, change in bladder status), diazepam (adverse effects include drowsiness, weakness, ataxia, depression, and the possibility of addiction or physical dependence), and dantrolene (adverse effects include weakness, liver function abnormalities or hepatitis) (Young & Delwaide, 1981a, b). Drugs may also be used to treat bladder incontinence or retention. Bethanechol acts to increase the tone of the detrusor muscle and aid urination; its side effects include flushing, salivation, and abdominal discomfort. Propantheline and oxybutinin inhibit detrusor action; their side effects include all those of anticholinergics—dry mouth, blurred vision, tachycardia, confusion, and constipation. Antibiotics and urinary antiseptics are frequently used. Occasionally, tricyclic antidepressants and anticonvulsants may be prescribed for the paresthesias associated with MS.

Surgery can be considered in the management of many different areas. Intention tremor may be helped by selective thalamotomy if it is unilateral or significantly interferes with function. Dorsal rhizotomies and similar procedures might be used to control spasticity or severe parethesias. Orthopedic tendon release might be considered to correct long-standing contractures. Urologic surgery may address the problem of urinary incontinence and retention or impotence. Plastic surgery may be necessary to heal deep and nonhealing pressure sores.

Physical therapy, or at least a regular program of stretching and exercise, is necessary for almost all patients to prevent worsening of spasticity, contractures, and the cardiovascular deconditioning and osteopenia associated with inactivity. There is no evidence that exercise in moderation has any deleterious effect on the disease process and much evidence that it enhances the general condition and well-being of the patient. Various mobility devices, including bracing, supports, and manual and electric wheelchairs, can assist in maintaining ambulation or independence in mobility. Occupational therapists can provide advice on structuring activities of daily living to minimize fatigue and can supply assistive devices as needed. Driving aids such as hand controls can help to prolong independence in these areas.

Speech Characteristics

In 1868, Charcot described a characteristic triad of signs—nystagmus, intention tremor, and scanning speech—which he termed *disseminated sclerosis*, today called *multiple sclerosis*. Scanning speech referred to the prolonged phonation of words with slow and slurred articulation. However, as large groups of individuals with MS were studied, it became apparent that dysarthria was not a universal characteristic of MS. Ivers and Goldstein (1963) completed a retrospective study of 144 individuals with MS and reported that dysarthria was present in 19 percent. In their sample, dysarthria was a presenting symptom only in 2 percent of the patients. Darley, Brown, and Goldstein (1972) evaluated 168 patients with MS who were referred to the neurology department in the Mayo Clinic. Speech samples were perceptually analyzed, and they reported that 41 percent of the sample demonstrated overall speech performance that was not essentially normal in terms of the impact on the listener. Beukelman, Kraft, and Freal (1985) reported on a survey of 656 individuals with MS. When a self-report technique was utilized, 23 percent reported a "speech and/or communication disorder." Perhaps the difference in the prevalence data reported in these studies resulted from the different methods used. In the reported studies, the prevalence of dysarthria in MS ranges from 19 percent to 41 percent, depending on who makes the judgment and how the population is sampled.

Obviously, severity of dysarthria in this population also varies. In the study by Beukelman and colleagues (1985) four percent of the respondants claimed to have communication so severely impaired that strangers were unable to understand them. Twenty-eight percent of this severely communicatively impaired group reported that they used augmentative communication approaches.

Other Communication Problems

Although dysarthria is the most common communication problem observed in individuals with MS, aphasia has been infrequently reported. Olmas-Lau, Ginsberg, and Geller (1977) summarized the literature and reported that:

> In several large reported series of multiple sclerosis patients, aphasia have been absent. . .Other authors have rated the incidence of aphasia from 1 to 3 percent. . . .

Poser (1978) reported two cases of aphasia in 812 individuals with MS. Although aphasia appears to be present in some cases of MS, Kraft (1981) points out that in the MS population intellectual dysfunction might be mislabeled as aphasia, because it also can affect language performance.

Perceptual Characteristics

Although "scanning speech" was included as an early symptom of MS by Charcot, there have been few careful studies of the dysarthria characteristics associated with this disease. Farmakides and Boone (1960) reviewed the case histories of 82 MS patients referred for speech therapy. They reported six characteristics that generally contribute to the dysarthria pattern—nasal voice quality, weak phonation and poor respiratory cycle, changes in pitch, slow rate, intellectual deterioration, and emotional liability.

Darley and colleagues (1972) rated the speech dimensions of 69 individuals with MS. They found that the perceptual speech patterns were consistent with a mixed dysarthria with both ataxic and spastic components. They summarize the speech characteristics as follows:

> The most prominent speech deviations in MS are impaired control of loudness, harshness, and defective articulation. Impaired use of vocal variability for emphasis, impaired pitch control, hypernasality, inappropriate pitch level, and breathiness are observed with lesser degrees of frequency.

MYASTHENIA GRAVIS

Medical Aspects

Myasthenia gravis is an autoimmune disorder that is characterized by abnormal fatiguability and weakness of skeletal muscles. The cause of this weakness is a defect in neuromuscular transmission. In the normal neuromuscular unit, the terminal axon of a motoneuron displays complex branching; the membrane of the muscle and plate shows a similarly complex array of clefts. This arrangement increases the amount of surface area that can be involved in transmission and thereby increases the strength of the chemical stimuli that crosses the unit. Acetylcholine (ACh) is the chemical produced by the neuron which fits into the receptor on the end plate and allows for depolarization and contraction. An enzyme, acetylcholinesterase (AChE), breaks the ACh molecule into component parts and causes the receptors to become available again for the next impulse. Myasthenia gravis is caused by the presence of a circulating ACh receptor (AChR) antibody which interferes with this binding capacity. There seem to be three different mechanisms by which this antibody interferes with normal transmission. The first is via direct interference with the AChR function by blocking it; this type of antibody is present in approximately 30 percent of patients with myasthenia gravis (Seybold, 1983) The second mechanism is the binding of the AChR antibody to another part of the receptor where it activates a complement which then destroys the cell membrane. This results in the "simplification" of the end-plate with a loss of surface area. The last mechanism concerns the cross-linking of two receptor molecules by an antibody molecule. This essentially accelerates the breakdown of receptor molecules beyond the body's capacity to produce new ones (Lisak, 1983). That different pathways exist to produce the disease suggests that different subgroups of patients exist and may benefit from different treatment approaches.

Population Characteristics and Natural Course

Myasthenia gravis has a prevalence of about one per 20,000 in the United States. Congenital and juvenile myasthenia are rare; however, some infants born to myasthenic mothers may show a transient form of the disorder. Females are affected about twice as often as males in young adulthood. After age 40, a slight preponderance of affected males may be seen. No genetic link is known (Seybold, 1983), and the natural history of myasthenia is essentially unknown. Prior to the introduction of anticholinergic medications in the 1930s, almost all patients who were recognized as having Myasthenia gravis were severely ill with a very high mortality rate. After 1934, all patients have been treated with the available drugs, so the untreated course of the disease is unclear (Grob, Brunner, & Namba, 1981). In the 1940s and 1950s the overall mortality rate was greater than 30 percent; by the 1970s, this had decreased to 3.3 percent due to the advent of improved artificial ventilation in 1960 (Cohen & Younger, 1981). The most common initial symptoms involve the extraocular muscles (ptosis, diplopia, and blurring of vision). Other presenting symptoms include leg weakness, generalized fatigue, difficulty in swallowing, slurred and nasal speech, difficulty in chewing, weakness of the face, arms, or neck, and trunk weakness or shortness of breath (Grob et al., 1981). Muscle weakness may not be present in the well-rested patient but can usually be elicited after exercise. Muscle atrophy is rare. Weight loss is most often due to difficulty in chewing or swallowing. Crises, due to the myasthenia process itself or to overmedication, usually manifest as acute respiratory insufficiency, aphonia, and immobility.

At onset, about 40 percent of patients will have only ocular signs and symptoms; within seven months about 60 percent of these will progress to generalized myasthenia gravis (Grob et al., 1981). The disease has an unpredictable course; spontaneous remissions can occur in any patient. Most patients show a fluctuating course with a particular muscle group primarily affected (Seybold, 1983). The maximal level of weakness for patients with generalized disease is reached within one to three years (Grob et al., 1981).

The disease symptoms can be exacerbated by environmental (bright light, heat), physical (pregnancy, viral illnesses, surgery), and emotional factors. The majority of patients with "idiopathic" crises had dysarthria or dysphagia at the time of occurrence, thereby predisposing them to aspiration (Cohen & Younger, 1981).

Other organ system disorders are frequently associated with myasthenia gravis. Thymomas are present in at least 10 percent of patients; thymic hyperplasia is extremely common in younger patients. Other autoimmune diseases, including thyroid disease, rheumatoid arthritis, systemic lupus erythematosus, and pernicious anemia, can be seen more often than in the normal population (Seybold, 1983).

The clinical signs and symptoms are sometimes sufficient to make the diagnosis of myasthenia gravis; more often, laboratory and pharmacologic testing are necessary. A blood test for the AChR antibody is the simplest; however, since a large percentage of patients will not have a detectable level, a negative test does not rule out myasthenia gravis. Pharmacologic testing involves the intravenous injection of short-acting cholinesterase inhibitors which inhibit the breakdown of ACh; a positive test will result in improved muscle strength or phonation for several minutes. Electrical testing for myasthenia gravis involves the fact that repetitive stimulation of a normal neuromuscular junction will produce action potentials with unchanging amplitudes. In the patient with myasthenia gravis, however, the muscle response amplitude decreases at least 10 percent between the first and the fifth responses. Testing under conditions of ischemia, heat, exercise, or after exposure to curare will increase the sensitivity of the test. A last method to be used in specialized testing centers involves single-fiber electromyography. In a normal muscle, the time interval between the firing of two terminal branches of a motor unit is variable, a characteristic called *jitter*. In a disease of the neuromuscular junction, jitter is increased and actual blocking of neuromuscular transmission can often be seen (Seybold, 1983).

Medical Management

The mainstay of therapy for myasthenia gravis has been the use of anticholinesterase drugs to improve muscle strength. Neostigmine (Prostigmin) and pyridostigmine (Mestinon) are the most frequently used. If a sustained release form is not used, the patient must take medication every two to six hours. Adjuvant drugs such as ephedrine are sometimes used to potentiate the AChE drugs. An excess of these drugs blocks AChR sites and produces a crisis identical to a myasthenic crisis with respiratory insufficiency and muscle weakness. Side effects are due to the action at both muscarinic receptor sites (smooth muscle and glands) and on nicotinic sites (skeletal muscles). They include abdominal cramps, diarrhea, nausea and vomiting, pupillary miosis, and increases in bronchial secretions, salivation, sweating or lacrimation, fasciculations, and muscle spasm. Patients will often take small doses of atropine, propantheline (Pro-Banthine) or diphenoxylate (Lomotil) to counteract these adverse effects (Kess, 1984).

Thymectomy is the accepted treatment for adolescent or young adults with generalized disease and for all patients with thymoma. Although no consistent immunologic changes can be detected in patients after thymectomy, it appears that the remission rate is higher (Seybold, 1983).

Steroids, in the form of prednisone, are often used during an exacerbation. The actual therapeutic effect is unknown, but it is felt that they may have a direct faciliatory effect on neuromuscular transmission or may decrease the production of AChR antibody. Adverse effects include those usually found with steroids: cataracts, gastrointestinal bleeding, infections, aseptic necrosis of bone, osteoporosis, myopathies, and psychoses (Kess, 1984; Seybold, 1983).

Immunosuppressants or cytotoxic drugs have recently been used; whether steroids or immunosuppressants are more effective is not known. Azathioprine (Imuran) has the side effects of hepatitis, thrombocytopenia, leukopenia, infections, nausea and vomiting, and alopecia; the severe adverse effects have been uncommon in the doses used for myasthenia gravis. Delayed malignancies due to immunosuppressant therapy have also been reported (Kess, 1984).

Plasmapheresis is used in the critically ill patient, presumably to remove the AChR antibody acutely. There have been reports of improvement, however, in patients without detectable antibody levels. Plasmapheresis is quite costly and without long-term benefits; antibody production may actually rebound after treatment (Lisak, 1983).

Other less exotic measures can be taken to improve the symptoms of myasthenia gravis. Advice should be offered to the patient regarding energy conservation while performing daily living activities. The home or work environment can be adjusted to require less use of affected muscle groups. Dietary advice is helpful to improve swallowing and nutritional status. Speech/language pathologists, in addition to treating dysarthria, can offer assistance for communication devices during periods of crisis or decreased ability to speak. Patients should avoid certain types of drugs (sedatives, narcotics, aminoglycoside antibiotics such as gentamicin, quinidine, or quinine products, barbiturates, muscle relaxants, cathartics) and should inform physicians or dentists of their disease as well as checking all over-the-counter drugs for these ingredients (Kess, 1984).

Speech Characteristics

The severity of the speech characteristics demonstrated by individuals with myasthenia gravis is dependent on the severity of the syndrome, the effectiveness with which the symptoms are controlled with medications, and the fatigue level at the moment. According to Grob (1958), 15 percent of persons with myasthenia gravis have bulbar involvement that causes the symptoms and signs of dysarthria. Generally, the speech symptoms result from weakness of the muscles of the soft palate, pharynx, tongue, and larynx (Walton, 1977). This weakness is usually reflected in increasing hypernasality, deterioration of articulation, increasing dysphonia, and reduction of loudness level. Speech may become unintelligible (Darley et al., 1975).

Speech abnormalities may be the initial symptom of myasthenia gravis. Wolski (1967) reported a case study of a 14 year old girl with myasthenia gravis whose presenting symptoms were hypernasality and nasal emission. Aronson (1971) reported a case study of a 20 year old woman with myasthenia gravis who demonstrated a mild, breathy dysphonia, which had been previously diagnosed as a symptom of a psychogenic condition. Aronson presented this case study to "alert the clinician to the fact that voice changes can be one of the first and only signs of early neurologic disease" (p. 115).

As was mentioned earlier in this chapter, the primary approach to treatment of persons with myasthenia gravis is pharmacological. Generally, an anticholinesterase drug is administered. Usually, speech symptoms are affected by the drugs if a positive effect is observed in other aspects of the disorder. Behaviorial speech treatment is usually not a routine aspect of the treatment program. Some individuals with severe residual speech problems will benefit from instruction in communication interaction, and a palatal lift may be helpful in reducing velopharyngeal insufficiency in some individuals (Gonzalez & Aronson, 1970).

REFERENCES

Adam, M., (Ed.). (1986). *Amyotrophic lateral sclerosis: A teaching manual for health professionals.* Kirkland, WA: ALS Health Support Services.

Alajouanine, T., Scherrer, J., Sabouraund, O., & Gremy, F. (1958). Etude oscillographique de la parole cerebelleuse. *Revue Neurologique, 98,* 708–714.

Amico, L.L., & Antil, J.P. (1981). Amyotrophic lateral sclerosis. *Postgraduate Medicine, 70,* 50–61.

Arnason, B.G.W. (1982). Multiple sclerosis: Current concepts and management. *Hospital Practice, 17*(2), 81–89.

Aronson, A. (1971). Early motor unit disease masquerading as psychogenic breathy dysphonia: A clinical case presentation. *Journal of Speech & Hearing Disorders, 36,* 115–124.

Aronson, A. (1980). Definition and scope of communication disorders. In D. Mulder

(Ed.), *The diagnosis and treatment of amyotrophic lateral sclerosis*. Boston: Houghton Mifflin.

Behrman, S., Carroll, J.D., Janota, A., & Matthews, W.B. (1969). Progressive supranuclear palsy: Clinico-pathological study of four cases. *Brain, 92,* 663–678.

Beukelman, D.R. (1983). Treatment of hyperkinetic dysarthria. In W.H. Perkins (Ed.), *Dysarthria and apraxia*. New York: Thieme-Stratton.

Beukelman, D.R., Kraft, G., & Freal, J. (1985). Expressive communication disorders in persons with multiple sclerosis: A survey. *Archives of Physical Medicine & Rehabilitation, 66,* 675–677.

Berry W.R., Darley, F.L., Aronson, A.E., & Goldstein, N.P., (1974). Dysarthria in Wilson's disease. *Journal of Speech & Hearing Research, 49,* 405–408.

Bianchine, J.R. (1976). Drug therapy of Parkinsonism. *New England Journal of Medicine, 295*(15), 814–818.

Blumenthal, H., & Miller, C. (1969). Motor nuclear involvement in progressive supranuclear palsy. *Archives of Neurology, 20,* 362–367.

Boshes, B. (1966). Voice changes in parkinsonism. *Journal of Neurosurgery, 24,* 286–288.

Brain, W., & Walton, J. (1969). *Brain's diseases of the nervous system*. London: Oxford University Press.

Brooke, M.H., Florence, J.M., Heller, S.L., Kaiser, K.K., Phillips, D., Gruber, A., Babcock, D., & Miller, J.P. (1986). Controlled trial of Thyrotropin Releasing Hormone in amyotrophic lateral sclerosis. *Neurology, 36,* 146–151.

Buck, J.F., & Cooper, I.S. (1956). Speech problems in parkinsonian patients undergoing anterior choroidal artery occlusion or chemopallidectomy. *Journal of the American Geriatric Society, 4,* 1285–1290.

Bundy. S., Harrison, M., & Martsden, C. (1975). A genetic study of torsion dystonia. *Journal of Medical Genetics, 12,* 12–19.

Burke, B., Fahn, S., & Gold, A. (1980). Delayed-onset dystonia in patients with "static" encephalopathy. *Journal of Neurology, Neurosurgery, Psychiatry, 43,* 789–797.

Caligiuri, M. (1985). *The influence of rigidity and hyperreflexia on speech labial kinematics in Parkinson's disease.* Unpublished doctoral dissertation, University of Wisconsin, Madison.

Canter, G. (1963). Speech characteristics of patients with Parkinson's disease: I. Intensity, pitch, and duration. *Journal of Speech & Hearing Disorders, 28,* 221–229.

Canter, G. (1965a). Speech characteristics of patients with Parkinson's disease: II. Physiological support for speech. *Journal of Speech & Hearing Disorders, 30,* 217–224.

Canter, G., (1969b). Speech characteristics of patients with Parkinson's disease: III. Articulation, diadochokinesis, and overall adequacy. *Journal of Speech & Hearing Disorders, 30,* 217–224.

Carrow, R., Rivera, V., Mauldin, M., Shamblin, L. (1974). Deviant speech characteristics in motor neuron disease. *Archives of Otolaryngology, 100,* 212–218.

Cartwright, G.E. (1978). Diagnosis of treatable Wilson's disease. *New England Journal of Medicine, 298,* 1347–1350.

Charcot, J. (1877). *Lecture on diseases of the nervous system*. London: New Sydenham Society.

Cohen, M.S., & Younger, D. (1981). Aspects of the natural history of myasthenia gravis: Crisis and death. *Annals of the New York Academy of Sciences, 377.*

Cooper, I. (1969). *Involuntary movement disorders.* New York: Harper & Row.

Crane, G.E. (1968). Tardive dyskinesia in patient treated with major neuroleptics: A review of the literature. *American Journal of Psychiatry, 124,* 40–48.

Cummings, J.L., & Benson, D.F. (1983). *Dementia: A clinical approach.* Boston: Butterworths.

Darley, F.L., Aronson, A.E., & Brown, J.R. (1969a). Differential diagnostic patterns of dysarthria. *Journal of Speech & Hearing Research, 12,* 246–269.

Darley, F.L., Aronson, A.E., & Brown, J.R. (1969b). Clusters of deviant speech dimensions in dysarthria. *Journal of Speech & Hearing Research, 12,* 462–496.

Darley, F.L., Aronson, A.E., & Brown, J.R. (1975). *Motor speech disorders.* Philadelphia: W.B. Saunders.

Darley, F.L., Brown, J.R., & Goldstein, N.P. (1972). Dysarthria in multiple sclerosis. *Journal of Speech & Hearing Research, 15,* 229–245.

de la Torre, R., Mier, M., & Boshes, B. (1960). Studies in parkinsonism. IX Evaluation of respiratory function: preliminary observations. *Quart. Bull. Northwestern University Medical School, 34,* 332–336.

DeLisa, J., Mikulic, M.A., Miller, R.M., & Melnick, R.R. (1979). Amyotrophic lateral sclerosis: Comprehensive management. *American Family Physician, 19,* 137–142.

Dworkin, J., Aronson, A., Mulder, D. (1980). Tongue force in normals and in dysarthric patients with amyotrophic lateral sclerosis. *Journal of Speech & Hearing Research, 23,* 828–837.

Eldridge, R. (1970). The torsion dystonias: Literature review and genetic and clinical studies. *Neurology, 20*(2), 1–78.

Ellison, G.W., Visscher, B.R., Graves, M.C., & Fahey, J.L. (1984). Multiple sclerosis. *Annals of Internal Medicine, 101,* 514–526.

Emery, A., & Holloway, S., (1982). Familial motor neuron diseases. In L. Rowland (Ed.), *Human motor neuron diseases.* New York: Raven.

Ewanowski, S. (1964). *Selected motor-speech behavior of patients with parkinsonism.* Unpublished doctoral dissertation, University of Wisconsin.

Fahn, S. (1984). The varied clinical expression dystonia. *Neurologic Clinics, 2,* 541–553.

Fahn, S., & Jankowic, J. (1984). Practical management of dystonia. *Neurologic Clinics, 2*(3), 555–569.

Farmakides, M., & Boone, D. (1960). Speech problems of patients with multiple sclerosis. *Journal of Speech & Hearing Disorders, 25,* 385–390.

Fischer, B.H., Marks, M., & Reich, T. (1983). Hyperbaric-oxygen treatment of multiple sclerosis. *New England Journal of Medicine, 308*(4), 181–186.

Gonzalez, J.B., & Aronson, A.E. (1970). Palatal lift prosthesis for treatment of anatomic and neurologic palatopharyngeal insufficiency. *Cleft Palate Journal, 7,* 91–104.

Goldstein, N.P., Tauxe, W.N., McCall, J.T., Gross, J.B., & Randall, R.V. (1969). Wilson's disease (hepatolenticular degeneration): Treatment with penicillamine and changes in epatic trapping of radioactive copper. *Archives of Neurology, 24,* 391–400.

Golper, L., Nutt, J., Rau, M., & Coleman, R. (1983). Focal cranial dystonia. *Journal of Speech & Hearing Disorders, 48,* 128–134.

Grewel, F. (1957). Dysarthria in post-encephalitic parkinsonism. *Acta Psychiatr. Neural. Scand., 32,* 440–449.

Grob, D., (1958). Myasthenia gravis: Current status of pathogenesis, clinical manifestations, and management. *J. Chron. Dis, 8,* 536–566.

Grob, D., Brunner, N.G., & Namba, T. (1981). The natural course of myasthenia gravis and effect of therapeutic measures. *Annals of the New York Academy of Sciences, 377*.

Gubbay, S.S., Kahana, E., Zilber, N., & Cooper, G. (1985). Amyotrophic lateral sclerosis: A study of its presentation and prognosis. *Journal of Neurology, 232*, 295–300.

Hallpike, J.F., Adams, C.W.M., & Tourtelotte, W.W. (Eds.). (1983). *Multiple sclerosis; pathology, diagnosis and management*. Baltimore: Williams & Wilkins.

Hanson, W.R., & Metter, E.J. (1983). DAF speech rate modification in Parkinson's disease: A report of two cases. In W.R. Berry (Ed.), *Clinical Dysarthria*. Austin, TX: PRO-ED.

Hanson, W.R., & Metter, E.J. (1983). DAF speech rate modification in Parkinson's disease: A report of two cases. In W.R. Berry (Ed.), *Clinical Dysarthria*. San Diego: College-Hill Press.

Hanyu, N., Oguchi, K., Yanagisawa, N., & Tsukagnoshi, H. (1981). Degeneration and regeneration of ventral root motor fibers in amyotrophic lateral sclerosis. *Journal of Neurological Sciences, 55*, 99–115.

Hauser, S.L., Dawson, D.M., Lehrich, J.R., Beal, M.F., Kevy, S.B., Propper, R.D., Mills, J.A., & Weiner, H.L. (1983). Intensive immunosuppression in progressive multiple sclerosis. *New England Journal of Medicine, 308*(4), 173–180.

Heck, A. (1964). A study of neural and extra neural findings in a large family with Friedreich's ataxia. *Journal of Neurological Sciences, 1*, 226–255.

Herz, E. (1944a). Dystonia. I. Historical review: Analysis of dystonic symptoms and physiologic mechanisms involved. *Archives of Neurology & Psychiatry, 51*, 305–318.

Herz, E. (1944b). Dystonia. II. Clinical classification, *Archives of Neurology & Psychiatry, 51*, 319–355.

Hiller, H. (1929). A study of speech disorders in Friedreich's ataxia. *Archives of Neurology & Psychiatry, 22*, 75–90.

Hirano, A., & Iwata, M. (1979). Pathology of motor neurons with special reference to amyotrophic lateral sclerosis and related diseases. In T. Tsubaki, & Y. Toyokura (Eds.), *Amyotrophic lateral sclerosis*. Baltimore: University Park Press.

Hirose, H., Kiritani, S., & Sawashima, M. (1982). Velocity of articulatory movements in normal and dysarthric subjects. *Folia Phoniatricia, 34*, 210–215.

Hirose, H., Kiritani, S., Ushijima, T., Yoshioka, H., & Sawashima, M. (1981). Patterns of dysarthria movements in patients with parkinsonism. *Folia Phoniatricia, 33*, 204–215.

Hoehn, M.M., & Yahr, M.D. (1967). Parkinsonism: Onset, progression, and mortality. *Neurology, 17*(5), 427–442.

Hogg, J.E., Massey, E.W., & Schoenberg, B.S. (1979). Mortality from Huntington's disease in the United States. *Avd. Neurol, 23*, 27–35.

Hughes, J. (1982). Pathology of amyotrophic lateral sclerosis. In L. Rowland (Ed.), *Human Motor Neuron Disease*. New York: Raven.

Hunker, C., & Abbs, J. (1984). Parkinsonian resting tremor and its relationship to movement initiation delays. *SMCL Reprints*, spring-summer, 103–122.

Hunker, C., Abbs, J., & Barlow, S. (1982). The relationship between parkinson rigidity and hypokinesia in the orofacial system: A quantitative analysis. *Neurology, 32*, 749–756.

Hunker, C., Bless, D., & Weismer, G. (1981). Respiratory inductive plethysmography: A clinical technique for assessing respiratory function for speech. Paper presented at the Annual Convention of the American Speech-Language-Hearing Association, Los Angeles.

Ivers, R., & Goldstein, N. (1963). Multiple sclerosis: A current appraisal of symptoms and signs. *Proceedings of the Staff Meetings of the Mayo Clinic, 38*, 457–466.

Joanette, Y., & Dudley, J. (1980). Dysarthria symptomatology of Friedreich's ataxia. *Brain & Language, 10*, 39–50.

Kammermeier, M. (1969). *A comparison of phonatory phenomena among groups of neurologically impaired speakers*. Unpublished doctoral dissertation, University of Minnesota.

Kelly, P.J., & Gillingham, F.J. (1980). The long-term of stereotaxic surgery and L-dopa in patients with Parkinson's disease. *Journal of Neurosurgery, 53*, 332–337.

Kess, R. (1984). Suddenly in crisis: Unpredictable myasthenia. *American Journal of Nursing, 8*, August.

Kim, R. (1968). The chronic residual respiratory disorder in post-encephalitic parkinsonism. *Journal of Neurology, Neurosurgery, & Psychiatry, 31*, 393–398.

Klawans, H.L., & Ringel, S.P. (1971). Observations on the efficacy of L-DOPA in progressive supranuclear palsy. *Europ. Neurol., 5*, 115–129.

Klawans, H.L., Goetz, C.G., & Perlik, S. (1980). Presymptomatic and early detection in Huntington's disease. *Ann. Neurol, 8*, 343–347.

Kraft, G. (1981). Multiple sclerosis. In W. Stolov & M. Clowers (Eds.), *Handbook of Severe Disability*. U.S. Government Printing Office, 111–118.

Kreul, E. (1972). Neuromuscular control examination (NMC) for parkinsonism: Vowel prolongations and diadochokinetic and reading rates. *Journal of Speech & Hearing Research, 15*, 72–83.

Lang, A.E., & Blair, R.D.G. (1984). Parkinson's disease in 1984: An update. *Can Med Assoc Journal, 131*, 1031–1037.

Lawyer, R., & Netsky, M. (1953). Amyotrophic lateral sclerosis: Clinicoanatomic study of 53 cases. *Archives of Neurology & Psychiatry, 69*, 171–192.

Leanderson, R., Persson, A., & Ohman, S. (1970). Electromyographic studies of the function of facial muscles in dysarthria. *Acta Otolaryngology*, (Suppl. 263), 89–94.

Lebrun, Y., Devreux, F., & Rousseau, J. (1986). Language and speech in a patient with a clinical diagnosis of progressive supranuclear palsy. *Brain & Language, 27*, 247–256.

Lisak, R.P. (1983). Myasthenia gravis: Mechanisms and management. *Hospital Practice, 3*, March 18.

Logemann, J.A. & Fisher, H.B. (1981). Vocal tract control in parkinson's disease: Phonetic feature analysis of misarticulation. *Journal of Speech & Hearing Disorders, 46*, 348–352.

Logemann, J.A., Fisher, H.B., Boshes, B., & Blonsky, E.R. (1978). Frequency and co-occurrence of vocal tract dysfunctions in the speech of a large sample of parkinson's patients. *Journal of Speech & Hearing Disorders, 43*, 47–57.

Ludlow, C.L., & Bassich, C.J. (1983). The results of acoustic and perceptual assessment of two types of dysarthria. In W.R. Berry, (Ed.), *Clinical Dysarthria*. San Diego: College-Hill Press.

Marsden, C. & Harrison, M. (1974). Idiopathic torsion dystonia (dystonia musculorum deformans): A review of 42 patients. *Brain, 97*, 793–810.

Marsden, C., Harrison, M., & Bundy, S. (1976). Natural history of idiopathic torsion dystonia. *Advances in Neurology, 14*, 177–187.

Marttila, R.J. (1983). Diagnosis and epidemiology of Parkinson's disease. *Acta Neurol Scan*, (Suppl. 95-9-17).

Maxwell, S., Massengill, R., & Nashold, B. (1970). Tardive dyskinesia. *Journal of Speech & Hearing Disorders, 35*, 122–125.

McFarlin, D.E. (1983). Treatment of multiple sclerosis. *New England Journal of Medicine, 308*(4), 215–217.

McFarlin, D.E., & McFarland, H.F. (1982). Multiple sclerosis, Part I. *New England Journal of Medicine, 307*(19), 1183–1188.

Menkes, J.H. (1974). *Textbook of child neurology*. Philadelphia: Lea & Febiger.

Morris, J.G.L. (1982). The manager of Parkinson's disease. *Aust. N.Z. Journal of Medicine 12*, 195–205.

Mueller, P. (1971). Parkinson's disease: Motor-speech behavior in a selected group of patients. *Folia Phoniatr, 23*, 333–346.

Netsell, R., Daniel B., & Celesia, G. (1975). Acceleration and weakness in parkinsonian dysarthria. *Journal of Speech & Hearing Disorders, 40*, 170–178.

Olmas-Lau, N., Ginsberg, M., & Geller, J. (1977). Aphasia in multiple sclerosis. *Neurology, 27*, 623–626.

Portnoy, R.A. (1979). Hyperkinetic dysarthria as an early indicator of impending tardive dyskinesia. *Journal of Speech & Hearing Disorders, 44*, 214–219.

Poser, C.M. (1978). *Multiple sclerosis*. New York: Springer Verlag.

Poser, C.M. (Ed.). (1984). *The Diagnosis of Multiple Sclerosis*. New York: Thieme-Stratton.

Putnam, A., Hixon, T., & Stern, L. (1982). *Speech breathing function in Friedreich's ataxia*. A presentation at the 19th Annual Meeting of the Federation of Western Societies of Neurological Sciences, San Diego, CA.

Rajput, A.H., Offord, K.P. Beard, C.M., Kurland, L.T. (1984). Epidemiology of parkinsonism: Incidence, classification, and mortality. *Annals of Neurology, 16*, 278–282.

Ramig, L.A. (1986). Acoustic analysis of phonation in patients with Huntington's disease: Preliminary report. *Annals of Otology, Rhinology, & Laryngology, 95*(3), 288–293.

Rigrodsky, S., & Morrison, E. (1970). Speech changes in parkinsonism during L-dopa therapy: Preliminary findings. *Journal of the American Geriatrics Society, 18*, 142–151.

Samara, K., Riklan, M., Levita, E., Zimmerman, J., Waltz, J., Bergmann, L., & Cooper, I. (1969). Language and speech correlates of anatomically verified lesions in thalamic surgery for parkinsonism. *Journal of Speech & Hearing Research, 12*, 510–540.

Sarno, M. (1968). Speech impairment in parkinson's disease. *Archives of Physical Medicine & Rehabilitation, 49*, 269–275.

Saunders, C., Walsh, T., & Smith, M. (1981). Hospice care in the motor neuron diseases. In C. Saunders & J. Teller (Eds.), *Hospice: The living idea*. Edward Arnold Publishers.

Scheinberg, L.C. (1983). *Multiple sclerosis: A guide for patients and their families*. New York: Raven Press.

Seybold, M.E. (1983). Myasthenia gravis: A clinical and basic science review. *Journal of the American Medical Association, 250*(18), November 11.

Sobue, G., Matsouka, Y., & Maukai, E. (1981). Pathology of myelinated fibers in cervical and lumbar ventral spinal roots in amyotrophic lateral sclerosis. *Journal of Neurological Sciences, 50*, 413–421.

Steele, J.C. (1972). Progressive supranuclear palsy. *Brain, 95*, 693–704.

Steele, J.C., Richardson, J.C., & Olszewski, J. (1964). Progressive supranuclear palsy. *Archives of Neurology, 10*, 333–359.

Swash, M., Roberts, A.H., Zakko, H., & Heathfield, K.W.G. (1972). Treatment of involuntary movement disorders with tetrabenzine. *Journal of Neurology, Neurosurgery, & Psychiatry, 35*, 186–191.

Tandan, R., Bradley, W.G. (1985a). Amytrophic lateral sclerosis: Part 1. Clinical features, pathology, and ethical issues in management. *Annuals of Neurology, 18*, 271–280.

Tandan, R., & Bradley, W.G. (1985b). Amyotrophic lateral sclerosis: Part 2. Etiopathogenesis. *Annals of Neurology, 18*, 419–431.

Tohgi, H., Tsukagnoshi, H., & Toyokura, Y. (1977). Quantitative changes of nerves in various neurological diseases. *Acta Neuropathologica, 38, 95*, 101.

Walton, J. (1977). *Brain's disease of the nervous system* (8th ed.). London: Oxford University Press.

Weismer, G. (1984). Articulatory characteristics of parkinsonian dysarthria: Segmental and phrase-level timing, spirantization, and glottal-supraglottal coordination. In M. McNeil, J. Rosenbek, & A. Aronson (Eds.), *The dysarthrias: Physiology, acoustics, perception, management*, San Diego: College-Hill Press.

Wilson, S.A.K. (1912) Progressive lenticular degeneration: A familial nervous disease associated with cirrhosis of the liver. *Brain, 34*, 295–509.

Wilson, S.A.K., & Bruce, A.N. (1955). *Neurology* (2nd ed.). Baltimore: Williams & Wilkins.

Wolski, W. (1967). Hypernasality as the presenting symptom of myasthenia gravis. *Journal of Speech & Hearing Disorders, 32*, 36–38.

Yanagisawa, N., & Goto, A. (1971). Dystonia musculorum deformans: Analysis with eletromyography. *Journal of Neurological Sciences, 13*, 39–65.

Young, R.R., & Delwaide, P.J. (1981a). Drug Therapy: Spasticity, Part I. *New England Journal of Medicine, 304*(1), 28–33.

Young, R.R., & Delwaide, P.J. (1981b). Drug Therapy: Spasticity, Part II. *New England Journal of Medicine, 304*(2), 96–99.

Zentay, P.J. (1937). Motor disorders of the nervous system and their significance for speech. Part I. Cerebral and cerebellar dysarthrias. *Laryngoscope, 47*, 147–156.

CHAPTER 7

Assessment and Treatment Planning

Clinical issues: We regularly provide clinical training opportunities for student interns in speech pathology, medical students, and resident physicians in neurology and rehabilitation medicine. The impetus for this text has come at least in part from our attempts to help our students make the transition from student to practicing clinician, from readers of research literature to individuals responsible for making decisions about management of communication problems. Typically, our speech pathology interns come to us relatively well-versed in the normal aspects of speech production. With some guidance, they are soon able to meet a dysarthric individual, review the medical chart, and provide an outline for obtaining descriptive information at a number of levels. They may be able to provide information related to the movement disorder, about the aerodynamic aspects of speech production, and about how the speaker sounds. However, when asked to interpret this descriptive data or to outline how they would use it to make decisions about what to do clinically, student interns often have difficulty developing an intervention plan. They may ask the following types of questions:

- *How is assessment different from description?*
- *What aspects of speech are important to measure, given clinical time limitations?*
- *Is it best to assess using perceptual or instrumental measurement techniques?*
- *How can the information from the assessment be used to set treatment goals and to plan intervention strategies?*

OVERVIEW OF ASSESSMENT

Assessment is a process by which intervention decisions are made. The term *assessment* is not synonymous with *description*. Description may be defined as the characterization of features of a disorder. In dysarthria, description involves giving a detailed account of the disorder—the impairment, disability, and handicap. In Chapter 3 discussion was largely descriptive, including listings of the features that distinguished one type of neurogenic communication disorder from another and one type of dysarthria from another. Assessment involves a critical step beyond description. It is more than a process of simply gathering information; rather, it also involves interpreting descriptive information and estimating the significance, importance, and value of that information to provide management directions.

Critical Assessment Points

The specific goals and outcomes of assessment may vary from situation to situation. McNeil and Kennedy (1984) list the following reasons for assessing a dysarthric speaker:

- to detect or confirm a suspected problem
- to establish a differential disgnosis
- to classify with a specified disorder group
- to determine site of lesion or disease process
- to specify the degree or severity of involvement
- to establish a prognosis
- to specify more precisely the treatment focus
- to establish criteria for treatment termination
- to measure any change in the patient that accompanies treatment, lack of treatment, or exacerbation of the original etiological factor (p. 337).

The range of possible assessment questions and outcomes may be illustrated by describing the critical points in the management of individuals with a particular degenerative neuromotor disorder. For example, with amyotrophic lateral sclerosis (ALS), we typically assess these individuals at four critical points. The first occurs when the diagnosis is made. At that time, we determine the presence of a problem and verify that the dysarthria is consistent with the proposed medical diagnosis. We discuss with the dysarthric speaker and family the nature of the problem, verify that the dysarthria is currently not a handicap in communicative situations, and give general suggestions for handling communication interactions. The second critical point occurs after the individual has achieved some psychological acceptance of the presence of the disease. At this point, the individual with ALS is involved in an information-gathering phase regarding services available to them, including augmentative communication alternatives. Guidelines are provided for when to return for reevaluation. The guidelines for return are general and suggest the need for reassessment when speech problems begin to interfer with any aspect of daily activities. In most cases, this occurs when intelligibility is compromised in some situations. Thus, the third critical assessment point occurs when the dysarthria becomes severe enough to become a handicap to the individual. At this time, assessment is carried out in order to establish candidacy for treatment and to specify the treatment focus. This assessment may be followed by a brief period of training in an effort to maximize intelligibility. The fourth critical point occurs when speech is so severely involved that it must be augmented by other communication approaches. As an outcome of this assessment process, an augmentative communication system may be selected. The case of a dysarthric individual with a degenerative disorder serves to illustrate the varying purposes of assessment. At times, we assess to confirm the presence of this disorder, at times, to measure its severity. Still other times, we assess to direct our treatment or to identify the intervention approaches that may be effective or to make recommendations about alternatives to verbal communication.

Selecting and Interpreting the Measures

We have defined assessment in dysarthria as a process of obtaining the descriptive data and interpreting it so that clinical decisions can be made. The literature contains literally hundreds of measures that may be obtained from dysarthric speakers (see McNeil & Kennedy [1984] for a brief review). Because it is not possible, and may not be important, in the clinical setting to obtain all of these measures, the clinician must select only those measures that are critical to the decisions that need to be made.

A model for selecting and interpreting assessment data is useful. Perhaps the best way of presenting such a model is by way of analogue. Consider the demands placed on a baseball pitcher. Pitching, like speech, is a complex motor activity with a series of specific goals that define the successfulness of the pitcher. The first goal of the pitcher is to be accurate—to get the ball over the plate within the strike zone. In speech, the first goal of the speaker is also accuracy or intelligibility. For a pitcher, if accuracy is not achieved, then none of the other goals can be reached. However, if a pitcher is accurate, then other goals become important. For example, it is to the pitcher's advantage to combine speed with accuracy. Likewise in speech, if a dysarthric speaker is understandable, then it is advantageous to to speak rapidly. Clearly, unintelligible but rapid speech cannot be considered successful. For a pitcher, it is also highly advantageous to be controlled. Control involves making subtle modifications that move the ball from one location in the strike zone to another. In speech, this subtle type of control may be analogous to the modifications needed to produce natural prosody, including appropriate stress patterning, intonation, and rate/rhythm adjustments. Thus, it is advantageous for a speaker to combine intelligibility with naturalness. In short, the overall goals of pitching are in many ways similiar to the overall goals of speech—accuracy, speed, and control.

Carrying the analogue one step further, suppose that a coach is called upon to improve the faulty performance of a pitcher. The coach would, of course, be interested in the overall measures of successfulness that we have just described. These measures would be used as an index of the severity of the problem. However, knowing the overall adequacy is not sufficient to know how to intervene with the troubled pitcher. The pitching coach would also need to know what has gone wrong with the process of pitching. This cannot be done simply by studying the outcomes, rather it must be done by studying the pitching movements themselves. The coach needs to know how the pitcher has thrown the ball. With a highly trained eye, the coach observes the components of the pitching process, watching all aspects of the delivery—the stretch, the wrist action, the release, and the follow-through. Most of the time, the coach observes the components as part of an integrated movement rather than in isolation. The pitching coach cannot usually make recommendations for modification of pitching style solely on the basis of watching the pitcher perform a series of isolated nonpitching movements—seeing how high the pitcher can kick, checking wrist flexibility, or monitoring the maximum arm strength and movement velocity. Likewise, the speech/language pathologist watches the complex activity of speech with an eye on the relative contribution of the various components. What is the level of respiratory support during connected speech? How does the speaker handle breath groups? What are the characteristics of phonation, velopharyngeal timing, or oral articulatory movements?

After viewing the pitcher in action, the coach will then identify a few features that may contribute to the problem. Suppose that the coach suggested a higher kick and modified wrist position at the time of delivery of the ball. Successfulness of the intervention is not measured solely by seeing whether or not the suggested modifications have been made. Rather, success must be measured relative to the pitcher's overall goals. Do the modifications in pitching style improve the accuracy, speed, and control of the pitch? Similarly, for the speech/language pathologist, if the goal of intervention is to increase respiratory support for pressure consonants and to achieve more vigorous bilabial movements, the first task is to train the speaker to perform the speech act differently. Once that has been accomplished, then the clinician verifies the success of the treatment by determining whether or not the speaker is any closer to the overall goals of intelligible, rapid, and natural-sounding speech.

In summary, clinicians have available to them several different types of assessment data. Some of the data are related to the impairment and describe what has gone wrong with the components of the speaking process. Other data relate to the disability and serve as an overall index of speech adequacy. Although on the surface these types of data may seem incompatible, they may indeed be complementary. While describing different aspects of the disorder of dysarthria, both types of information are needed for making management decisions.

ASSESSMENT OF THE DISABILITY

Although speech intelligibility, rate, and naturalness are all important indicators of the level of disability in dysarthria, only intelligibility will be discussed in this chapter. Approaches to the assessment of speaking rate can be found in Chapter 13 and assessment of naturalness in Chapter 14.

Intelligibility as an Overall Index of Disability

Intelligible speech may be viewed as a primary goal of dysarthric speakers. Achieving this goal is a prerequisite for other aspects of speech performance, including naturalness. A variety of reasons have been suggested for the clinical measurement of speech intelligibility and speaking rate (Yorkston, Beukelman & Traynor, 1984). First, measures of speech intelligilibity, when accompanied by measures of speaking rate, provide a useful index of the severity of the overall disability. They provide a comprehensive indicator of all components of speech production including not only oral articulatory performance, but also respiratory, phonatory, and velopharyngeal performance, which are frequently impaired in dysarthric individuals. Second, reduced intelligibility and speaking rate are nearly universal consequences of dysarthria, regardless of the underlying neuromotor impairment. Even mildly dysarthric speakers can be distinguished from nonimpaired individuals on the basis of speaking rate (Yorkston & Beukelman, 1981). Third, intelligibility appears to be closely related to other aspects of the impairment, disability, and handicap. For example, work of Platt, Andrews, Young, and Neilson (1978) indicated that measures of single word intelligibility and ratings of prose intelligibility correlated well with diadokokinetic rates, phonemes correctly identified, and judgments of speech handicap. A close relationship between transcription intelligibility scores and information transfer were also reported (Beukelman & Yorkston, 1979). Finally, we use speech intelligibility as our primary measure of disability because the results of this type of assessment are easily communicated to the speakers and families. Intelligibility measures can be understood without a detailed knowledge of the physiology of the speech process. Intelligibility is usually the first area of assessment that we consider because the dysarthric individual nearly always views the dysarthria from this functional point of view.

Factors That Influence Measurements of Intelligibility

Considering the importance of intelligibility, care must be taken when measuring this aspect of disability in the clinical setting. The research literature summarized elsewhere (Yorkston & Beukelman, 1981; Yorkston, Beukelman, & Traynor, 1984) cites numerous examples of how intelligibility scores can be changed depending on the speakers' task, the transmission system, and the judges' task. Table 7-1 contains a summary of a series of studies examining issues related to measurement of intelligibility in dysarthric speakers.

Speakers' Task

The speaking task or the message format has an influence on intelligibility scores. For example, with dysarthric speakers, recording of single words results in different intelligibility scores than does recording sentences. Further, there is an interaction between severity of dysarthria and performance on these two speaking tasks (Yorkston & Beukelman, 1978). For severely dysarthric individuals, intelligibility scores tend to be higher for single words than for sentences. For mildly dysarthric individuals, the opposite is the case, with sentences receiving higher scores than single words. Thus, for mildly involved speakers, sentences appear to provide contextual cues to aid the listeners. For the more severely involved, these contextual cues may not be present or sentence production tasks may simply be too demanding in the presence of poorly controlled and coordinated respiratory, laryngeal, and articulatory systems.

Spontaneous speech scores may also be different from scores on a sentence production task. Frearson (1983) obtained samples of spontaneous speech and sentence productions from 20 dysarthric adults, including flaccid, spastic, and hypokinetic dysarthric speakers. T-test comparison of intelligibility scores indicates that sentences read aloud were more intelligible than spontaneous speech. However, speaking rate and rate of intelligible speech were not significantly different for spontaneous speech versus sentence productions.

Research in the field of audiology has documented that spondaic words and phonetically balanced monosyllables generate different intelligibility scores. Intelligibility scores for dysarthric speakers may vary depending on word selection. Tikofsky and Tikofsky (1964) and Tikofsky (1970) proposed a list which contained 50 different words of 9 difficulty levels. Although specific words in this list varied in difficulty, rank-ordering of severity was similar across word lists.

Still another important speaker variable is rate. The effects of rate control on dysarthric speech will be discussed in detail in Chapter 13. Briefly, the intelligibility scores for some speakers will vary depending on their rate of speech (Hanson & Metter, 1980; Yorkston & Beukelman, 1981). Because modification of a dysarthric speaker's rate often becomes a critical issue in

TABLE 7-1.
A Summary of Studies Examining Issues Related to Intelligibility Measurement in Dysarthria Speakers

Comparison	Results	References
Speakers' Task		
Different words & words lists	Words vary in difficulty, different word lists & orderings rank speakers similarly	Tikofsky & Tikofsky (1964) Tikofsky (1970)
Single words vs. sentences	Interaction between severity & speakers' task: for severely involved, intelligibility is higher for single words; for mildly involved, it is higher for sentences.	Yorkston & Beukelman (1978)
Sentence production vs. spontaneous speech	Intelligibility scores higher for sentence production; speaking rate, rate of intelligible, speech, & communication efficiency ratio no significant differences.	Frearson (1983)
Judges' Task		
Transcription vs. completion vs. multiple choice juding format	Lowest scores on transcriptions, intermediate on completion, highest on multiple choice (all rank-ordered speaker similarly)	Yorkston & Beukelman (1978)
Estimates vs. objective judging modes	Mean scores similar dispersion much greater for estimates	Yorkston & Beukelman (1978)
Naive judges' transcription vs. speech pathologists' estimates	Speech pathologists overestimate transcription scores	Beukelman & Yorkston (1980)
Estimate of judges unfamiliar & familiar with the passage	Estimates of intelligibility increase with increasing familiarity for moderately severe dysarthric speakers	Beukelman & Yorkston (1980)
Judges with increasing familiarity with master pool and randomly generated word lists	Slight but consistent increases in scores with increasing familiarity	Yorkston & Beukelman (1980)
Judges with increasing familiarity with the dysarthric speaker	No familiarization effect.	Yorkston & Beukelman (1983)

treatment, it is useful to (1) use tasks that sample connected speech, and (2) report speaking rates in conjunction with intelligibility scores.

Transmission System

Intelligibility tasks involve a speaker producing a message that is transmitted to a listener who in some way judges that sample. Thus, in addition to the message produced by the speaker, the transmission system may influence intelligibility scores. In most clinical and research work, high-quality audio-recordings are made and played to the listener under optimal conditions. It is reasonable to assume that intelligibility scores for some speakers would change if live voice or video-tape were used as the transmission medium.

Judges' Task

Intelligibility scores may be influenced by the task that the judge is being asked to perform. In a study by Yorkston and Beukelman (1978), three different response formats were compared: (1) word and sentence transcription in which listeners were asked to write down the words that had been spoken, (2) word and sentence completion in which listeners were asked to complete sentences from which a single word had been deleted, and (3) multiple choice tasks in which listeners were asked to select, from ten options, the utterance being produced. Results indicated that although all formats produced scores that rank-ordered speakers in a similiar way, the actual intelligibility scores differed from task to task. Transcription judging formats were associated with the lowest intelligibility scores, completion formats with intermediate scores, and multiple choice tasks with the highest scores. As a second phase of the same study, estimates of intelligibility were compared with objective judging modes in which judges' responses could be scored as either correct or incorrect. Results indicated that although the mean scores across a large group of judges were similiar for estimates and objective modes, the dispersion of judges' scores was much greater when estimating intelligibility. Differences between judge estimates of intelligibility for some moderately severe dysarthric speakers were as large as 90 percent, covering nearly the entire possible range.

The judges in the previous study had not been speech/language pathologists. Therefore, in a later study (Yorkston & Beukelman, 1980), estimates made by speech/language pathologists were compared with transcription intelligibility scores of naive judges. Once again, estimates of intelligibility were not consistent with transcription intelligibility scores. In this case, speech/language pathologists, who were familiar with the message being spoken, consistently overestimated the transcription scores. These overestimates were large for the moderately involved speaker. In the same study, the initially naive judges were made progressively more familiar with the passage being spoken. Estimates of intelligibility made by initially naive judges increased with increasing familiarity with the passage. Consistent with the results obtained from the speech/language pathologist judges, this effect was the largest for the moderately involved speaker.

Estimates of intelligibility appear to be problematic in clinical measurement for a number of reasons. First, the dispersion of individual judges' responses was large. Second, estimates of intelligibility appear to be influenced by judge familiarity with the message. Third, estimates would need to be averaged across large groups of judges before they appeared to correspond to transcription scores. In order to circumvent some of these problems, the use of a random message selection process was explored as a means of controlling judge familiarity with the speech sample and, at the same time, generate multiple responses that could be objectively scored. The technique utilizes samples randomly generated from a master pool. Results of Yorkston and Beukelman's 1980 study of single word intelligibility indicated slight, but consistent and predictable, increases in scores following an extensive period of familiarization with the master pool.

Clinical Measurement of Speech Intelligibility

Although speech intelligibility and rate provide information essential for clinical management of dysarthric speakers, their measurement is not straightforward. Because intelligibility can be so easily influenced, care must be taken to control as many of the factors described in the previous section as possible. Assessment of Intelligibility of Dysarthric Speech (Yorkston & Beukelman, 1981b) and Computerized Assessment of Intelligibility of Dysarthric Speech (Yorkston et al., 1984) were designed to provide a clinician-judged technique for measuring intelligibility in the clinical setting. These tools provide an objective measure of sentence and single word intelligibility during a reading or imitative speaking task. In developing these clinical tools, task selection involved a number of decisions. Some were based on research evidence; others on the basis of ease of clinical administration. The following are some general considerations that guided speaker and judge task selection.

Standardized Speaker Tasks

Two speaker tasks, single word and sentence production, were selected for a number of reasons. Sentences varying in length from 5 to 15 words were chosen, because it was felt that they more closely approximated the demands of ordinary speaking situations than did single words. Further, the use of sentence stimuli also allows the simultaneous measurement of speaking rate, a critically important variable for some dysarthric speakers. Speaking rate should be considered in a number of clinical decisions, for example, reduction of speaking rate may be an important intervention technique. A measure of intelligibility combined with speaking rate (intelligible words per minute) is a useful means of distinguishing mildly dysarthric from normal speakers (Yorkston & Beukelman, 1981a). Single words also are included in the assessment protocol because some severely dysarthric individuals are unable to produce long sentences. Further, a comparison of intelligibility scores on single word tasks with scores obtained from the sentence production task may provide some general information regarding appropriateness of speaking rates.

Control of Judge Familiarity

Because ability to repeatedly administer and judge similiar speaking tasks is one of the primary requirements of a clinical measurement tool, an attempt was made to control judge familiarity with the sample. This was done in two ways: (1) a randomized sample selection procedure ensures that although the judges have a general familiarity with the sample being produced, they do not know the specific words or sentences being spoken; (2) all samples are selected, recorded, and scored by an examiner who does not participate in judging the intelligibility samples.

Judges' Tasks

Because research reported earlier suggested that objective measures are less subject to interjudge differences than estimates of intelligibility, all tasks require a response from the judge that can be scored as correct or incorrect. Two different judging formats (multiple choice or transcription) are available for the single word task. Many severely dysarthric speakers may receive intelligibility scores of near zero when a transcription judging format is used. Therefore, when quantifying the changing performance of severely dysarthic speakers, an "easier" intelligibility task must be used. A multiple choice judging format was selected for this purpose.

Assessing Intelligibility in Natural Settings

Thus far, the discussion has focused on obtaining and interpreting carefully controlled measures of intelligibility in the clinical setting. Information about intelligibility of speech in natural situations is also important for clinical management. Berry and Sanders (1983) have listed the environmental variables that may impact intelligibility in natural settings, including the situation (learned expectations surrounding the message—where, when, who, why, and what), noise, lighting, distance, resonance, and posture. They have suggested that clinicians cannot assume that dysarthric speakers and their listeners are aware of and will learn to control these variables. In order to assess intelligibility in natural settings, Berry and Sanders interviewed the dysarthric speaker and key informants regarding selected environmental variables. A partial listing of items from the Situational Intelligibility Survey are listed in Table 7-2. Information for such interviews provides the clinician with an estimate of the severity of handicap that results from the dysarthria.

ASSESSING THE IMPAIRMENT

Physiologic Approach

During assessment of the impairment, focus is placed on the speech production process. The clinican asks:

- What aspects of the speech motor activity are impaired?
- How has the weakness, slowness, discoordination or abnormal tone of the speech musculature affected the respiratory, laryngeal, velopharyngeal, or oral articulatory components?

The physiologic approach to understanding motor speech disorders provides a framework for this type of assessment (Netsell, 1973, 1984, 1986, Rosenbek & LaPointe, 1985). Figure 7-1, adapted from Netsell (1973), contains a number of vocal tract components that warrant attention during assessment. Netsell and Daniel (1979) have defined the term *functional component* as "a structure (or number of structures) that work to generate or value the speech air stream" (p. 502).

TABLE 7-2.
Selected Items for the Situational Intelligibility Survey

People have trouble understanding me, him/her:
everywhere
in noisy places
in dark places
when strangers are the listeners
in group conversations
when watching TV/listening to the radio
in stores
in restaurants/night spots
on the phone
while in a car

From Berry, W.R., & Sanders, S.B. (1983). Environmental Education: The Universal management approach for adults with dysarthria. In W.R. Berry (Ed.), *Clinical dysarthria*. San Diego: College-Hill Press.

Items are scored using the following scale: 0—All the time; 1—Occasionally; 2—Never.

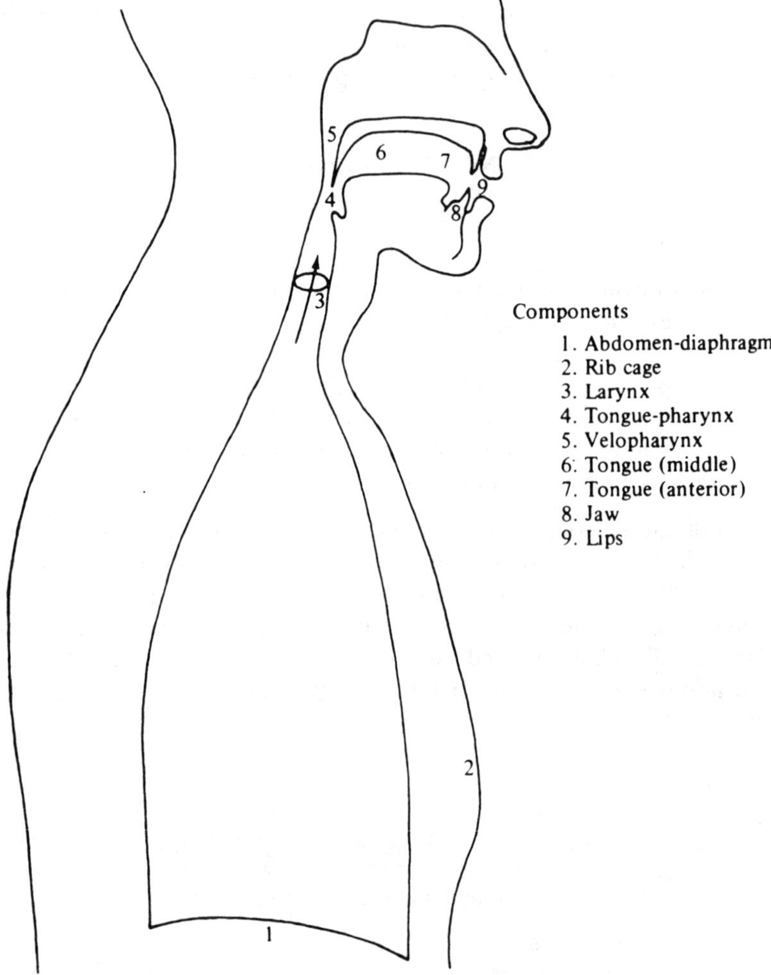

Figure 7-1. A line-drawing representation of the speech production mechanism (Adapted from Netsell, 1973).

Although this model provides a useful focus to organize both perceptual and instrumental measures of speech performance, to evaluate each point in isolation would seriously oversimplify the complex process of speech production. In dysarthria the impairment is almost never restricted to a single point. Rather, impairments of varying levels of severity may occur in various components. Further, vocal tract components do not function independently of one another (Hardy, 1967). Numerous examples of this interdependence are cited throughout this text. Consider the function of the muscles and structures of respiration as a pump to provide breath support for speech. The adequacy of respiratory support may be effected by the efficiency of all of the "upstream" valves. Thus, inadequate laryngeal, velopharyngeal, or oral articulatory valving interact with poor respiratory support to create a cumulative negative effect. An appreciation of the remarkable ability of speakers to compensate for abnormalities at single points in the speech production mechanism has been provided (Fletcher, 1985). However, a speaker's ability to compensate for impairment at multiple points is much more poorly understood. Clinical experience suggests that relatively mild impairment in multiple speech components may be more devastating than severe impairment of some single components. Better understanding of the interaction between speech components in dysarthric speakers is clearly needed.

Selecting the Tasks and Measurement Approaches

Armed with the physiologic model that allows the clinician to focus on specific aspects of the speech production process, tasks that adequately sample the behaviors of interest and approaches for measuring those behaviors must be selected. In terms of task selection, performance has been measured in a variety of tasks, including connected speech (with specially constructed sentences and paragraphs), speech-like tasks (repetition of selected syllables, e.g., /papapa/), tasks that involve only one or two selected components (sustained phonation), and tasks that focus on a single component (panting rates as a measure of respiratory system performance). The relation among measures obtained from speech, speech-like, and nonspeech tasks await more careful study. Research points to some differences between speech and nonspeech tasks (Hixon & Hardy, 1964). Clinical experience suggests that some speakers perform differently depending on the tasks. For example, at times, traumatically brain-injured speakers will perform adequately on simple nonspeech tasks, but will demonstrate severe impairment on more complex speaking tasks.

Once the task has been selected, the clinician decides how to measure performance on that task. Generally, the tools for measuring the function of the each of the speech components are categorized as either perceptual or instrumental. Perceptual measures are those that rely on the trained eyes and ears of the clinician. Instrumental approaches to assessment, on the other hand, employ a series of devices that provide information about the acoustic, aerodynamic, movement, or myoelectric aspects of speech production. A more detailed description of the assessment of the various speech components is contained in later chapters. For this general discussion, the reader should be aware that each of the speech components can be assessed with a number of different perceptual and instrumental approaches. For example, when assessing the respiratory system in the clinical setting, perceptual measures of performance might include ratings of breath group length and loudness of samples of connected speech as well as visual observations of the presence of clavical breathing. Among the instrumental approaches to the measurement of respiratory function are the acoustic measures of intensity and utterance duration. Aerodynamically, respiratory performance may be assessed by estimating the subglottal air pressure generated by the speaker. Respiratory inductive plethysmography (commerically available as the Respitrace) is an instrumental means of obtaining information about the rib cage and abdominal components of the respiratory system and lung volume exchange. This instrumentation can be used to study the timing of breathing for speech, the relative contributions of rib cage and abdominal components during speech, and the lung volume level at which utterances are produced. When so many approaches to the measurement of a given phenomenon are available, then the question of which assessment tools are the best is raised. There is no simple answer, therefore, the clinical advantages and disadvantages of each are outlined in the following discussion.

Perceptual Measures

The "ears of a trained clinician" are wonderful integrators that seek to categorize the phenomenon they hear. At times, this ability is a real asset; at other times it is problematic. When measures of overall speech disability are needed, clinicians will usually turn to perceptually derived measures. This is quite logical when the phenomenon being measured is considered. Measures of disability reflect overall aspects of speech—intelligibility, naturalness, rate, and general articulatory adequacy. Thus, an integrative function of perceptual measures is needed. Measurement of impairment may be slightly different. Here, the integrative nature of perceptual measures may be a disadvantage. Speech scientists caution against making inferences about physiological phenomena from perceptual measures alone. The principle of motor equivalence suggests that a single perceptual end-product may be the result of one of a number of physiological events. For example, what the listener hears as imprecise articulatory movements may be the consequence of lack of movement as in rigidity, slow movement, or incoordinated movement. Perceptual measures are of limited use in determining the contributors to the problems. Rosenbek and LaPointe (1985) summarize some disadvantages of perceptual approaches to the assessment of dysarthria:

- trained judges are required
- difficult it is to separate premorbid characteristics (age, medical, and social history) from those that are related to the neurologic problem
- symptoms may be present under some conditions and not others
- certain symptoms influence others (e.g., severe articulation problems may influence judgments of hypernasality)
- the same symptoms may be the result of very different underlying conditions

Instrumental Observations

The instrumental approach to speech impairment measurement also presents problems for the clinician. Unlike the perceptual measures just discussed, some instrumental measures do not lend themselves to measurement of integrative activities. Simultaneous measures of multiple aspects of speech production are technically difficult to obtain and interpret. On the other hand, instrumental measures "bring us closer to events in the peripheral speech mechanism . . . [and] leave us guessing less about the neuromuscular deficits underlying the perceptual symptoms" (Rosenbek & LaPointe, 1985, p. 112).

Selectivity is critical to the appropriate clinical use of instrumentation. Given sufficient equipment and time, the clinician could instrumentally measure an almost endless number of aspects of dysarthria. However, the usefulness of a given measure of dysarthric performance may depend upon the answer to two questions:

- Can this measure be obtained accurately and reliably in the clinical setting?
- How important is the measure?

For purposes of illustration, these questions will be applied to the clinical measurement of vital capacity in dysarthria. Vital capacity can be reliably and relatively easily measured in the dysarthric population, and in most cases, these measures would reveal a problem in dysarthric speakers in the form of reduced function relative to the normal population. However, consider the clinical importance of vital capacity—it is an important decision-making variable in relatively few dysarthric speakers. Thus, the clinician must distinguish the important from the easy, straightforward, and perhaps, the trivial.

A Clinical Compromise

Earlier in this chapter, assessment was defined as a process of placing importance on our information as we decide what is important and what is not. Admittedly, the assessment process is heavily dependent on subjective opinions, judgments, and hunches. Many of the opinions that we provide in this discussion await research verification. In the following section, we will describe the clinical compromises we have reached in response to the pressures of limited time, equipment, and knowledge.

We begin our assessment with the integrative measures that give general information quickly. The tools used in this level of assessment are perceptual and the tasks typically sample connected speech. Thus, we begin with perceptual measures and a physiologic approach to focus our listening. The first level of perceptual assessment is conducted to identify speech components where impairment may occur. Table 7-3 contains a listing of perceptually

TABLE 7-3.
Perceptually Based Indicators of Component Impairment in Connected Speech

Respiratory Function

- abnormal loudness
- excess loudness variability
- short breath group lengths
- complaints of fatigue with extended speaking
- failure to initiate phonation
- claviclar breathing
- audible air wastage prior to initiation of utterance
- failure to match breath group with syntax of the utterance
- lack of variability in length of breath groups

Laryngeal Function

- abnormal loudness level
- excessive loudness variation
- alternating loudness
- monoloudness
- loudness decay
- harsh voice
- breathy voice
- strain-strangled voice
- hoarse (wet) voice
- pitch breaks
- breathy voice (transient)
- failure to distinguish voiced from voiceless consonants
- continuous voicing
- audible air wastage prior to initiation of utterance
- failure to initiate phonation

Velopharyngeal Function

- nasal emission
- hypernasality
- hyponasality
- short phrases
- inability to produce pressure consonants
- problems with voiced/voiceless distinctions

Oral articulation

- imprecise consonants
- irregular articulatory breakdowns
- prolongation of phonemes
- distortion of vowels

derived signs of impairment in each of the components. Readers will note that many of these features are among those used in the Mayo Clinic studies (Darley, Aronson, & Brown, 1969a, b). Others are obtained through visual examination or through speaker reports. Some features are common to more than one speech component. Admittedly, these lists may not be exhaustive, however, they serve to focus attention on component impairment.

Once an impairment in a specific speech component is suspected or has been identified, we ask a series of questions in an effort to more accurately describe the nature and severity of the problem. The results of the general perceptual assessment allow the clinician to formulate questions that will lead to a more detailed analysis of component function. These detailed questions are most frequently answered with instrumentally based measures. Although the specific questions vary considerably from speaker to speaker, the questions generally fall into one of two categories:

- What is the nature and severity of the component impairment?
- What can be done about it?

Nature of the Impairment

One of the chief objections to perceptually derived assessment approaches is that they generally provide little information about the nature of the problem. Once an impairment has been identified it must be examined in detail in order to formulate a treatment plan. For example, many dysarthric individuals speak with short phrases, producing only a few syllables or words per breath group. This speech characteristic is easily identified perceptually. However, an understanding of the underlying problems that may be responsible for this is best obtained instrumentally. A number of different problems may result in short breath groups. In some speakers, the problem may be primarily one of respiratory insufficiency. If this is the case, the speaker may be unable to generate adequate subglottal air pressure for more than a second or two. Simple instrumental techniques for measuring a speaker's ability to sustain an adequate level of subglottal air pressure are described in Chapter 9. In other cases, respiratory function may not be the primary problem; rather, the respiratory signs may be secondary to impairments in other speech components. Short breath groups may occur in dysarthric individuals who are attempting to compensate for spasticity in the laryngeal musculature. These individuals must "overdrive" their respiratory component in order to produce phonation. The function of the respiratory system in these indivduals can be documented by aerodynamically estimating subglottal air pressure during the production of voiceless stop consonants (see Chapter 11 & Netsell, Lotz & Shaughnessy, 1984). Often these individuals generate much greater than normal subglottal air pressure.

In still other cases, short phrase length may be the result of impairment in multiple rather than single speech components. Frequently, dysarthric individuals exhibit impairment in all of the components. The perceptual feature of short phrases may be the result of mild to moderate respiratory support problems coupled with velopharyngeal incompetency. Thus, moderate difficulty in generating adequate breath pressure may be exaggerated by air wastage from an incompetent velopharyngeal port. Instrumentally, this type of problem may be documented by obtaining simultaneous aerodynamic measures of intraoral air pressure and nasal air flow (see Chapter 11). These measures can be used to make inferences about the timing of velopharyngeal closure and, coupled with information about respiratory support, may provide an explanation for the perceptual measures. A gross estimate of the relative contribution of the respiratory versus the velopharyngeal components can be obtained by asking the individual to perform speech and nonspeech maneuvers with the nares occluded and then documenting changes in performance.

Finally, other dysarthric individuals speak with short phrases for reasons not related to their current level of physiological support. Examples of such cases frequently occur in recovering traumatically head-injured speakers. Despite the fact that short phrases are a characteristic of their habitual speech, these individuals may demonstrate the motor control to perform in a much more normal fashion. When assessed instrumentally, they may exhibit respiratory support adequate for extended utterances. No other speech component may markedly contribute to the tendency to produce short phrases. When instructed, these individuals can produce nearly normal breath group lengths. In such cases, we speculate that these head-injured individuals are continuing to use a respiratory pattern that they learned when their impairment was much more severe, even though their respiratory control has increased and they no longer need to use a "one-word-at-a-time" approach. What once was a useful compensatory behavior may now be maladaptive.

In summary, by reviewing the list of perceptual features related to each of the components, the reader will realize that as with short phrases, many of the features may have multiple underlying causes. Perceptual means are used to identify the problems and generate clinical hypotheses about the underlying causes. Instrumental means are used to confirm or reject these hypotheses. Armed with a thorough understanding of normal aspects of speech and vocal tract impairment assessement, some possible explanations can be posed.

An understanding of why a perceptual feature is occurring is obviously important for treatment planning. Consider the differing treatment approaches for each of the speakers just described, all of whom share the common characteristic of speaking with short phrases. For the speaker with insufficient respiratory support, treatment might focus on increasing the ability to sustain adequate breath pressure either prosthetically or by training. For the speaker who uses short phrases to compensate for increased laryngeal tone, training to improve respiratory support is not needed. Rather, the laryngeal problem must be managed, perhaps through the prescription of antispasticity medications. For the speaker whose moderate respiratory support problems are exaggerated by inadequate velopharyngeal function, fitting a palatal lift may be appropriate to compensate for the velopharyngeal problem. For the speaker who has recovered physiological support but has maintained an abnormal respiratory pattern, behavioral training may be appropriate to change the maladaptive pattern. Thus, different speakers with a common perceptual feature would each be managed differently, depending on the underlying nature of the problem.

Identifying Features That Can Be Modified

The first phase of assessing the impairment is conducted using perceptual means to identify speech features that are disrupted and to pose clinical hypotheses that offer an explanation of the perceived features. The second phase of assessment involves the use of instrumental means to verify those hypotheses; thus, to better understand why the perceptual features are present. The third phase of assessment involves identifying those aspects of the impairment where change is possible and where change will result in important reduction in overall disability. This phase is necessary because it is possible to know what has gone wrong and why, and yet have no apparent means of changing that feature.

Unlike previous phases of assessment where the clinician focused observations on the speaker's habitual performance, during the third phase the focus is on instructed or modified performance. The comparison between modified and habitual performance gives an indication of the potential value of various intervention techniques. This discussion will not involve listing tasks or techniques that can be used with all speakers, as no such list exists. Rather, the process is illustrated with an example of two speakers who both exhibited perceptually identified characteristics related to velopharyngeal port dysfunction, including nasal emission, hypernasality, imprecise production of "pressure" consonants, and short breath group units. Although these speakers exhibited similiar perceptual features, results of the instrumental assessment suggested that different underlying problems may have caused the velopharyngeal dysfunction in each of these speakers. Results of aerodynamic studies in the first speaker suggested that this individual never achieved closure at habitual speaking rates and loudness levels. Behavioral intervention techniques appeared to have no effect. Instructions to slow the speaking rate did not result in improved performance, and instructions to speak louder or softer (to increase or decrease subglottal air pressure) resulted only in proportional increases or decreases in nasal emission as measured by increases in the volume velocity of nasal air flow and intraoral air pressure. When asked to produce contrastive phoneme pairs in single words (/mat/ versus /bat/ versus /pat/) and to "make them as different as possible," the speaker was unable to successfully distinguish nasals from plosives or voiced from voiceless plosives.

Despite the apparent ineffectiveness of behavioral techniques, aerodynamic closure of the velopharyngal port by occluding the nares had beneficial effects. The precision with which the speaker produced pressure consonants was judged to be improved with the nares occluded. With the nares occluded, the speaker was able to generate 5 cm water pressure during the stop phase of voiceless plosives. In summary, this speaker with consistent velopharyngeal incompetency in the presence of adequate respiratory support for speech appeared not to be able to modify the problem behaviorally. However, performance was improved by occluding the velopharyngeal port. The outcome of the assessment was a recommendation that the patient be fitted with a palatal lift.

Result of a perceptual analysis of the speech of the second individual also indicated a velopharyngeal dysfunction. However, unlike the first speaker who was consistently incompetent no matter what he was instructed to do, the second speaker's performance varied considerably, depending on the task. For example, he was able to achieve closure more consistently when speaking at a slowed rather than at his habitual speaking rate. Listeners were able to distinguish nasal from nonnasal productions when the speaker was producing single words, although these distinctions were not present during extended samples of connected speech. In summary, this patient appeared to be able to behaviorally modify the adequacy of velopharyngeal function along with other articulatory behaviors. Therefore, the outcome of this assessment was the recommendation for a period of therapy, focusing on slowing speech rate in an effort to increase velopharyngeal function and articulatory precision.

TREATMENT PLANNING

Assessment has been described as the process of gathering pertinent data about the impairment (the underlying neuromotor problem), the disability (the decreased functional ability resulting from the impairment), and the handicap (the inability of the individual to perform expected roles). Decisions about the clinical course of action are made on the basis of that information. Thus, treatment planning in many respects can be viewed as the outcome of the assessment process. Decisions about the management of dysarthric speakers are made at a number of levels. The first level involves the most general decisions about goals of treatment. These decisions are based primarily on two types of information—the severity of the disability and the handicap experienced. The second level of decisions, discussed later in this chapter, involves the selection of specific treatment approaches. These approaches are selected so that the general goals of intervention can be reached. Selection of intervention techniques is heavily dependent upon an understanding of the pattern of impairment. The following section will describe a framework for making decisions about the general goals of treatment and about specific intervention approaches to achieve those goals.

Goals of Treatment

Because of the chronic nature of the underlying neuromotor impairment, "normal" speech is rarely a realistic goal for dysarthric individuals. Therefore, the clinican must find another framework for setting realistic treatment goals. In the following sections, we discuss intervention goal setting for severely, mildly, and moderately involved dysarthric speakers.

Severely Involved Speakers

The general goals of treatment for a dysarthric speaker vary with the severity of the disability. For severely involved speakers whose intelligibility is so reduced that they are unable to communicate verbally in ordinary situations the general goals of treatment involve establishing a functional means of communication, using augmentative communication approaches. The selection of an appropriate communication augmentation approach will be discussed in Chapter 8. For the speaker with a degenerative disorder, an augmentative communication approach must be selected with an increasing level of impairment in mind. For the recovering or stable dysarthric speaker, a second goal is to establish the motor control prerequisites for future speech development so that a transition to independent use of speech can be made.

Moderately Involved Speakers

For those moderately involved speakers who are able to use speech as their sole means of communication, but who are not completely intelligible, the general goal of treatment is maximizing intelligibility. The term *compensated intelligibility* (Rosenbek & LaPointe, 1985) aptly describes the goal of this phase of intervention. Achieving compensated intelligibility may take a variety of forms, depending on the speaker and the nature of the underlying impairment. For example, it may include an effort to control speaking rate for some individuals with coordination problems or may involve prosthetically managing an impaired component of the speech mechanism as it does with palatal lift fitting for individuals with little or no velopharyngeal movement.

Mildly Involved Speakers

For the mildly involved dysarthric speaker, general treatment goals are based both on the severity of the disability and the handicap resulting from it. Speech of mildly dysarthric individuals is characterized as intelligible but less efficient and natural than normal. For some speakers, this mild reduction in speech efficiency poses no problem. Such speakers are able to function adequately in all necessary communication situations. However, for those individuals who are handicapped by their disability, intervention may be warranted. The general treatment goals for dysarthric individuals with mild disabilities include maximizing communication efficiency and speech naturalness while maintaining intelligibility.

Approaches to Treatment

Once the general goals of treatment have been established, the selection of specific treatment approaches is based on the severity of the disability and the pattern of vocal tract involvement. Approaches to intervention with dysarthric individuals can be grouped into a few options. Development of a treatment plan involves the selection of options appropriate for the particular dysarthric individual.

Supplementing Speech with Augmentative Communication Approaches

The anarthric or severely dysarthric individual may experience such an extensive disability that natural speech alone does not serve as a functional means of communication. Augmentative communication strategies are required to meet some or all communication needs. During the past 10 years, the number of alternative communication options has increased. These options range from the "light" technology of alphabet/word boards to sophisticated computer-based systems with multiple output options. A detailed discussion of these systems of communication is beyond the scope of this book, however, this material is presented in detail elsewhere (Beukelman, Yorkston, & Dowden, 1985; Blackstone, 1986).

For some dysarthric speakers, natural speech can meet some, but not all, communication needs. In such cases, speech is supplemented with one or more augmentative communication approaches. For example, some severely dysarthric individuals use speech for greetings. In this type of communication, the timing of message delivery may be more critical than message intelligibility. These individuals may also speak with those partners who are very familiar with their speech and lifestyle. However, with partners who have difficulty understanding them, they may point to the first letter of each word as the word is spoken. They may use systems such as portable typewriters to communicate with strangers and to resolve communication breakdowns with everyone. For a more detailed discussion of intervention with severely involved dysarthric individuals, see Chapter 8.

Reducing the Impairment

At times, dysarthria treatment involves a direct attempt to reduce the degree of impairment or to increase the physiological support for speech in selected components. These activities may involve normalizing muscle tone and/or increasing strength and movement precision. A thorough understanding of normal and disordered aspects of speech production is needed when taking this approach to treatment. Not only must the impairment be carefully described; impairments noted in various components must also be placed in a hierarchy so that initial treatment can focus on the most fundamental of the impairments. For a discussion of such hierarchies see Netsell (1984) and Rosenbek and LaPointe (1985). Generally, these techniques have as their goal the normalization of function. Their rationale is that reducing the impairment will produce a corresponding improvement in functional ability or a decrease in disability. Netsell and Daniel (1979) present an excellent case report of the use of this approach. Numerous examples of treatment tasks whose goals are reduction of impairment will be found in later chapters.

Behavioral Compensation

Compensatory approaches to treatment, unlike those aimed at a reduction of impairment, do not have normalization of function as their primary goal. Rather, many of the behavioral compensatory techniques encourage the dysarthric individual to move away from the normal range of functioning in selected parameters in order to minimize the overall disability. Rate control is an example of such a compensatory technique. Despite the fact that the majority of dysarthric individuals speak at rates slower than normal, clinicians frequently attempt to slow rate still further in an effort to increase intelligibility. Rate control techniques will be reviewed in Chapter 13. Examples of other behavioral compensations are found in certain aspects of respiratory training. Some speakers with reduced respiratory support are trained to shorten breath groups beyond their already relatively short habitual length. Behavioral compensation is also seen in prosody training. Normal speakers signal stress by subtle adjustments of the parameters of fundamental frequency, intensity, and duration adjustments. Dysarthric speakers may be trained to select only certain parameters to signal stress patterning. They may be asked to limit use of fundamental frequency and intensity and to use only increased segment duration to signal stress. Thus, many of the treatment techniques that will be described in later chapters fall into the category of behavioral compensation. These techniques, rather than seeking normalcy in speech production, involve strategies to offset selected aspects of the impairment.

Prosthetic Compensation

Prosthetic compensation is frequently employed to supplement or replace component function. In contrast to behavioral compensation where the speaker is trained to produce speech in a modified manner, prosthetic compensation employs a mechanical or electronic device to offset certain aspects of the impairment. Palatal lifts have been used extensively to compensate for velopharyngeal incompetence in dysarthric speakers. Another prosthetic compensation is the use of a delayed auditory feedback device to control the excessively rapid speaking rate of certain parkinsonian dysarthric speakers. A third example of prosthetic compensation is the use of respiratory paddles or abdominal binders. An amplification system to compensate for reduced loudness levels is yet another example of a prosthetic compensatory device. One advantage of prosthetic over behavioral compensation is the immediacy of the effect. With prosthetic compensatory techniques, little training is usually required, therefore, these techniques are particularly useful for individuals with degenerative disorders.

Elimination of Maladaptive Behaviors

Earlier, dysarthria was defined as a motor speech impairment resulting from abnormalities in movement rates, strength, precision, and coordination. In the clinical setting, it is useful to attempt to separate the problem into at least two aspects. The first reflects the direct result of the underlying impairment. The second reflects an attempt to compensate for that impairment. As mentioned earlier, compensatory adjustments can be beneficial. For example, consider the case of an adult with a sudden onset of ataxia. A wide-based gait may be seen to compensate for reduced balance, just as a reduced speaking rate may be a compensatory response to discoordination of the speech mechanism. However, compensatory efforts are not always beneficial. Consider the dysarthric speaker who overdrives a poorly controlled respiratory system in an effort to compensate for reduced velopharyngeal function or increased laryngeal tone. The effort to compensate for the defective component may have the effect of increasing vocal harshness and reducing breath group length. Thus, the compensatory effort does nothing to increase the overall adequacy of speech.

Maladaptive compensatory behaviors may be a response to current physiological problems. However, they may also be over-learned behaviors that once were adaptive but are no longer needed. We have seen a number of indviduals with brain injury who exhibit respiratory compensatory patterns that are maladaptive. For example, some began to speak following their injury by producing a single word or syllable per breath. Years later, we find ourselves attempting to train them to use an extended breath group for which they now have the physiologic capability. Another example of maladaptive compensation can be found in an individual who pauses for breath to meet his physiologic respiratory requirements without regard to the linguistic aspects of the utterance.

Interaction Enhancement Strategies

Communication effectiveness involves both the speaker and the listener. Traditionally, dysarthria treatment has focused primarily on the speaker with the listener being ignored or receiving a few minutes of counseling.

Increasingly, we are involving the frequent listeners in interaction training activities with our dysarthric clients. Appropriate interaction strategies cannot be assumed, and both the speaker and the listener often need guidance in developing these strategies. A more detailed discussion of interaction training can be found in Chapter 8.

Communication Skill Maintenance

As in many areas of motor activity, skill maintenance is often required if an individual is to perform maximally. The goal of this phase of treatment must be carefully explained to the speaker and his important listeners. Previous treatment may have been oriented toward improving performance. When speakers fail to see continued improvement, they will mistakenly believe that the "practice" is not working or is unimportant. We usually limit maintenance training activities to a brief time period (10 minutes) once or twice a day. Often activities include a short passage to be read aloud with notations regarding the practice objectives, such as phrase, respiratory, or articulatory patterns.

Reducing the Handicap

In Chapter 1, *handicap* was defined as a disadvantage that limits the fulfillment of a role that is normal or desired for that individual. Perhaps the most frequently employed means of reducing the handicap is to reduce the impairment or the disability. However, the handicap may also be reduced by changing the attitudes of those in the environment. At times, dysarthric speakers are able to participate more fully in social, educational, or vocational activities when their listeners are well informed about the nature of the disorder and appropriate interaction techniques.

Evaluating the Treatment Plan

Treatment planning is a process in which general goals are established and specific methods selected to achieve those goals. Treatment plans for dysarthric speakers are individualized based on communication needs, level of disability, and nature of the underlying motor impairment. Because of this individualization, treatment plans vary considerably. However, a number of general principles are used to evaluate the adequacy of our treatment plans.

Attention to Present Communication Needs

The principle of attention to present communication needs suggests that one of the primary concerns of treatment should be to maximize the speaker's current ability to communicate. At least a portion of each training session should be devoted to developing those skills. For the severely involved dysarthric speaker, this may involve training in the use of an augmentative communication approach. With the recovering speaker, this approach may initially serve temporarily as a replacement to speech when motor control problems are so severe that no functional speech is possible. Later, as recovery occurs, the augmentative system may be used to supplement speech when the speaker cannot be understood. For the moderately involved speaker, attention to present communication needs may take the form of attempts to maximize speech intelligibility through prosthetic compensation. Another general approach designed to maximize present communication is interaction training. This general category of tasks includes training both dysarthric speakers and their listeners in such skills as topic identification and repair of communication breakdowns.

Preparation for the Future

The principle of preparation for the future suggests that in addition to maximizing current communication skills, treatment plans should include steps appropriate for the predicted changes that may occur in the impairment, disability, or handicap. Preparation for the future can take a number of forms. First, it may involve establishing a hierarchy of treatment. When multiple speech components are involved, it may not be prudent to intervene at all levels at one time. Rather, the clinician must decide where to begin. If, for example, the clinician believes that poor respiratory control is limiting all other aspects of speech, then work in this area would have high priority. Second, preparation for the future may involve selecting specific treatment approaches based on the predicted natural course of the disorder. For example, we rarely utilize techniques that fall under the heading of "Reducing the Impairment" when developing a plan for an individual with a degenerative disorder. Instead, many of the techniques we select will involve prosthetic compensation. These techniques usually have immediate impact and require little training for the user. Third, planning for the future may involve an effort to prevent future problems. There are a number of patterns that are appropriate to compensate for severe motor control or coordination problems that may be counterproductive if continued as impairment severity decreases. For example, severely dysarthric individuals are often taught to produce one word at a time or to use an alphabet board to indicate the first letter of each word as it is produced. Although this compensatory pattern may be needed early in recovery, if the pattern persists as neuromotor recovery occurs, it becomes maladaptive, interfering with natural prosodic patterns. Of course, it would be ideal to simply avoid training patterns that may in the future be maladaptive. In clinical practice, this is not always possible. Therefore, the experienced clinician, aware of potential maladaptive patterns, can train the speaker to move away from them as soon as they are no longer appropriate.

Minimal Intervention

The priniciple of minimal intervention suggests that treatment should attempt to change the motor activity only so far as is needed to achieve treatment goals. This principle, when applied to training the complex motor act of speaking, suggests that the clinician does not always need to "start from the ground up" in all cases. Consider, for example, the mildly involved dysarthric speaker who is intelligible but is not normal in terms of the naturalness of speech. In this case, naturalness may be enhanced by training the speaker to make slight modifications in his breath patterning or to make slight durational adjustments. The clinician does not typically begin with the basics, that is, the clinician does not typically attempt to increase the speaker's capabilities in all components of speech. For example, respiratory/phonatory control is not extended by training the speaker to extend phonation time, and articulatory precision is not increased by asking the speaker to produce more rapid diadokokinetic movements.

The principle of minimal intervention has implications for rate control as well. Generally, the more rigid the rate control technique, the more it disrupts speech naturalness. Minimal intervention implies that if rigid techniques are not needed, they should not be employed. Rather, the clinician should employ the least restrictive rate control techniques that produce the desired result.

Attention to Principles of Motor Learning

The distinction between *cognitive learning* and *motor learning* has important implications for training dysarthric speakers. This distinction can be illustrated with examples from the sport of tennis. Learning the basic rules and strategies of tennis is an example of cognitive learning and can occur, at least on a basic level, in a brief period of time. The learner, having been told only once or twice, will have learned enough to play the game—at least from a cognitive view point. Learning to produce a good backhand stroke involves an entirely different type of learning. Learning complex motor activities may require thousands of repetitions before a player is first able to adequately perform them, then be able to "hit the groove" and repeat the adequate performance time after time at will. Modifying speech is an example of an extremely complex motor learning task. The nature of motor learning dictates a number of approaches to training. Adequate performance of a specific task one time or 10 times or even 100 times may not be enough to establish a consistently successful pattern. Therefore, massed practice often is required. This is not always easily accomplished within the time limitations of treatment sessions. When possible, it is highly desirable to structure ordinary communication situations so that they too offer the possibility of practice. For example, a severely dysarthric individual who is not sufficiently understandable to communicate independently via speech may be afforded valuable practice by supplementing speaking efforts with an alphabet board. Thus, in using a system in which the speaker indicates the first letter of each word as it is spoken, many individuals are able to speak functionally earlier in the course of their recovery than would have been possible if a supplementary system had not been used. Still another example of the need for massed practice of motor learning tasks is in the area of rate control. An individual with ataxic dysarthria may learn cognitively in a very brief period of time that a slow rate is best. The motor learning required to speak consistently at an appropriate rate may require an extensive period of training.

Motor learning is also heavily dependent upon knowledge of results. In other words, motor activities are learned more efficiently if the learner receives immediate and precise feedback about how well the activity was performed (see Weismer & Cariski [1984] for an excellent review). Information regarding the adequacy of a speech motor activity can be provided to the client in a number of ways. The speaker can be taught to listen and judge the adequacy of his or her own speech. The clinician can provide qualitative information, generally rating the adequacy of the production. Knowledge of results for speech can also take the form of feedback about whether or not the utterance has been understood by the listener. See Chapter 8 for a discussion of intelligibility drills that are based on this type of feedback.

REFERENCES

Berry, W.R., & Sanders, S.B. (1983). Environmental education: The universal management approach for adults with dysarthria. In W.R. Berry (Ed.), *Clinical dysarthria*. Austin, TX: PRO-ED.

Beukelman, D.R., & Yorkston, K.M. (1979). The relationship between information transfer and speech intelligibility of dysarthric speakers. *Journal of Communication Disorders, 12,* 189–196.

Beukelman, D.R., & Yorkston, K.M. (1980). The influence of passage familiarity on intelligibility estimates of dysarthric speech. *Journal of Communication Disorders, 13,* 33–41.

Beukelman, D.R., Yorkston, K.M., & Dowden, P. (1985). *Augmentative communication: A casebook of clinical management.* San Diego: College-Hill Press.

Blackstone, S. (Ed.). (1986). *Augmentative communication: An introduction.* Rockville, MD: American Speech Language & Hearing Association.

Darley, F.L., Aronson, A.E., & Brown, J.R. (1969a). Differential diagnostic patterns of dysarthria. *Journal of Speech & Hearing Research, 12,* 246–269.

Darley, F.L, Aronson, A.E., & Brown, J.R. (1969b). Clusters of deviant speech dimensions in the dysarthrias. *Journal of Speech & Hearing Research, 12,* 462–496.

Fletcher, S.G. (1985). Speech production and oral motor skill in an adult with an unrepaired palatal cleft. *Journal of Speech & Hearing Disorders, 50,* 254–261.

Frearson, B. (1983, November). *A comparison of Assessment of Intelligibility of Dysarthric Speech sentence list and spontaneous speech intelligibility scores.* A research paper submitted in partial fulfillment of the requirements for B.App.Sci (Speech and Hearing Science), Western Australian Institute of Technology.

Hanson, W.R., & Metter, E.J. (1980). DAF as instructional treatment for dysarthria in progressive supranuclear palsy: A case report. *Journal of Speech & Hearing Disorders, 45,* 268–276.

Hardy, J. (1967). Some suggestions for physiological research in dysarthria. *Cortex, 3,* 128–156.

Hixon, T.J., & Hardy, J. (1964). Restricted mobility of the speech articulation in cerebral palsy. *Journal of Speech & Hearing Disorders, 29,* 293–306.

McNeil, M.R., & Kennedy, J.G., (1984). Measuring the effects of treatment for dysarthria; Knowing when to change or terminate. In J.C. Rosenbek (Ed.), *Seminars in Speech and Language.* New York: Thieme-Stratton, *5*(4), 337–358.

Netsell, R. (1973). Speech physiology. In F.D. Minifie, T.J. Hixon, & F. Williams (Eds.), *Normal aspects of speech, hearing and language.* Englewood Cliffs, NJ: Prentice-Hall.

Netsell, R. (1984). Physiological studies of dysarthria and their relevance to treatment. J.C. Rosenbek (Ed.), *Seminars in language.* New York: Thieme-Stratton, *5*(4), 279–292.

Netsell, R. (1986). *A neurobiologic view of speech production and the dysarthrias.* San Diego: College-Hill Press.

Netsell, R., & Daniel, B. (1979). Dysarthria in adults: Physiologic approach to rehabilitation. *Archives of Physical Medicine & Rehabilitation, 60,* 502.

Netsell, R., Lotz, W., & Shaughnessy, A.L. (1984). Laryngeal aerodynamics associated with selected vocal disorders. *American Journal of Otolaryngology, 5,* 397–403.

Platt, L.J., Andrews, G., Young, M., & Neilson, P.D. (1978). The measurement of speech impairment of adults with cerebral palsy. *Folia Phoniatrica, 30,* 50–58.

Rosenbek, J.C., & LaPointe, L.L. (1985). The dysarthria: Description, diagnosis and treatment. In D.F. Johns (Ed.), *Clinical management of neurogenic communication disorders.* Boston: Little, Brown.

Tikofsky, R.S. (1970). A revised list for the estimation of dysarthric single word intelligibility. *Journal of Speech & Hearing Research, 13,* 59–64.

Tikofsky, R.S., & Tikofsky, R.P. (1964). Intelligibility measures of dysarthric speech. *Journal of Speech & Hearing Research, 7,* 325–333.

Weismer, G., & Cariski, D. (1984). On speakers ability to control speech mechanism output. Theoretical and clinical implications. In N.J. Lass (Ed.), *Speech and language: Advances in basic research and practice* (Vol. 10). New York: Academic Press.

Yorkston, K.M., & Beukelman, D.R., (1978). A comparison of techniques for measuring intelligibility of dysarthric speech. *Journal of Communication Disorders, 11,* 499–512.

Yorkston, K.M., & Beukelman, D.R. (1980). A clinician-judged technique for quantifying dysarthric speech based on single word intelligibility. *Journal of Communication Disorders, 13,* 15–31.

Yorkston, K.M., & Beukelman, D.R. (1981a). Communication efficiency of dysarthric speakers as measured by sentence intelligibility and speaking rate. *Journal of Speech & Hearing Disorders, 46*(3), 296–300.

Yorkston, K.M., & Beukelman, D.R. (1981b). Assessment of intelligibility of dysarthric speech. Tigard, OR: C.C. Publications.

Yorkston, K.M., & Beukelman, D.R. (1983). The influence of judge familiarization with the speaker on dysarthric speech intelligibility. In W. Berry (Ed.), *Clinical dysarthria*. Austin, TX: PRO-ED.

Yorkston, K.M., Beukelman, D.R., & Traynor, C.D. (1984). *Computerized assessment of intelligibility of dysarthric speech.* Austin, TX: PRO-ED.

CHAPTER 8

Transition to Speech With Severely Dysarthric Individuals

Clinical Issues: Our consultation request from the outpatient physician read as follows: "Please see this 21 year old (1 year post onset closed head injury) who is not speaking at all. Does he need an augmentative communication system or speech treatment?" After evaluating this patient, we began to appreciate the complexity of this young man's communication problems. The evaluation revealed severely reduced respiratory support, phonation initiated only occasionally when the speaker was supine, no velopharyngeal closure during speech but movement during sustained vowel production, and the ability to mouth some words with observable modification of tongue position and labial movements. He consistently responded to and initiated interactions by mouthing words. These attempts were almost never understandable. When his listeners indicated that they did not understand, the young man would persist in repeating the same utterance until he was told to use his alphabet board. Then he would accurately spell out the message letter-by-letter. The following questions appear to be pressing clinical concerns:

- *What factors related to the selection of communication approaches must be considered in responding to the physician's question?*
- *Should the speech/language pathologist focus on speech training when the probability is small that this individual will regain completely understandable speech?*
- *How long does work continue to reestablish speech?*
- *When all speech components are involved, where should initial treatment efforts be focused?*

- *How important are the communication problems not related to dysarthria, and how should they be handled?*

Planning an intervention program for individuals such as the young man described previously, provides an excellent example of the challenge of developing programs that consider both current communication needs and future development. The individuals discussed in this chapter differ from each other in a number of ways—etiology, age of onset, and pattern of underlying neuromotor deficits. However, they are all severely communicatively disordered and none are independent communicators in all situations using natural speech. The majority of these individuals fall into one of two general groups. The first group consists of traumatically brain-injured individuals. As outlined in Chapter 5, this population is young, often exhibiting severe motor limitations in the form of mixed dysarthria. At times, management begins early in the course of recovery of these individuals, when changes are rapidly occurring. In these cases, a traditional program of daily speech treatment may be appropriate. However, at other times, management begins years after onset. Intervention may then involve home practice programs developed and monitored by the clinician through periodic reevaluations of communication status. At times, important changes in speech motor control come years after onset and necessitate long-term follow-up. The second group of individuals described in this chapter are those with brain stem cerebrovascular accidents (CVAs) (Beukelman & Yorkston, 1978). Although their preserved cognitive ability may allow them to make more adjustments to their impairment than is typical for the traumatically brain-injured, at times they may benefit from the same series of treatment techniques.

ESTABLISHING COMMUNICATION

Selection of Augmentative Approaches

Because the first goal of treatment with the severely dysarthric recovering speaker is to reestablish communication, development of augmentative approaches may take precedence over direct speech treatment in early intervention. During this early phase, the clinician may select an appropriate augmentative communication approach after the communication needs and capabilities of the individual have been determined. The assessment process involves evaluation of cognitive, language, and motor control abilities. A detailed discussion of the selection of augmentative communication systems is not permitted here. Sources for this information exist elsewhere (Beukelman, Yorkston, & Dowden, 1985; Yorkston & Dowden, 1984; Yorkston & Karlan, 1986). A word regarding terminology is warranted. In the augmentative communication field, the term *system* encompasses the multiple communication techniques used by the nonspeaking individual. Vanderheiden and Lloyd (1986) have defined the term as follows:

> The communication system for a disabled individual, therefore, should not be a single technique, or aid, but rather a collection of techniques, aids, and strategies (some aided, some not) that the individual uses interchangeably. (p. 52)

Thus, the augmentative communication system used by severely dysarthric individuals may contain a number of components, including devices or aids and, to whatever extent possible, natural speech.

The augmentative communication approaches that we select for different individuals with severe, sudden-onset dysarthria may vary widely in technical sophistication. For some individuals with severe cognitive limitations accompanying their motor control deficits, the system may be as simple as a "yes/no" signal technique. For other cognitively intact individuals, who are experiencing a course of steady and relatively rapid recovery, the approach may be a simple alphabet board upon which they can indicate their messages in a letter-by-letter fashion. This augmentative approach is viewed as transitional, used until the motor control to support functional speech has been reestablished. For still other individuals whose course of recovery is slow, approaches may be more technologically sophisticated with display, print, or speech synthesis options. These systems are selected in order to serve the user's communication needs for extended periods of time or indefintely, should return of speech not occur.

Speech in Conjunction With Augmentative Approaches

After the augmentative communication system is in place, other aspects of management can be addressed. It is a mistake to consider management complete when an appropriate communication aid has been selected for a severely dysarthric individual. An aggressive attempt to reestablish speech is warranted for a number of reasons. First, intelligible speech is obviously far superior in terms of rate, efficiency, and flexibility to any augmentative approach. Further, natural speech need not be completely intelligible in order to facilitate communication in a number of important ways. We were made especially aware of the utility of marginally intelligible speech when we studied the interaction strategies used by a severely dysarthric young man named Marvin. His skill in using severely distorted speech allowed him to function much more rapidly and effectively than would have been the case if he had been restricted to the use of his augmentative communication device. At the time of the study, Marvin was a 26 year old individual with athetoid cerebral palsy who had used a sophisticated, electronic communication augmentation system (Wilson, 1981) for approximately two years. Marvin activated the system by tapping out Morse code on switches mounted on either side of his head. The system translated the Morse code into orthographic English. Messages were spoken, printed, or perhaps most importantly for interaction, displayed on a marquee for his listener to read. Marvin accurately spelled messages in a letter-by-letter fashion. However, as with so many of the spelling-based communication augmentation systems, his rate was extremely slow—approximately five to eight words per minute. Marvin's natural speech was extremely limited, with intelligibility less than 10 percent when measured with a standard single-word production task (Yorkston & Beukelman, 1981).

Marvin had volunteered to participate in a research project focusing on the interaction skills of individuals who were proficient users of augmentative communication systems. As part of the project, samples of interaction between the individual using an augmentative communication system and a normal listener were video-taped. Of particular interest were the patterns of interaction between the two participants—who was producing the larger proportion of words, who was initiating, who was simply responding to the partner's initiations, and who was exhibiting the most conversational control. Marvin's first meeting with the experimenter was at the time of the video-taping. During this meeting, Marvin used his augmentative communication device almost exclusively, except for greetings. After the purpose of the research was explained and the interaction tasks described, he asked, "May I speak?" He was told that he should communicate as he normally would. It was assumed that he would depend almost exclusively on his device because his speech was so difficult to understand and he used his device so accurately and effectively.

Marvin and his communication partner were asked to participate in a direction-giving task. Marvin was to provide instructions to his partner about how to reproduce a colored, geometic design similiar to one that appears in Figure 8-1. The partner, who was unable to see the geometric pattern, was free to ask questions about the task but not to look at the stimulus card. A detailed description of this and other tasks used to obtain samples of interaction in the clinical setting can be found Farrier, Yorkston, Marriner, and Beukelman (1985).

Marvin began this task by spelling out complete words using Morse code. Soon he began to spell out only a portion of the words and, at times, to say the words. One of the advantages of the Morse code system was that Marvin did not need to view a display because the system is based on a previously learned code. In effect, he was free to watch his partner during communication. Marvin proved to be a master at knowing when his partner was understanding and following the content of his message and when the partner

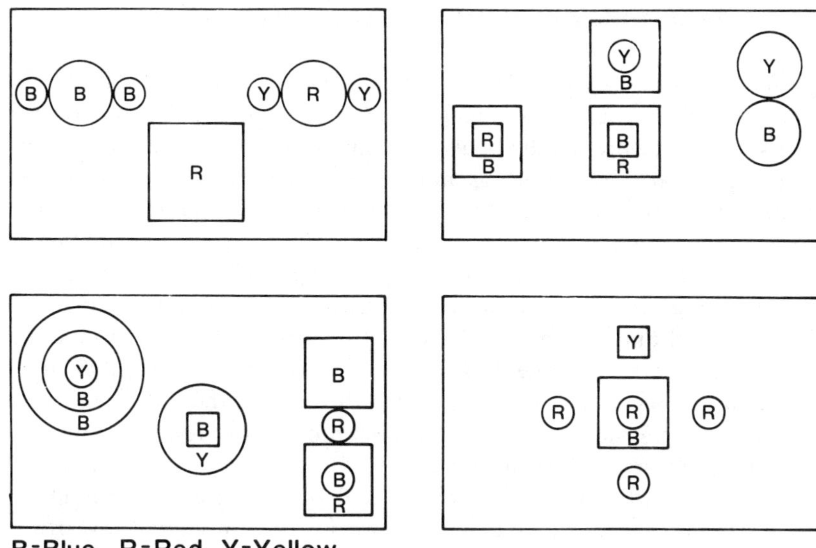

Figure 8-1. Examples of geometric shapes used in the direction giving task.

was not. Marvin would say or spell a portion of a word and then would pause, waiting for his partner's response. Often the partner would guess or confirm what she believed the message to be. Marvin would always signal if the partner's guess had been correct. As the interaction progressed, the communication style changed. Marvin began using the augmentative communication device less and began speaking more. Because this task included such a limited vocabulary, Marvin appeared to be training his partner to recognize severely distorted words from within that closed set. If the partner had been attempting to understand the words without the context of the task, almost none of the words would have been understood. After five minutes of interaction, Marvin was using natural speech almost exclusively and, what may be even more remarkable, his partner was understanding him.

We will return to Marvin's case later. At that time, we will describe more specifically how Marvin managed the communication interaction. We will also compare and contrast Marvin's performance with an individual with dysarthria of similiar severity but who did not have Marvin's subtle communication skills. The point to be made here is that even severely limited speech can serve an important function. This means that work on speech should not be abandoned once an augmentative communication device is in place, nor should work on speech be abandoned in cases in which the probability of the development of completely understandable speech is poor.

ESTABLISHING PHYSIOLOGIC SUPPORT FOR SPEECH

When working with severely dysarthric speakers, clinicians at times find themselves following principles different from those which may be appropriate for less severely involved individuals. Usually, with the less severely involved, we attempt to work on speech as an integrated activity. Research related to factors facilitating learning of complex motor activities lends support to this approach. Although an attempt is made to understand the contribution of speech components to overall performance, training would typically not involve drills focusing on the isolated components of respiration, phonation, velopharyngeal function, and oral articulation. For example, we would not train individuals to generate 5 cm of water pressure for 5, then 10 or 15 seconds, until they achieved "normal" performance and then assume that the speaker would transfer these skills to speech production. Rather, training to improve respiratory performance might involve such activities as increasing the number of words per breath group or maintaining adequate loudness throughout an entire utterance. When working with severely dysarthric speakers, it may be inappropriate to focus on speech as an integrated activity. These individuals may not be able to perform an activity as complex as speech unless it is separated into less-demanding units. The development of intervention strategies to establish physiological support for speech are critically important when treating the improving or stable individual with severe dysarthria. We will discuss intervention strategies in detail in later chapters, therefore, we will review each speech component only briefly in the following section.

Respiration and Phonation

The selection of a starting point for intervention with severely dysarthric speakers may be problematic because it is not unusual to find severe impairment in all of the components of speech. In situations where all speech components are severely impaired, task selection decisions may be based on the principle of "peripheral dependencies" (Netsell & Rosenbek, 1985). One corollary of this principle suggests that intervention should begin with the component whose change will have the most general effects on the others. In our clinic, the starting point is often the respiratory/phonatory component. We have found that inability to produce consistent, voluntary phonation is the barrier that prevents many severely dysarthric individuals from regaining some measure of functional speech. Without some minimal level of respiratory/phonatory control, speech cannot be functional, regardless of the relative adequacy of the "upstream" speech components. See Chapter 9 and Chapter 10 for a detailed discussion of training of the respiratory/phonatory system. Such topics as training of the coordination of speaking and breathing, increasing respiratory support for speech, and early strategies to initiate phonation will be presented there.

Velopharyngeal Management

Once a minimum level of respiratory support and phonatory function has been achieved, then the velopharyngeal component may be the next focus of intervention. The velopharyngeal mechanism may be managed prosthetically with a palatal lift. See Chapter 11 for a complete discussion of candidacy and fitting sequence for palatal lifts. Although palatal lifts may not result in an immediate improvement in speech for the severely involved individual, early fitting is desirable for a number of reasons. First, prosthetically managing an impaired speech component makes the speaking task an easier one. Early management of the velopharyngeal port also prevents the development of bad habits or maladaptive behaviors. Often, in an attempt to build up sufficient intraoral air pressure in the presence of an inability to close off the oral from the nasal airway, a dysarthric speaker will "overdrive" the respiratory mechanism by generation of maximal levels of subglottal air pressure in a compensatory effort. This tendency to overdrive the respiratory mechanism has certain negative consequences. For example, it may result in harsh voice quality and unnecessarily short breath groups. If the velopharyngeal port is managed early in the course of recovery, then the severely dysarthric speaker may make better use of marginal respiratory support (Netsell & Daniel, 1979).

Oral articulatory precision may also be improved by velopharyngeal management. When a speaker with an incompetent velopharyngeal mechanism makes an adequate oral articulatory gesture in the production of the bilabial /p/, the end-product will be acoustically unacceptable. The sound may be perceived as the nasal /m/ or as a nasal emission. On the other hand, with an adequately fitted palatal lift, the same oral articulatory gesture will result in an acoustically and perceptually acceptable sound. Thus, in many cases, appropriate velopharyngeal management will mean that training in other aspects of articulation can proceed with greater speed and probability of success.

Oral Articulation

Early training of oral articulation is reviewed in detail in Chapter 12. The articulation drills described in that chapter may be effective as the first speaking activities in treatment. Once a dysarthric individual is able to produce a voice consistently, lists of words the speaker can produce are developed. Words are included on this list if the clinician can distinguish among the words in that closed set. Words are selected so that their production is within the physiologic capability of the individual. When possible, an attempt is made to select words that meet the communication needs of the individual. With one severely involved flaccid dysarthric individual, the initial word list contained only three words, "my," "Hi," and "I'm." A "deck" of 20 cards was created, each containing one of these three words. The deck was shuffled and presented to the dysarthric individual, whose task it was to produce the syllable with sufficient precision to allow the clinician to "understand" the word. In this simple example, the presence or absence of bilabial movement was sufficient for that understanding. Later, as improvement continued, a greater range of vowel and consonant combinations were added in order to increase the demands of the task. After one month of daily, 30 minute sessions, the list had grown to 20 words (See Table 8-1.) Two new words were added each session in which the clinician successfully understood 80 percent or more of the words in the current deck. Words were selected not only on the basis of ease of production but also on utility of the word for the speaker. A printed word list was mounted on the lapboard of his wheelchair. The speaker was encouraged to say words on this list in ordinary communication situations after he had indicated to his listener that the word he was attempting to produce was in the closed set. The availability of the closed set increased the probability of the listener's understanding.

ALPHABET BOARD SUPPLEMENTATION OF SPEECH

The training tasks just described involve the establishment of physiological support for speech. This phase of treatment may be thought of as an investment in the future, because the changes that are brought about in the speech component functions may not have an immediate impact on speech intelligibility or naturalness. In order to move from early speech drills to functional use of speech in natural communication situations, an alphabet board supplementation approach is often helpful. In this approach, speech is supplemented with an alphabet-number board similiar to the one presented in Figure 8-2. The dysarthric individual points to the first letter of each word as the word is spoken. The listener repeats each word after the dysarthric speaker. If the listener's guess is correct, the speaker continues by pointing to the first letter of the next word as that word is spoken. However, if the listener's guess is incorrect, the speaker indicates "no" and repeats the word

Table 8-1.
An Example of a Word List Developed for an Individual with Brain Stem CVA for Speech Intelligibility Drills.

bye	hi	mine	room
down	I'm	more	Roy
eat	in	nap	up
ham	Larry	no	more
hello	me	pillow	why

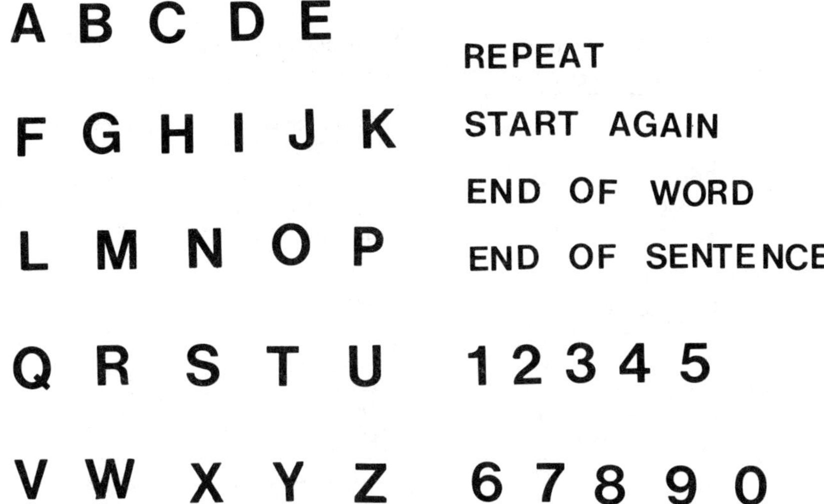

Figure 8-2. An alphabet-number board with selected "control" phrases.

in question. The dysarthric speaker spells out the entire word on the alphabet board if the listener does not understand the word after one repetition.

Case Presentations

The impact of the alphabet board supplementation approach on speech intelligibility and rate was documented for two severely dysarthric individuals (Beukelman & Yorkston, 1977). Speaker N was a 61 year old man with severe primarily flaccid dysarthria as the result of a brain stem CVA. Speaker H was a 17 year old high school student who had suffered a brain stem injury in a motor vehicle accident. Both of these individuals had sufficient language and spelling skills to support a letter-by-letter spelling approach. Table 8-2 contains measures of speaking rate and sentence intelligibility obtained in three listening conditions. In the Unaided Speech condition, the subjects spoke without the aid of the spelling board. In the Alphabet Supplementation condition, the subjects identified the initial letter of each word as they spoke. In the Spelling Board Concealed condition, the speech samples recorded for the Alphabet Supplementation condition were presented to the subjects; however, the portion of the video monitor showing the spelling board was concealed. Thus, in this condition the subjects were unable to benefit from knowledge of the initial letter of the word despite the fact that the speech sample itself was the same as in the Alphabet Supplementation condition.

Results differed for the two speakers. For both, the alphabet board supplementation approach had the effect of reducing their overall speaking rate.

TABLE 8-2.
Percentage of Intelligible Words in Sentences and Speaking Rates for Speakers N and H under Three Listening Conditions

	Speaker N	Speaker H
Unaided Speech		
Intelligibility	16%	32%
Speaking Rate	39 wpm	86 wpm
Alphabet Supplementation		
Intelligibility	65%	75%
Speaking Rate	18 wpm	28 wpm
Spelling Board Concealed		
Intelligibility	18%	53%
Speaking Rate	18 wpm	28 wpm

From Beukelman, D.R., & Yorkston, K.M. (1977). A communication system for the severely dysarthric speaker with an intact language system. *Journal of Speech & Hearing Disorders*, *42*, 265–270.

For Speaker N, rate was reduced from 39 to 18 words per minute (wpm). For Speaker H, rate was reduced from 86 to 28 wpm. However, rate reduction alone did not have an important impact on the intelligibility scores of Speaker N. Unaided speech was 16 percent intelligible whereas speech that was reduced in rate but not supplemented with initial letter identification (Spelling Board Concealed condition) was just 18 percent intelligible. Intelligibility appeared to improve because the listener benefited from the letter identification. When listeners were able to see the initial letters, intelligibility scores for Speaker N improved to 65 percent, a change of nearly 50 percent from habitual (Unaided Speech condition). For Speaker H, however, rate reduction alone appeared to improve intelligibility somewhat. Intelligibility scores improved from 32 to 53 percent in the Unaided Speech condition as compared to the Spelling Board Concealed condition. Intelligibility was further improved when the listeners were given information about the initial letter of the words. In the Alphabet Supplementation condition intelligibility scores were 75 percent.

In the experimental conditions described here, intelligibility was never greater than 75 percent even when the subjects were using the alphabet supplementation approach. This is probably an underestimation of their performance in natural communication situations. In natural settings listeners are aided by situational context and are not asked to understand a series of unrelated sentences. Further, in a conversational situation, dysarthric speakers are able to resolve communication breakdowns by either repeating or spelling the entire word. No such opportunity for breakdown resolution was possible during the experimental tasks.

Candidacy

Generally, candidates for the alphabet supplementation approach are severely dysarthric individuals who are using an alphabet-based augmentative communication approach. These individuals have some speech, but reduced intelligibility limits the usefulness of that speech in natural communication situations. The requirements for successful use of the alphabet supplementation approach can be divided into five areas.

Speech

Minimal speech production requirements are needed for successful use of the alphabet board supplementation approach. Individuals using this approach must be able to achieve consistent, voluntary phonation. Because the first letter of each word is identified for the listener, often treatment initially focuses on vowel differentiation and later on the inclusion of final consonants for individuals who are being trained to use the alphabet board supplementation approach.

Approach to Letter Identification

Most frequently, the dysarthric individuals using this approach point to letters on an alphabet board. In cases where the dysarthric individual is unable to indicate letters by direct selection, other options are available. Some speakers with minimal hand function indicate letter selection via a head-mounted light pointer (See Figure 8-3). Other individuals who use alphabet-based typing systems, such as the Canon Communicator or the Sharp Memowriter, may turn off the devices and use them as an alphabet board while speaking.

Spelling

Individuals using the alphabet supplementation approach must have spelling skills that are sufficient to correctly identify initial letters of words. Although no data are available that suggest minimal grade levels, our experience has shown that this is not a demanding spelling task. Musslewhite (personal communication, 1986) has modified the approach for children as young as five years of age. She teaches children to indicate initial sounds of words as they speak. Orthographic symbols representing initial sounds are accompanied by other symbols more meaningful for the child. For example, the sound /s/ is accompanied by a line drawing of a snake.

Language

Dysarthric individuals who use spelling-based devices or alphabet boards must make a number of changes in their communication style as they make the transition to the alphabet board supplementation approach. It is usually

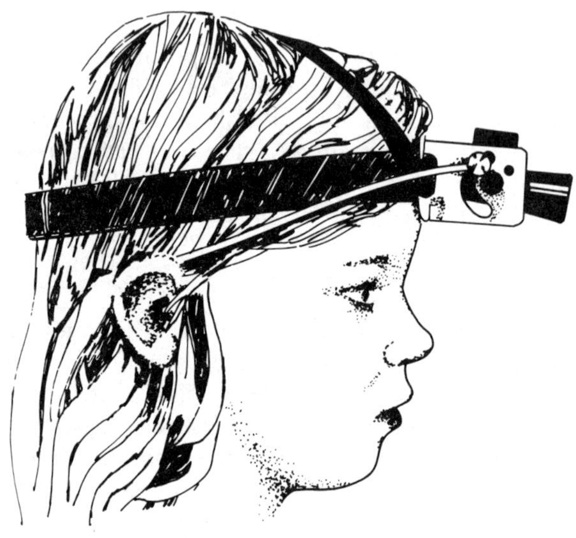

Figure 8-3. A head-mounted light pointer used for letter identification when hand function is poor.

appropriate for individuals who are completely dependent on letter-by-letter spelling approaches to be highly telegraphic in their utterances. Because communication rates are slow but messages are highly understandable, proficient users of such systems will increase efficiency by providing only content words and letters and allowing their partners to fill in the rest of the message. Individuals making the transition to the alphabet board supplementation approach need to learn to do just the opposite. They are more likely to be understood if they produce grammatically complete utterances in order to increase the redundancy of their message. Often, some instruction and practice is needed in order to develop the ability to change from one style to the other when appropriate.

Interaction Skills

Many dysarthric individuals prefer to use the alphabet board supplementation approach because it is much more rapid than a letter-by-letter spelling approach. However, the price that is paid for this increase in communication rate is often a reduction in intelligibility. For communication partners who are good readers, a spelling-based approach to communication may approach 100 percent intelligibility. Severely dysarthric speech, even when it is supplemented, is typically less than 80 percent intelligible. Therefore, users of this approach must be skilled at "managing" their listeners and resolving communication breakdowns. A review of Figure 8-3 indicates that four control phrases appear on the alphabet-number board. These include "end of sentence," "end of word," "start again," and "repeat." These phrases are used to facilitate the resolution of communication breakdowns. Instructions to new listeners, outlining the speaker's and listeners' roles in interaction, are mounted on the back of the board. One typical set of instructions appears in Figure 8-4. It has been our experience that some dysarthric individuals prefer to have their communication partners repeat each word after them. These speakers indicate that it is less fatiguing for them to resolve the breakdowns as they occur, rather than waiting for the end of the utterance only to find that the listener has misunderstood the first or second word. Word-by-word repetition is unnatural for many listeners and some less severely dysarthric speakers find it easier to complete the entire sentence before the listener repeats it. Some cognitively limited dysarthric individuals have difficulty switching from the communication styles used with the alphabet board to supplement speech to the communication style used with the alphabet board to spell out words in their entirety when resolving breakdowns. For such individuals, we have recommended the use of two different alphabet boards—one with black letters on a white background and the other with white letters on a black background. By training the speaker to use a different board for different communication tasks, confusion resulting from task shifting can be minimized.

Advantages of the Approach

If the dysarthric individual meets the general requirements just outlined, use of the alphabet board supplementation approach has a number of advantages. First, this approach is more rapid than letter-by-letter selection using an augmentative communication device. In the cases of the two brain-stem

To help you understand me, I will point to the first letter of each word as I speak. Please say each word after me. I'll let you know if you are right or wrong. If you don't understand a word, let me know and I will repeat it or spell it for you. Please don't finish the sentences for me unless I ask you to do so. Thank you for your patience.

Figure 8-4. Instructions Mounted on the Back of Alphabet-Number Boards for Communication Partners

injured speakers described earlier, Speaker N increased his communication rate from four wpm using the alphabet board to 18 wpm using the supplemented speech. Speaker H increased his communication rate from 6 to 28 wpm. The second advantage of this approach is obvious: it improves speech intelligibility as compared to unaided speech. This improvement may be brought about by a reduction in speaking rate, by the linguistic information provided by the initial letter of each word, or by a combination of both. The final advantage of the approach is perhaps the most important one for the severely dysarthric individual who is making the transition to speech. This approach allows for the continual practice of speech at a point earlier in recovery than would be otherwise possible. At times, the importance of practice is underestimated. New motor learning does not occur efficiently without extensive practice. Two daily, 30 minute practice sessions simply may not be enough to establish a new motor pattern or restore an old one. The speaker not only may benefit from the continual practice but also may benefit from the immediate feedback from listeners about the intelligibility of production.

TRAINING INTERACTION SKILLS

Treatment is often focused on the motor control impairment of dysarthric individuals and only casual attention is given to the communication handicap experienced by these individuals. This may be, at least in part, because we assume that an individual with intact language skills and extensive premorbid experience as a normal speaker will automatically adopt all of the appropriate interaction strategies needed to manage communication situations. However, years of normal communication which is rapid, precise, efficient, and intelligible may do little to prepare the individual for a sudden onset of severely dysarthric speech. In short, strategies for conversational interaction when speaking at 170 to 200 wpm with near-perfect intelligibility may no longer be successful when speech is 10 percent intelligible at a rate of 30 wpm. Thus, interaction skills of severely dysarthric individuals need to be evaluated. Some severely dysarthric indivduals are exceptionally skilled communicators, whereas others need to be taught even the most elementary breakdown resolution strategies. We have attempted to learn from the skilled in order to develop techniques for training the less skilled.

Clinical Measurement of Interaction Skills

Interviews

Clinicians can obtain information about a dysarthric speaker's interaction skills in a number of ways. The informal interview may be an easy means of obtaining basic information about dysarthric speakers' judgments of their own intelligibility. This process can also help to identify breakdown resolution strategies dysarthric speakers find beneficial. Berry and Sanders (1983) have added some structure to the interview process in the Situational Intelligibility Survey. At times, dysarthric speakers grossly over- or underestimate their intelligibility as compared to standard clinical measures. Clinically, it is important to understand the reasons for such discrepancies. Some severely dysarthric speakers appear to have developed strategies for taking full advantage of their residual speech, including reliance on semantic context, partner familiarity, and any number of factors that facilitate getting their message across in natural settings. For these individuals, differences between their own estimates of intelligibility in natural settings and standard intelligibility scores, which minimize contextual factors, reflect successful compensatory strategies. However, in other cases, overestimates of intelligibility may reflect the speaker's poor judgment and failure to monitor communication interaction. Information from interview and standard clinical measures of intelligibility can serve as a starting point for counseling and intervention.

In-Clinic Observations of Interaction

In addition to the general information obtained from the interview, useful information about communication interaction skills may be obtained from structured tasks performed in the clinical setting. Use of a direction-giving task was described earlier in this chapter. Marvin, the 26 year old cerebral-palsied individual with severely dysarthric speech, was discussed as an illustration of successful use of speech in a structured communication situation. The direction-giving task was a simple one. The dysarthric speaker was presented a card with a variety of colored geometric shapes drawn on it. The speaker's task was to give directions to the listener, who was unable to see the original design. Listeners had all the materials needed to reproduce the design and were told that they were free to interact in any way they chose in order to complete the task. They could simply listen to the dysarthric speaker and follow directions, they could ask confirmatory questions, or they could ask for new information from the dysarthric speaker.

In-clinic tasks that sample interaction skills are useful for a number of reasons. First, they allow for the sampling of a large number of communication turns in a relatively short period of time. The direct observation of interactive behaviors in natural settings is so time consuming that it is not usually feasible in clinical practice. Second, because the materials used in the task are easy to generate, an essentially unlimited source of material is available for both assessment and training. Further, the material can be tailored to meet the needs of the dysarthric individual. The number and complexity of the shapes is dependent upon the speaker's skills and can be varied easily to alter the difficulty level of the task. Finally, because the communication partner is naive regarding the actual content of the message, there is the opportunity to assess communication breakdowns and resolution strategies.

The analysis of performance on this task may take a number of forms, including simple observation and verbal descriptions of the performance, checklists, or tallies of the number of occurrences of specific behaviors. At times, we video-tape the interaction and then view the tape along with the dysarthric speaker and the listeners. In this way, pertinent behaviors can be described and discussed and, if necessary, more appropriate strategies developed.

Case Presentations

In order to illustrate the use of the direction-giving task, the performance of two severely dysarthric speakers will be described. These speakers were selected as examples because they are similiar in the severity of their motor speech disability but differ greatly in their interaction skills. The first individual, Tom, was a 24 year old traumatically brain-injured individual with severe dysarthria. His speech was approximately 10 percent intelligible on a single word production task. Spelling, word finding, and grammatical formulation skills were all sufficient to allow him to use a spelling-based augmentative communication device. He had sufficient motor control to use a Canon Communicator with his left hand. His communication rate using this device was approximately 8 wpm. Tom had been taught to use the alphabet board supplementation approach described earlier, but he would only speak when specifically requested to do so. When asked why he did not speak more, he indicated that "speech is too hard," and that "people don't listen."

Observation of performance on the direction-giving task helped to explain why communication interaction in natural settings was so difficult for Tom. His performance was an excellent example of the consequences of poor interaction skills. In one condition he was told that he could communicate with the system of his choice, either the Canon Communicator, supplemented speech, or any combination of speaking and typing. When given his choice, he used the Canon Communicator exclusively. His communication strategy was a simple one. For approximately the first 12 minutes of the task, he typed, in a letter-by-letter fashion, a lengthy series of instructions to the partner. During this long interval, Tom did not look at his partner or in any way interact with her. He simply attended to his message preparation task while his partner sat and waited. If this were a natural communication situation, she would have probably excused herself and returned at some later time. At the end of the 12 minutes, Tom handed the tape with his printed message to his partner who read it in its entirety. Then she read it again, this time tearing it into shorter units. From this point on in the interaction, she took complete control of the situation. With each short unit, she asked a number of confirmatory questions before reproducing the geometric shape. Tom responded adequately but rarely elaborated a response. Although Tom and his partner successfully completed the direction-giving task, Tom initiated only one communication exchange—the first one. After the first message, he merely responded to his partner's initiations.

The task was next repeated with different geometric patterns. This time, because we were interested in Tom's ability to resolve communication breakdowns, he was asked to use the alphabet board supplementation approach in which he pointed to the first letter of each word as he spoke the word. Again, his breakdown resolution strategies were stereotyped and not always effective. When his partner indicated that she was unable to understand a word, Tom had only one breakdown resolution strategy: to repeat the word. If this failed, he would persist and repeat the word again and again. This would continue until his partner would take charge and indicate to him that she wasn't understanding, and to please spell out the word.

Marvin, on the other hand, is an excellent example of a skilled communicator. Marvin's speech was similar in terms of severity to that of Tom's. However, because Marvin had considerably less hand function than Tom, he used a head switch to tap out Morse code that was translated by his communication device into orthographic English. In contrast to Tom, Marvin maintained a good deal of control over the communication interaction. Over the course of the 20 minute interaction, he used his speech more and more. By the end of the interaction, he almost exclusively relied on his speech, resorting to the Morse code system only to resolve some breakdowns that he could not resolve verbally. After the taping session, we interviewed Marvin about his performance. Many of his statements were an accurate reflection of what we saw in the interaction. For example, he indicated that he watched his partner carefully and that he knew when she was not understanding his speech. Because his augmentative communication device was based on Morse code, he did not have to view a keyboard or array when preparing messages. In this way, his eyes were free to monitor the behavior of his partner.

Other statements appeared to contradict the clinician's impressions. For example, when asked why he spoke sometimes and used his augmentative communication device at other times, his response was, "Some words are easier to say than others and I take the easy way out." A review of a portion of the transcript of the interaction revealed that Marvin was making decisions about which words to speak and which to communicate via Morse code on the basis of a more complex set of factors than simply the articulatory difficulty of the words. This point can best be illustrated by describing how Marvin communicated one short message, "In the circle there's a yellow square." The following is the sequence of interactions leading to successful communication of that message. The colons represent pauses which Marvin appeared to intersperse throughout the interaction so that his partner could confirm the understanding of the message. Text in capital letters was communicated via the Morse code device; text in lower case was spoken.

Marvin—IN THE circle:
Partner—in the circle
Marvin—there's a yellow square:
Partner—I didn't understand that
Marvin—THERE
Partner—there's
Marvin—Y:
Partner—yellow
Marvin—S:
Partner—square, there's a yellow square

Reviewing this series of exchanges, you can see that Marvin's control was achieved in a number of subtle ways. In the first line, he used Morse code to produce the relatively simple words "in the," yet he spoke the word "circle." He appeared to be violating his own rule of speaking only the words that were easy to pronounce. However, if the phrase is analyzed in a slightly different way, it is apparent that he was using a different, but effective, strategy. By producing the words "in the" using his most understandable communication mode, the augmentative communication device, the listener was able to predict that the next word must be either an adjective or a noun. Further, within the confines of this task, there were a relatively small number of options. Thus, Marvin had used syntactical structure to increase the listener's chances of understanding his severely distorted speech. The word "circle" was successfully understood and Marvin then continued to speak the entire next phrase, "there's a yellow square." A review of the entire transcript suggested that once he had been successful, he continued to speak until there was a communication breakdown. Marvin tolerated a relatively high frequency of communication breakdowns. When the entire transcript was analyzed, approximately 20 percent of the words he spoke were not understood by his partner the first time. It appears that this relatively high breakdown frequency was not frustrating for Marvin's communication partner because he so quickly and effectively resolved breakdowns. What was gained in terms of communication efficiency appeared to be worth the price of regular communication breakdowns.

The cases presented here represent the ends of the continuum, one extremely skilled and the other not. Table 8-3 contains a listing of some of the features that distinguished the two communicators. Perhaps the most striking difference is the fact that Marvin effectively utilized severely distorted speech, while Tom made no attempt to do so. Marvin appeared to do this in order to increase overall communication rate. His ability to resolve communication breakdowns quickly and effectively may have been a factor important to the success of his communication. Tom, on the other hand, did not modify his behavior when faced with a communication breakdown, and breakdowns were frustrating and disruptive for both him and his listener. In an effort to prevent breakdowns, Tom appeared to adopt two strategies. First,

TABLE 8-3.
A Summary of the Differences in Interaction Styles Between Marvin and Tom.

	Marvin	Tom
Uses speech	yes	no
Sacrifices accuracy for speed	yes	no
Alters behaviors when breakdowns occur	yes	no
Chunks information	yes	no
Watches partner's reaction	yes	no*
Changes mode dependent on the message	yes	no
Uses abbreviation	yes	no*
Pauses for predictions	yes	no*

*Indicates strategies difficult for Tom to use because of the features of his augmentative communication devices.

he used only a completely intelligible communication mode, the Canon Communicator. Second, he allowed his partner to control the interaction by initiating most of the utterances. In this way, he could take on the role of a responder and could consistently be quite understandable.

Marvin had a number of other strategies with which he increased the likelihood of successful communication. For example, he gave his partners information in processable units and confirmed their understanding of each unit before proceeding to the next. Finally, Marvin used a number of techniques to pick up the pace of the interaction. Use of speech was one of the most effective rate-enhancing strategies, there were also others. For example, once terms had been introduced so that Marvin and his partner had shared information, Marvin would begin to use abbreviations rather than complete words. He would also allow partner prediction, which, when successful, enhanced communication rate.

It is interesting to speculate about the underlying reasons for the differences we observed between Marvin and Tom. One important factor is the etiology of the motor speech disorder. Marvin was congenitally impaired and thus had had 26 years to develop his interactional skills. Tom, on the other hand, had normal speech prior to his brain injury. He was approximately one year post onset when his interaction skills were evaluated. Further, Tom's brain injury resulted in cognitive problems that no doubt interfered with his ability to handle complex, rapidly moving interactional exchanges. Although he did not exhibit the specific language deficits seen in aphasic individuals, he illustrated the kind of language problems that Holland (1982) described as problems with the function rather than the form of language.

Improving Interaction Skills

It may not be realistic to think that training in effective interaction strategies can bring all severely dysarthric individuals to the level of skill exhibited by Marvin. However, training may provide the less skilled with some basic techniques for managing communication situations. We divide interaction training into three categories: (1) those techniques designed to reduced the probability of communication breakdowns, (2) those techniques designed to resolve or repair breakdowns once they occur, and (3) those techniques designed to improve the skills of the communication partner. Each category of techniques will be discussed in turn.

Techniques for Preventing Breakdowns

Only recently have authors begun to focus on identifying environmental variables that might influence successful communication in natural settings. Berry and Sanders (1983) outlined an educational program to help dysarthric individuals identify factors that may interfere with speech intelligibility. Their program, called Environmental Education, is based on the principles of aural rehabilitation in which situation, noise, lighting, and distance are among the factors evaluated. The goal of the program is to optimize each of these factors in order to increase intelligibility.

Another important approach for preventing communication breakdowns is to train the dysarthric speaker to use multiple approaches to communication. We all use multiple communication approaches. The key is to select the approach that best fits the situation. Once again, the case of Marvin can serve as an illustration of the effective selection of multiple approaches. Marvin, despite his severe physical limitations, had at least eight approaches to choose from in any communication situation. These choices included speech, verbal letter-by-letter spelling, gestural eye-gaze and head nods, speech supplemented with letters generated via his Morse code device, word abbreviations displayed on his Morse code device, complete words either displayed on the device or printed out, and synthesized speech via his Morse code device. A number of factors appeared to influence Marvin's selection of communication approaches. The first factor related to the message itself. For social greetings,

Marvin typically used speech. Greetings require prompt delivery but high levels of intelligibility are not necessary, since the context of the situation typically gives the listener additional cues so that the message can be understood. Thus, speech is better suited for this task than, for example, the slower but more intelligible printing of a complete message with his Morse code device.

For conversation control messages, such as "Wait, it's my turn now," "Did you understand?" 'I have something to tell you," Marvin used eye-gaze and head gestures. For severely dysarthric speakers, we often find that the control techniques should be delivered nonverbally, so that the partner does not confuse the control technique with the message. Routine instructions to his care-givers were usually printed out or displayed on the Morse code device. These types of memos do not demand rapid delivery, yet intelligibility is important. For topic introductions, Marvin typically used his Morse code device. Once the topic had been introduced via his most intelligible approach, he switched to a more rapid but less intelligible approach, such as speech. For a more complete discussion of the "trade-offs" among rate, accuracy, and message flexibility, see Dowden and Beukelman (in press).

Marvin also selected his communication approach depending on his listeners. He typically used speech when interacting with familiar listeners. On the other hand, he would routinely use Morse code at least initially with strangers. Finally, Marvin selected different approaches for breakdown resolution than for initial attempts at communication. He may have verbally spelled letter-by-letter to resolve communication breakdowns for familiar partners and used the Morse code device to resolve breakdowns with less-familiar partners.

Training breakdown resolution strategies

Communication breakdowns are a fact of life for severely dysarthric speakers. Yet, with the exception of a study we will subsequently report, we are aware of no systematic investigations of how dysarthric speakers handle these breakdowns. Ansel, McNeil, Hunker, and Bless (1983) studied the response to communication breakdown of a group of adult cerebral-palsied individuals. Subjects were selected to represent a range of severity and a number of a different types of dysarthria. Each subject was engaged in a 25 minute conversation. Twelve times during each conversation, the experimenter indicated a communication failure by saying, "What?" 'Excuse me?" or "I'm sorry?" Responses to these failures were analyzed for both verbal adjustments and adjustments in voice intensity of their speech. Results indicated that these speakers did not systematically alter intensity when faced with a breakdown. Further, the majority of their verbal adjustments fell into one of four categories, including total repetition, partial repetition of a phrase, partial repetition of a phrase with elaboration, and total repetition with elaboration. Results also indicated that responses were not different for multiple as opposed to single experimenter queries. As is often the case with initial research in a new area, this work brings up many unanswered questions. For example, why did these speakers not respond differently to a series of apparent communication failures than they did to a single question? Ansel and her colleagues suggest that the key may be in the nature of the query. The examiner was purposefully nondirective in the question. Thus, no specific cues were given to the dysarthric speaker about the nature of the misunderstanding. Had more specific cues been given, responses of the dysarthric speakers may have been altered. However, it may also be the case that these individuals simply do not have well-established breakdown resolution strategies that are responsive to changing communicaton situations. Clearly, resolution of communicaton breakdowns is an important area of future research.

Clinically, we often teach dysarthric speakers and their listeners to use a specific series of steps to resolve communication breakdowns. First, as soon as a breakdown has occurred, listeners signal that they have not understood. They are encouraged to do this gesturally, so as not to interrupt the dysarthric speaker, who has the floor. Thus, the dysarthric speaker can decide whether to stop and repair immediately or continue on the hope that the partner will understand once more context has been provided. Next, the partners confirm what they know or think they know rather than attempting to guess at the completion of the message. In this way, the dysarthric speaker can be specific in the repair. Many severely dysarthric speakers find it most efficient to use two levels of repair strategies. First, they simply repeat the misunderstood portion of the utterance, at times elaborating a portion of it. If that fails to resolve the communication breakdown, they use a communication approach that they know will be intelligible. This typically means that they use the slow but accurate approach of spelling the message out letter-by-letter.

Listener Training

Throughout this discussion of interaction training, the importance of the role of the listener has been indicated. Some ways in which listeners can facilitate the resolution of communication breakdowns have just been reviewed. We believe that there are two levels of training for communication partners—one involving the training of primary listeners and the other involving training of strangers with whom the dysarthric speaker may interact during the course of daily activities.

Direct and extensive training may be warranted for primary listeners. This includes training of communication breakdown resolution strategies as well as recognition of the environmental factors described by Berry and Sanders (1983) that have an impact on intelligibility. Elderly listeners may have particular difficulty understanding the dysarthric speakers. If this is the case, the partner is encouraged to have an audiological evaluation to rule out the possibility of a hearing loss or to have an existing hearing problem treated appropriately.

Although it is feasible to train a small number of primary listeners, training is not possible for all of the individuals that the dysarthric speaker may encounter in ordinary communication situations. For this reason, the dysarthric speaker must be provided with the means to instruct strangers. Usually this takes the form of written instructions on a card or on the back of an alphabet board. This card provides a simple description of the problem and a set of rules for listeners' behavior. Individualization of these instructions with the help of the dysarthric individual is more effective than providing long lists of general rules.

SPECIAL CONSIDERATIONS

Long-Term Management of the Recovering Speaker

Clinicians who manage the communication programs of severely dysarthric individuals, especially those recovering from head injury, are faced with a number of dilemmas. The first dilemma is predicting the future. The parents of young brain-injured individuals for whom we have selected augmentative communication devices may ask the legitimate question, "Does this mean that you think our child will never speak again?" We usually respond by saying that we do not know enough about the recovery of motor function in young brain-injured individuals to say with confidence that speech will "never" return. However, the sustained inability to communicate interferes with cognitive and academic rehabilitation programs necessary for the recovery of the brain-injured individual. The following analogue is often helpful in aiding the family to make decisions about the allocation of resources. If a family is considering whether to place their limited savings in high-risk but high-payoff investments or low-risk and modest-payoff investments, many investment counselors will suggest that the majority of savings be placed in the "sure thing" but that a portion be placed in the "long-shot" with high risk and high payoff. An investment in an augmentative communication approach may be considered the safe investment that will provide the dysarthric individual with a guaranteed means of communication. Speech, on the other hand, can be considered the long-shot with tremendous payoff. However, if you invest all of your time and efforts into a long-shot that does not pay off, then you run the risk of being left with no effective means of communication. Depending on the risks that families are willing to take, they should allocate an appropriate portion of resources to an augmentative communication approach that will provide communication for today, and to speech that may pay great rewards in the future. Many traumatically brain-injured individuals have a long life expectancy, and their personal development plan over the years must be considered. If we fail to consider it, their families may reject us as insensitive or as individuals who have taken a position that contains no hope.

The second dilemma faced by a clinician is how to manage the long-term communication program within the constraints of a third party payer support. It is clear that intensive, regular professional training cannot continue for the years that may be needed. Instead, we recommend that families who wish to invest their time carry out a simple training program developed in consultation with the professional. These programs are usually designed to increase physiological support for selected speech components and may involve practice sessions of 10 to 15 minutes twice daily. Through these long-term efforts, families will either be able to see slow progress or will be better able to accept the fact that speech will not return, despite their best efforts.

Applying These Techniques in Degenerative Disorders

Thus far, this chapter has focused on the recovering dysarthric individual. However, several of the techniques described here are also appropriate for the severely involved individual with degenerative disorders. For example, in order to maintain functional speech for as long as possible, the alphabet board supplementation approach has been utilized successfully for periods of time with individuals that have ALS (Beukelman, Yorkston, & Dowden, 1985). Identification of difficulties with communication interaction and training to prevent and resolve communication breakdowns is also a critical element of management programs for the degenerative dysarthric individual. The only techniques described in this chapter that are perhaps inappropriate for the individual with a degenerative disorder are those whose goal is to increase physiological support for speech. These techniques are not typically utilized with this population for two reasons. First, because of the progressive nature of disorders such as ALS, techniques that focus on increasing physiological performance will fail. Nonspeech drills, even if their only goal is to maintain function, should be used only with extreme caution. We are aware of no documentation that would suggest that such drills have a beneficial effect. Second, fatigue may be such an overriding problem for some severely involved speakers that efforts to drill on speech components will only have the effect of reducing their physical reserves needed to support functional speech. Thus, individuals with degenerative disorders may expend their small energy resources for drill rather than actual communication.

REFERENCES

Ansel, B., McNeil, M., Hunker, C., & Bless, D. (1983). The frequency of verbal and acoustic adjustments used by cerebral palsied dysarthric adults when faced with communication failure. In W.R. Berry (Ed.), *Clinical dysarthria*. Austin, TX: PRO-ED.

Berry, W., & Sanders, S. (1983). Environmental education: The universal management approach for adults with dysarthria. In W. Berry (Ed.), *Clinical Dysarthria*. Austin, TX: PRO-ED.

Beukelman, D.R., & Yorkston, K.M. (1977). A communication system for the severely dysarthric speaker with an intact language system. *Journal of Speech & Hearing Disorders*, *42*, 265–270.

Beukelman, D.R., & Yorkston, K.M. (1978). A series of communication options for individuals with brain stem lesions. *Archives of Physical Medicine & Rehabilitation*, *59*, 337–342.

Beukelman, D.R., Yorkston, K.M., & Dowden, P.A. (1985). *Communication Augmentation: A casebook of clinical management*. Austin, TX: PRO-ED.

Dowden, P.A., & Beukelman, D.R. (in press). Rate, accuracy and message flexibility: Case studies in communication augmentation strategies. In L.E. Bernstein (Ed.), *The vocally impaired*. New York: Academic Press.

Farrier, L.D., Yorkston, K.M., Marriner, N.A., & Beukelman, D.R. (1985). Conversational control in nonimpaired speakers using an augmentative communication system. *Augmentative & Alternative Communication*, *1*, 65–73.

Holland, A.L. (1982). When is aphasia aphasia? The problem of closed head injury. In R. Brookshire (Ed.), *Clinical aphasiology: Conference proceedings*. Minneapolis: BRK Publishers.

Netsell, R., & Daniel, B. (1979). Dysarthria in adults: Physiologic approach rehabilitation. *Archives of Physical Medicine & Rehabilitation*, *60*, 502–508.

Netsell, R., & Rosenbek, J. (1985). Treating the dysarthrias. *Speech and language evaluation in neurology: Adult disorders*. New York: Gurne & Stratton.

Vanderheiden, G., & Lloyd, L. (1986). Communication systems and their components. In S. Blackstone (Ed.), *Augmentative communication: An introduction*. Rockville, MD: American Speech-Language-Hearing Association.

Wilson, W. (1981). *An alternative communication system for the severely physically handicapped*. (Grant #6007804512). Handicapped Media Services & Captioned Films Program, Department of Education.

Yorkston, K.M., & Beukelman, D.R. (1981). *Assessment of intelligibility of dysarthric speech*. Austin, TX: PRO-ED.

Yorkston, K.M., & Dowden, P.A. (1984). Non-speech language and communication systems—Adults. In A. Holland (Ed.), *Recent advances: language disorders*. San Diego: College-Hill Press, 283–312.

Yorkston, K.M., & Karlan, G. (1986). Assessment procedures. In S. Blackstone, (Ed.), *Augmentative communication: An introduction*. Rockville, MD: American Speech-Language-Hearing Association.

CHAPTER 9

Respiration

Clinical Issues: Both consultation requests gave evidence of respiratory impairment. In the first, we were asked to evaluate the speech of a 67 year old women with ALS and severely reduced vital capacity. In the second, we were asked to evaluate the speech of a 35 year old man with residual ataxia from a motor vehicle accident over 10 years ago. The physician had indicated that this man's speech sounded "explosive" and that he produced only one or two words per breath. Our evaluation of the woman with ALS confirmed a reduced vital capacity. In addition, she was only able to sustain phonation for approximately eight seconds, was unable to increase the loudness of her speech, and complained of fatigue after relatively brief periods of speaking. Yet, despite evidence of respiratory impairment, her conversational speech was remarkably good. It was adequately loud for face-to-face conversation, her breath group length was nearly normal, and inhalations occurred at locations appropriate for the syntax of the message. In short, she appeared to be handling a severely compromised respiratory system as well as she could. On the other hand, the man with ataxic dysarthria presented a very different pattern of respiratory impairment. Our evaluation began with a perceptual evaluation of his speech. His speech pattern was typical of ataxic dysarthria and was characterized by "excess and equal" stress patterning. His voice was excessively loud, somewhat harsh, and vowels were hypernasal. Irregular articulatory breakdowns occurred frequently. Perhaps the most unique aspect of his speech was his abnormal breath patterning. In both conversational speech and reading, he would inhale after every word and occasionally within words. His abnormal breathing pattern, in combination with a tendency to speak too rapidly for his level of motor control, not only increased the bizarreness of his speech but also reduced his speech intelligibility. A more detailed examination of his performance indicated that he was "overdriving" his respiratory system during speech. He was initiating each word at excessively high lung volume levels and generating excessive levels of subglottal air pressure for speech. Despite the abnormal pattern of breathing during speech, he could sustain loud phonation for over 15 seconds and could count from

1 to 23 with adequate loudness on a single breath. Clearly, he was not making optimum use of his respiratory system during speech. As we reviewed the results of these two evaluations, we asked the following questions:

- *Why were the respiratory impairments of these two individuals so different from one another?*
- *Why was the woman with ALS able to compensate so well for severe respiratory impairment?*
- *What intervention approaches might be useful in helping reduce the fatigue she was experiencing?*
- *Why did the man with ataxia develop such an unusual respiratory pattern for conversation and reading?*
- *How did his abnormal respiratory patterning affect other aspects of speech?*
- *What technique would be effective in teaching him to modify his abnormal breathing pattern during speech?*

The impact of respiratory impairment on dysarthric speakers is often complex to evaluate. Some individuals with severely compromised respiratory function do remarkably well during speech; others with apparently less impairment utilize unusual and maladaptive respiratory patterns. Some speakers are able to modify their respiratory function very well in response to training; others are remarkably rigid in their respiratory patterning. For some dysarthric speakers, the respiratory dysfunction is so severe that functional speech is precluded; for others, respiratory performance does not substantially interfere with speech. We will devote this chapter to the management of respiratory aspects of dysarthric speech. Unfortunately, the research literature related to the topic is not extensive, and this chapter contains more than its share of conjecture, approaches based on clinical hunches, and attempts to understand dysarthric speakers based on a model of what we know about the respiratory patterns of normal speakers.

With these cautions in mind, we believe that an understanding of the respiratory aspects of dysarthric speech is important in clinical management. The respiratory system is the source of aerodynamic energy for speech. If respiratory performance is severely impaired, adequate speech may be impossible. When it is less severely impaired, poor respiratory performance many have an impact on other speech components, most notably the phonatory system. Overall aspects of speech, such as naturalness, may also be impaired. Breath patterning is basic to speech naturalness because the breath group may be considered the unit upon which other aspects of prosody, such as intonation and stress patterning, are superimposed. (See Chapter 14 for a discussion of prosody.) An understanding of the respiratory component of dysarthric speech is needed in order to make appropriate intervention decisions. For selected dysarthric individuals, focus on respiratory performance during treatment is clearly beneficial. For some dysarthric individuals, intervention focuses on improving physiological support for speech. For others, intervention focuses on the development of optimal patterns of performance within the limitations of their current level of physiological support.

RESPIRATORY FUNCTION DURING SPEECH

Normal Speakers

Consistent Subglottal Air Pressure

Generally, the respiratory goal of a speaker is to generate steady subglottal air pressure with slight variations to support stress patterning. Normal speakers accomplish this goal efficiently. Functioning well within their physiological capabilities, they do not experience fatigue during ordinary speech tasks. Although respiration for speech appears to be quite simple, adequate respiratory support and patterning requires a high level of motor control. A detailed review of the literature describing normal respiratory function for speech is well beyond the scope of this chapter. However, an understanding of the basic respiratory goals for speech and how these goals are achieved is needed if one is to understand the respiratory impairments experienced by dysarthric individuals. Readers are referred to Hixon (1973, 1987), Hixon, Mead, and Goldman (1976), Folkins and Kuehn, (1982), and Weismer (1985) for excellent discussions of normal respiration for speech.

Achieving Respiratory Goals

The steady energy source for speech is reflected in the contour of the subglottal air pressure levels generated during an utterance. Subglottal air pressure refers to the air pressure generated below the vocal folds (see Figure 9.1). The subglottal air pressure level during speech is a reflection of the driving forces of the respiratory system and the resistance to airflow imposed by the glottal and supraglottal structures.

Subglottal air pressure is generated by the compression of the volume of air in the lungs. This compression results from a combination of two forces generated by the respiratory system. One of these forces is generated by muscular activity and the other by elastic recoil of the respiratory structures. The respiratory system has many of the characteristics of a spring. The passive forces of elastic recoil vary depending on the lung volume level; the larger

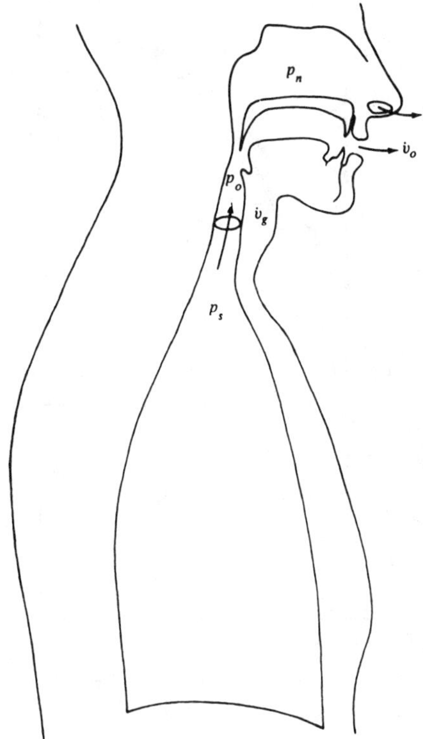

Figure 9-1. A mid-sagittal line drawing of the vocal tract showing pressures in nasal tract (P_n), oral (P_o), and subglottal region (P_s) and volume velocities in the glottis (V_g), and leaving the nasal (V_n) and oral tracts (V_o) (From Netsell, 1973).

the volume of air in the lungs (lung volume level) the larger the elastic recoil force. The elastic recoil properties of the respiratory system can be understood by examining what are known as *relaxation curves*. Two such curves for upright and supine positions are illustrated in Figure 9-2. This figure contains a plot of subglottal (alveolar) air pressures generated at various lung volume levels (expressed in a percentage of vital capacity). Examination of the figure suggests that if a speaker is asked to inhale to a high lung volume level, close the glottis, and then relax, high levels of subglottal air pressure are generated. For example, in the upright and supine positions, when the speaker inhales to 90 percent of lung volume level and then relaxes, over 30 cm water pressure is generated. At 70 percent lung volume level in the upright position, approximately 15 cm H_2O is generated by relaxation forces only. At 36 percent of lung volume level, the relaxation forces generate 0 cm H_2O.

Careful examination of Figure 9-2 also suggests that, for a given lung volume level, greater air pressures are generated in the supine as compared to the upright position. This occurs because, in the supine position, gravitational forces contribute to the net expiratory force of both the rib cage and abdomen. In the upright position, gravitational forces contribute to the

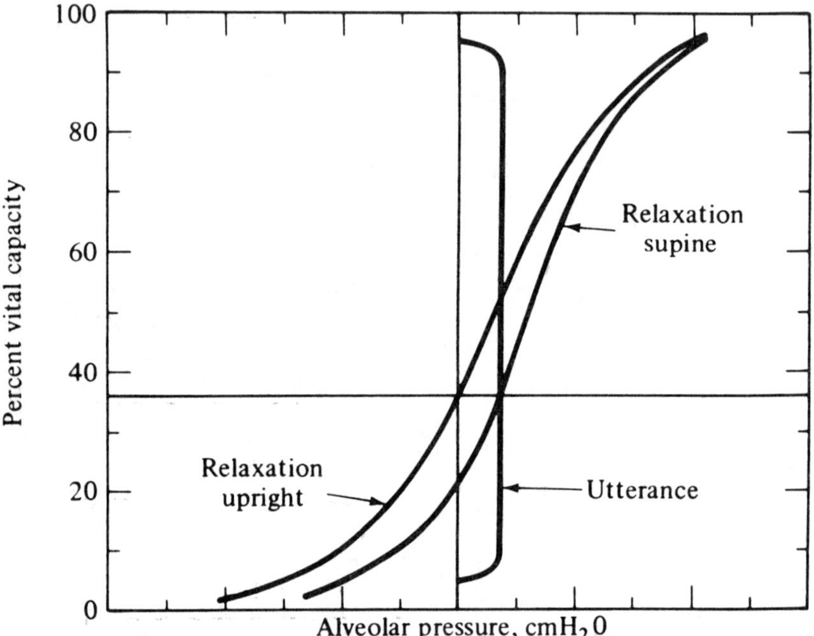

Figure 9-2. Subglottal air pressures generated at various lung volume levels (in percent of vital capacity) in supine and upright position (From Hixon, 1973).

expiratory forces of the rib cage and the inspiratory forces of the abdomen. This difference in elastic recoil force, as a function of posture, is important in management of the respiratory/phonatory components of severely involved dysarthric speakers. A more detailed discussion of the influence of position on respiratory function in severe dysarthria will be presented later in this chapter. Readers are referred to Hixon (1973) for a complete discussion of the effects of position on the resting expiratory level in normal speakers.

In addition to the elastic recoil forces, there are forces generated by the contraction of the respiratory muscles. Subglottal air pressure is generated by the interaction of the elastic recoil and contraction forces. Speech requires an essentially constant level of subglottal air pressure throughout an utterance in the presence of a declining lung volume level. Thus, a steadily changing relationship between muscular effort and passive respiratory forces is necessitated. This relationship is illustrated in Figure 9-3, which depicts the various contributions of passive respiratory forces and muscular effort as a function of lung volume level during a maximum sustained phonation task. Note that the target subglottal air pressure remains at a constant level of approximately 7 cm H_2O. At high lung volume levels, if left unchecked, these forces would generate greater than necessary subglottal air pressures.

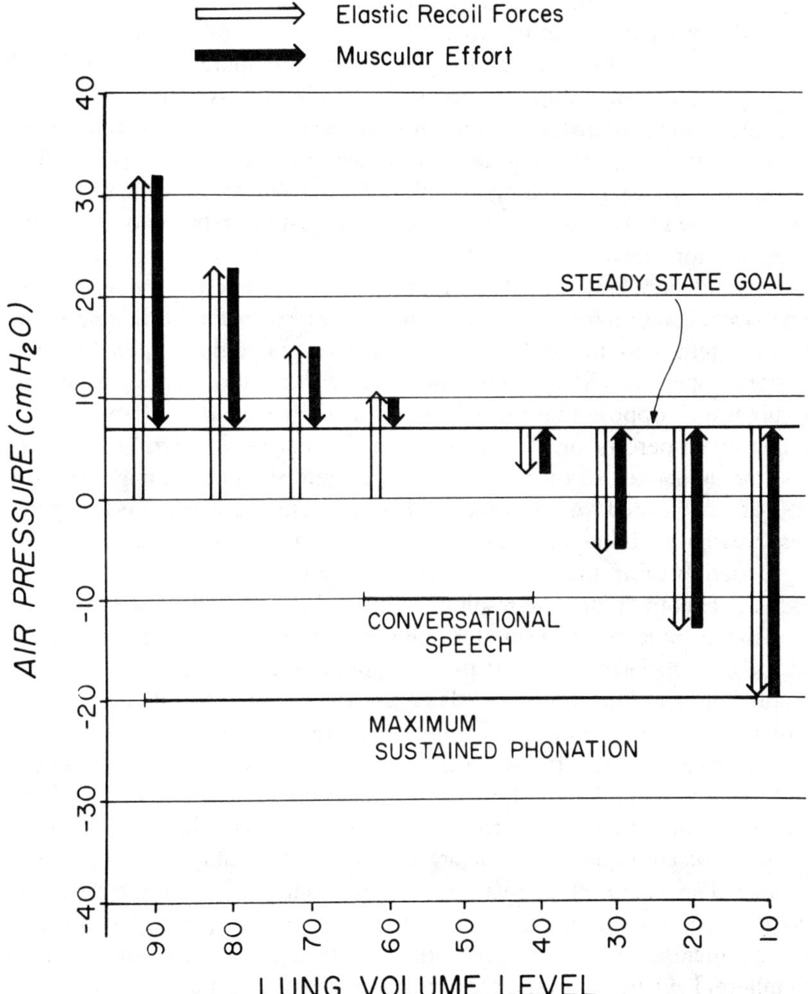

Figure 9-3. Relative contribution of elastic recoil and muscular forces needed in order to achieve a steady subglottal air pressure of 7 cm H_2O. Also noted are typical lung volume levels for conversational speech and maximum sustained phonation (Adapted from Hixon, 1973).

Therefore, at high lung volume levels, muscular activity must be in the inhalatory direction to counterbalance the excessive contribution of the exhalatory elastic recoil forces. As lung volume levels decrease, less and less inspiratory checking is necessary. At slightly less than 60 percent lung volume level, elastic recoil alone is no longer sufficient to generate adequate air pressure for speech. At that point and below, the active respiratory forces begin to act in the exhalatory direction in order to generate the appropriate level of air pressure. Thus, maximum sustained phonation, an apparently simple speech task, requires complex adjustments in the respiratory system.

Maximum sustained phonation in some respects is very unlike ordinary speech utterances. Speech typically is produced by normal speakers within a relatively narrow range of lung volumes (60 percent to 35 percent of vital capacity in the seated position) that allows adequate generation of subglottal air pressure for speech with a minimal expenditure of energy (Hixon, 1987). Note that in Figure 9-3, when speech is initiated at 60 percent of vital capacity, the passive relaxation forces, resulting from the elastic recoil of the respiratory structures, generate subglottal air pressure nearly equal to that required for conversational speech. There is little need for contraction of the inspiratory musculature to oppose these recoil forces, as there would be if speech were initiated at 80 percent or 90 percent of vital capacity. At high lung volume levels, the associated recoil forces would generate subglottal air pressures in excess of that needed for conversational speech. During speech, as compared to rest breathing, abdominal muscles to some extent are contracted throughout the production of an utterance. The active role of the abdomen throughout speech appears to "tune" the respiratory musculature for increased efficiency during the inspiratory and expiratory phases of respiration for speech. During loud speech associated with increased subglottal air pressure, normal speakers typically inhale to lung volume levels greater than 60 percent of vital capacity in order to efficiently initiate speech at a subglottal air pressure level similar to that which is generated by the elastic recoil forces of the respiratory structures.

Throughout the lung volume level range utilized for speech, the elastic recoil forces and muscular forces interact to compress the air within the respiratory system in order to generate a steady level of subglottal air pressure. The normal speaker is able to vary the relative contributions of the chest wall structures and the abdomen to the respiratory patterns for speech. For example, one might increase lung volume level primarily through expansion of the thorax with minimal expansion of the abdomen. On the other hand, another speaker might increase lung volume level primarily through expansion of the abdomen. Actually, most normal speakers utilize an integrated pattern of expanding and reducing thorax and abdominal shapes simultaneously. In summary, normal speakers are not only able to generate a steady level of subglottal air pressure, but are also able to do so in a highly efficient manner that is well within the mid-range of their physiological capabilities.

Dysarthric Speakers

Interpreting Perceptual Assessment Results

Several of the speech dimensions perceptually studied by Darley, Aronson, and Brown (1975) appear to be related to respiratory aspects of speech, including monoloudness, excess loudness variations, loudness decay, alternating loudness, forced inspiration-expiration, and short phrases. Although these perceptions may appear among the most deviant in at least some groups of dysarthric speakers, they are by no means universally present in dysarthria. For example, in flaccid dysarthria, often associated with decreased vital capacity and poor control of exhalation, only three respiratory dimensions (audible inspiration, short phrases, and monoloudness) appear among the most deviant speech dimensions. Further, appearance of these dimensions may not be entirely related to respiration but may also be a function of laryngeal and velopharyngeal inadequacy.

The work of Darley and colleagues was based solely on perceptual judgments made from a sample of connected speech. Inferences about respiratory performance from perceptual studies are problematic because they mistakenly result in both false positives and false negatives. False positives may occur when what perceptually appears to be respiratory impairment may indeed result from the dysfunction of some other speech component. For example, short phrases may reflect the presence of faulty laryngeal, velopharyngeal, or oral articulatory valving rather than a respiratory impairment per se (Hardy, 1966).

False negatives may be obtained when respiratory performance during speech appears to be perceptually adequate, but a careful examination of respiratory functioning reveals that speakers are accomplishing their respiratory goals only by making substantial modifications in normal respiratory patterning. Hixon, Putnam, and Sharpe (1983) illustrate this point with an excellent case study of a post-polio individual with flaccid paralysis of the rib cage, diaphragm, and abdomen. Respiratory function was impaired to the extent that respiration was usually assisted by one of the following devices: a positive-pressure respirator, a rocking bed, or a torso pneumobelt. This individual was able to spend brief periods "free breathing." Hixon and his colleagues studied breathing and connected speech activities during these periods. Although the connected speech of this dysarthric individual was judged to be "normal" by laypersons, it was accomplished using some remarkable compensatory maneuvers of the respiratory, laryngeal, and upper airway speech components. Respiratory compensation was described as follows:

> Connected speech was performed in breath groups begun by neck gestures that 'cocked' the breathing apparatus and stored recoil energy in it for use during ensuing expirations. Some breath groups were also extended through intermittent glossopharyngeal pumping. (p. 315)

In addition to these respiratory maneuvers, this individual used the respiratory support that he generated in a highly efficient manner. In fact, data indicated that the speaker used only 5 percent of his predicted vital capacity during speech in comparison to 20 percent typically used by normal speakers. He accomplished this by adopting a mildly strained-strangled voice quality and by making slight modifications in his oral articulatory patterning, including shortening fricative durations, substituting stops for fricatives, and producing intrusive glottal stops. Studies of cases such as this one provide valuable insights into effective strategies adopted by speakers without systematic training. The implication here is that these strategies may also serve as the focus for training in individuals who have not developed efficient compensations spontaneously.

Patterns of Respiratory Impairment in the Dysarthrias

Without careful evaluation of respiratory movements during speech production, clinicians may simply fail to appreciate the extent to which motor-impaired individuals deviate from normal respiratory patterning. In their 1975 work, Darley and colleagues write:

> The data concerning respiratory patterns in cerebellar disease remain inadequate and nondefinitive. Studies are needed that will provide direct measurement of respiratory function in a large number of subjects who represent a range of severity of physical involvement from mild to severe. Only through such studies can one confirm the existence of the respiratory aberrations whose occurrence is reasonably hypothesized. (p. 158)

Unfortunately, this statement remains true today and can certainly be extended beyond cerebellar diseases to nearly every type of dysarthria. On a more positive note, investigators are developing techniques and strategies for measuring respiratory aspects of dysarthric speech productions. However, there has been debate related to the specifics of measurement techniques (Abbs, 1985; Hixon & Hoit, 1984, 1985). The following parameters are becoming standard measures for describing respiratory function in clinical populations (Hixon, 1984):

1. An estimate of subglottal air pressure as an indicator of respiratory drive for speech
2. Air flow measured by the air volume entering or exiting the respiratory system per unit of time
3. Lung volume level measured as a percentage of vital capacity and used to describe levels at which selected respiratory and speech activities are being performed
4. Respiratory shape measured by anteroposterior diameter or circumference of the rib cage and abdomen and used as an indicator of respiratory system movements.

Realizing the existing literature is not adequate for comprehensive understanding of respiratory patterns in dysarthria, we will review some preliminary studies and case reports dealing with speech-related respiratory activities.

Several research groups have described the speech breathing characteristics of dysarthric speakers using the kinematic techniques described by Hixon

(1973, 1982). These studies suggest different patterns of respiratory impairment for individuals with differing underlying neuropathologies. For example, Putnam and Hixon (1984) studied 10 speakers with motor neuron disease (including four individuals with ALS). They found movement abnormalities suggestive of chest wall muscle weakness, particularly in the inspiratory direction. Yet, despite the fact that most of their speakers initiated speech tasks at low lung volume levels, all were able to:

> muster adequate volume displacement and, apparently, volume compression for the demands of conversation, inspite of the kinematic signs of chest wall muscle weakness or disordered control. (p. 64)

A different pattern of respiratory dysfunction has been noted in individuals with ataxic dysarthria. Hunker, Bless, and Weismer (1981) studied the respiratory patterns of a 69 year old woman with ataxic dysarthria who initiated speech at highly variable lung volume levels. She frequently continued speaking far below the normal lung volume level of 35 percent to 40 percent of vital capacity. She also demonstrated abrupt shifts in the relative volume displacement of the rib cage and abdomen. Hixon (1982) studied an ataxic 17 year old woman having moderate to severe paresis of the rib cage and diaphragm, and paralyzed abdominal muscles. During speech, her rib cage was smaller and the abdomen larger than they were during rest breathing at similar lung volumes. Apparently, this woman's paralyzed abdominal wall could not resist the downward force from the decreasing size of the chest wall. Thus, the muscular forces utilized to decrease the circumference of the chest wall resulted in an expansion of the abdominal circumference in addition to the compression of the air within the respiratory system.

Kim (1968) and Hunker and colleagues (1981) studied dysarthric speakers with Parkinson's disease. These speakers, unlike other dysarthric individuals reported here, had rather "inflexible" respiratory patterns during speech. Kim suggested that these patterns resulted from reduction in lung volume excursions, and Hunker and colleagues described a restricted use of chest wall movements to achieve lung volume displacements.

ASSESSMENT

Perceptual Indicators of Respiratory Inadequacy

Clinical assessment of respiratory function begins with the question, "Is respiratory function adequate for speech?" Because respiratory demands for conversational speech are minimal compared to the physiological capability of normal speakers, respiratory function that is not normal in all respects may be adequate to support conversational speech. At a preliminary level, we judge the adequacy of respiration for speech with perceptual judgments of connected speech. We are fully aware of the potential for failing to identify the presence of abnormal respiratory patterns in some speakers who may sound normal in terms of the respiratory aspects of speech. However, we need more basic research before the seriousness of this mistake can be evaluated. For the present, if the respiratory component of speech appears adequate to the trained eyes and ears of the clinician, our respiratory function evaluation stops. A number of visual-auditory characteristics may alert the clinician to potential respiratory impairment. If any of these characteristics appears, respiratory function is examined in depth.

Loudness

As was described earlier, the primary respiratory goal for speech is to generate an adequate, sustained energy source. An adequate loudness level for connected speech is a good indicator of the adequacy of respiratory support. However, reduced loudness may be the result of a variety of physiologic, psychologic, and social factors. Loudness is closely related to the level of subglottal air pressure being generated. As we listen to a sample of connected speech, we ask the following questions:

- Is the overall loudness level too high or too low?
- Is the loudness level consistent?
- Are sudden uncontrolled alternations in loudness present?
- Does loudness diminish over the course of a single breath group unit or over the course of extended speech?
- Can the speaker increase speech loudness (shout)?
- Can the speaker produce quiet phonation?
- Does the speaker complain of fatigue when speaking for extended periods of time at conversational loudness levels?

If the clinician identifies a loudness problem, then an in-depth examination of respiratory/laryngeal components during speech must be carried out. Particular attention should be given to the speaker's ability to produce adequate levels of subglottal air pressure.

Breath Patterning

In addition to the perceptual estimates of loudness, clinicians need to make judgments about breath patterning characteristics. Normal speech breathing is characterized by rapid inhalation and a prolonged period of exhalation. Typically, the ratio of inhalation to exhalation duration is approximately 1:6 for normal speakers. Figure 9-4 illustrates lung volume levels obtained as a normal speaker reads a passage. Note that this speaker inhales to slightly more than 60 percent of lung volume level, and depending on the utterance, speaks until she reaches approximately 35 percent of lung volume

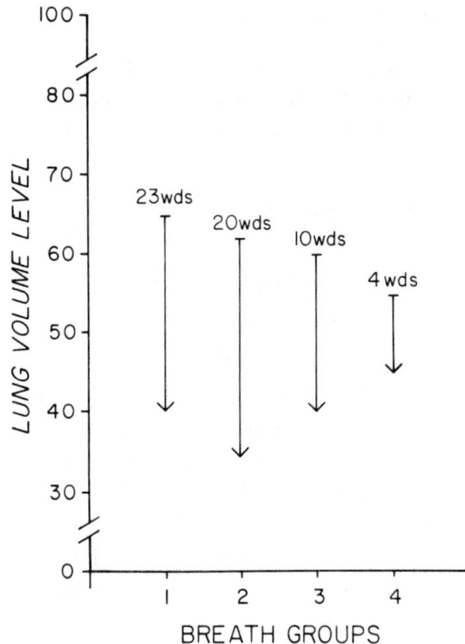

Figure 9-4. Lung volume levels for a normal speaker reading a paragraph. The following utterances correspond to breaths 1–4. (1) I pointed to the mountain covered with snow, but someone said, "Don't try to show him all that snow. Show Sam some snow." (2) I picked a handful of snow and began to show everyone, but they interrupted and said, "Show Sam some snow." (3) Pretending to be angry, I questioned, "Show Sam some snow? (4) What a ridiculous idea."

level. At that time, she inhales again. Note also that this speaker inhales to higher lung volume levels before beginning long utterances, and inhales to only 55 percent of lung volume level before initiating the final four-word utterance. Similiar data obtained during the speech of an ataxic dysarthric woman will be presented in the next section as part of a detailed description of the respiratory impairment seen in dysarthria.

Clinicians, during the initial perceptual evaluation, should listen for evidence suggesting an abnormal pattern or timing of inhalation and exhalation for speech. The following questions pertain to this aspect of speech:

- Does the speech respiratory pattern differ from the normal pattern of a quick inhalation phase followed by a prolonged exhalation?
- Does the speaker inhale to an appropriate lung volume level?
- At what point in the respiratory cycle does the speaker initiate an utterance?
- Is there a quick preparatory inhalation before the initiation of an utterance?
- Does the speaker use pauses for emphasis or do all of the pauses contain an inhalation?
- Is speech interrupted by sudden, forced inspiration or expiration sighs?
- Are exaggerated respiratory maneuvers, such as excessive elevation of the shoulders during inhalation, apparent during speech?

- Does the speaker appear to run out of air before inhaling?

In addition to movement patterns during inhalation and exhalation, the clinician may find evidence of respiratory dysfunction by examining the phrasing or breath group units produced during connected speech. The following questions relate to breath group units:

- How many words or syllables does the speaker produce on one breath?
- What is the duration (in seconds) of each breath group?
- Do breaths occur at syntactically appropriate locations in the utterance?

In order to identify abnormalities in this aspect of respiratory performance, it may be useful to first review data related to normal performance. Patterns of inhalation and exhalation were recorded during a paragraph reading task for groups of normal and dysarthric speakers (Beukelman, Yorkston, Dowden, & Minifie, 1986). The paragraph that these individuals read can be found in the Appendix of this chapter. Figure 9-5 illustrates data related to breath group lengths (in words) for five normal male adults ranging in age from 18 to 68. Mean length of breath groups ranges from 7.3 to 10.7 words. Perhaps more important than the mean number of words per breath group is the apparent flexibility within each of the these speakers. Consider the performance of the 68 year old speaker in Figure 9-5. Although his average number of words per breath group is 10.7, three of his breath groups contained only four words while two contained 17 words and one contained 19 words. In short, examination of the length of his breath groups indicates a highly flexible pattern.

For normal speakers, the location of inhalations during paragraph reading does not appear to be related entirely to physiological need, but rather to the syntactical constraints of the material being read. This point can be illustrated by examining the locus of breaths for normal speakers (Beukelman et al., 1986). We assigned a code after every word in the passage to indicate how "appropriate" it is to inhale at that location. Every inhalation was assigned one of the following codes:

4—At locations where most normal speakers inhaled
3—At locations where some normal speakers inhaled
2—At locations where no normal speakers inhaled; however, inhalations at these locations were judged to be grammatically permissible
1—At locations where no normal speakers inhaled; inhalations at these locations were judged to be grammatically impermissible (for example, between the words "the" and "story" in the phrase "This is the story of Sam's first day on the mountain")

Results of this coding for normal speakers appear in Figure 9-5. Note that the overwhelming majority of inhalations for normal speakers was assigned a code of 4, meaning that most normal speakers inhaled at that location.

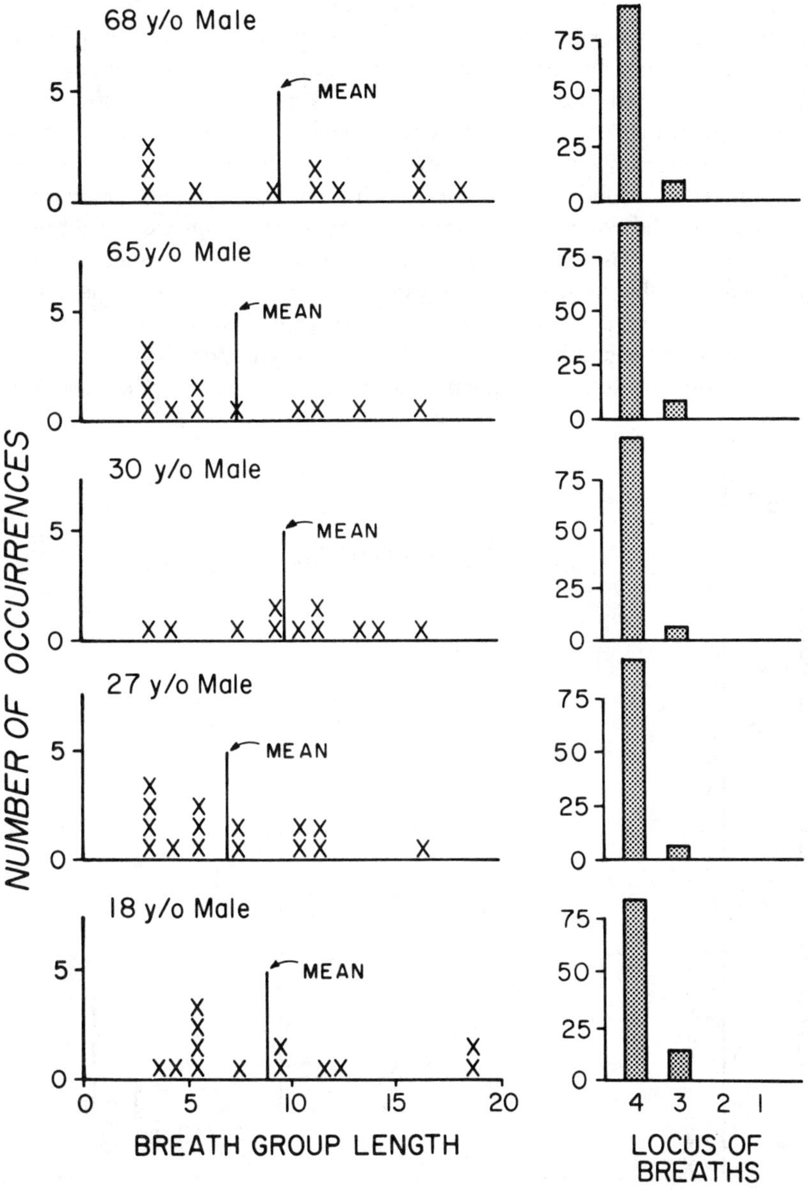

Figure 9-5. Breath group lengths (in words) and locus of breaths codes for five normal male speakers.

The performance of some dysarthric speakers is extremely different from the physiologically flexible, rule-governed performance of normal individuals. Figure 9-6 contains respiratory data during paragraph reading by a brain-injured speaker with predominately ataxic dysarthria. Examination of the figure suggests that most of the time this speaker inhaled after only one or two words. Because short breath groups are frequently associated with reduced respiratory support in dysarthric speakers, it is tempting to speculate that this speaker simply did not have the respiratory support for more extended breath groups. Although this may be the case for some dysarthric speakers, this individual was able to sustain phonation for more than 15 seconds and to count to over 20 on a single breath when instructed to do so. Clearly, he had the physiological capability to avoid grammatically impermissible locations for inhalation. Although this case may be extreme, many dysarthric speakers

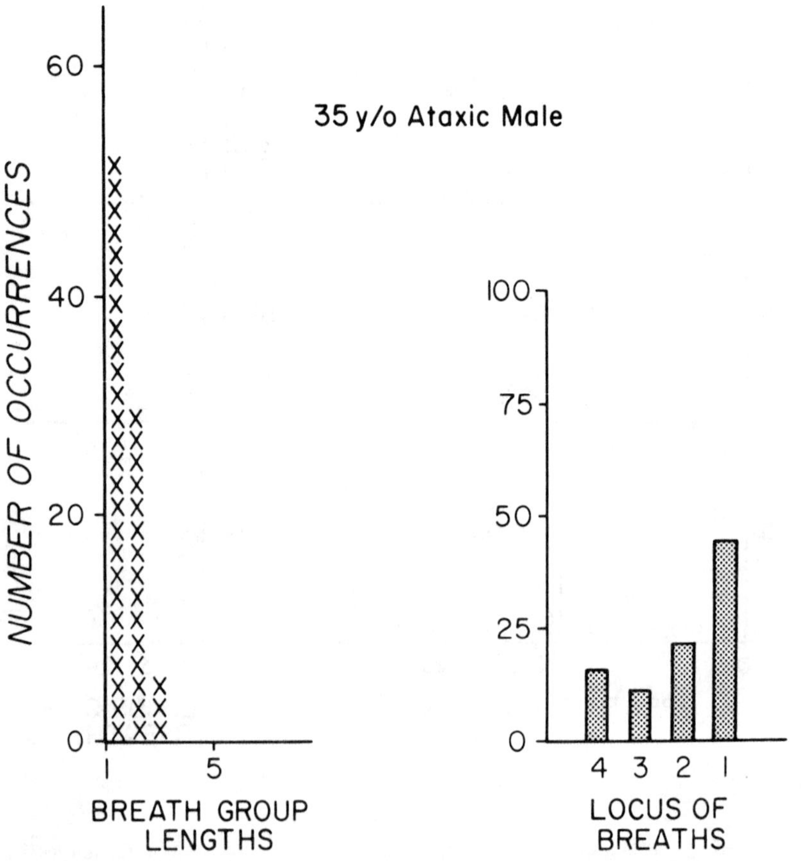

Figure 9-6. Breath group lengths (in words) and locus of breath codes for a predominantly ataxic dysarthric speaker.

disrupt the naturalness of their speech needlessly by taking breaths at grammatically impermissible locations.

In-depth Examination of Respiratory Impairment

Once the presence of inadequate respiratory support has been confirmed through perceptual evaluation, an attempt is made to examine respiratory function in depth. This is typically accomplished with instrumental measurement techniques. The perceptual analysis of respiratory function during connected speech alerts the clinician to a potential problem. A more detailed series of questions are addressed in the in-depth examination. These questions may include the following:

- Is the speaker achieving the primary respiratory goals of a steady energy source during speech?
- How are pressures being generated?
- Does impairment of other speech components contribute to the perception of inadequate respiratory function during speech?
- Is the respiratory impairment physiologically based or does the pattern appear to be related to learned maladaptive patterns?

Adequacy of Respiratory Support

We begin the in-depth evaluation of respiratory function by examining the energy source for speech. Measurement of subglottal air pressure is the most direct approach to access respiratory adequacy for speech. In speakers with tracheostomies, subglottal air pressure can be sensed through the tracheostomy tube or tracheostomy button. However, in speakers without tracheostomy, it is difficult to directly measure subglottal air pressure. Rather, subglottal air pressure levels are estimated by measuring intraoral air pressure during the stop phase of a voiceless stop consonant and estimating the corresponding level of subglottal air pressure. Consider the posturing of the speech mechanism structures during the stop phase of /p/ in the syllable "apa." The respiratory system provides the driving force for speech. The glottis is open for the voiceless phoneme /p/. The oral cavity is a sealed system, because the velopharyngeal port is closed and the lips are closed. Because the glottis is open and the remaining system is sealed, the oral and subglottal cavities can be considered to function as a single cavity from an aerodynamic point of view (Netsell, 1969; Smitheran & Hixon, 1981). During conversational speech, the normal adult's subglottal air pressure level averages between 7 and 10 cm of water pressure.

Although measurement of intraoral air pressure during the stop phase of the voiceless plosive /t/ or /p/ is a good estimate of subglottal air pressure for normal speakers, care must be taken in obtaining and interpreting these measures for dysarthric speakers. One cannot assume that reduced air pressure values for dysarthric speakers are always indicative of respiratory weakness or incoordination. Because subglottal air pressures generated by the compression of the respiratory mechanism may be acted upon by several of the speech valves, it is possible that impairment of the larynx, velopharyngeal mechanism, or oral articulators may also contribute to reduced air pressure values (Hardy, 1966).

If intraoral air pressure is to be used as an estimate of subglottal air pressure, both the velopharyngeal port and the anterior oral cavity must be completely sealed. Simultaneous sensing of nasal airflow through a full face mask is one way of verifying these seals. If nasal airflow is observed, a nose clip should used to obstruct the nasal airflow. If, on subsequent recordings, no airflow was recorded during the stop phase of the consonant, one would assume that the velopharyngeal port had been responsible for the air leak from the oral cavity under the previous condition. With the occlusion of the nasal airflow, one could estimate subglottal air pressure from the intraoral air pressure measure. A comparison of the level of intraoral air pressure measures with and without the nares occluded would provide some indication of the effect of velopharyngeal dysfunction on the speaker's ability to generate adequate air pressures for speech.

If, during the measurement of intraoral air pressure with the nares occluded, airflow was still present, one would assume that the oral seal was inadequate to prevent the escape of air from the oral cavity during the production of the voiceless stop consonant. An attempt would be made to sense intraoral air pressure during the production of a different voiceless consonant in an effort to find a consonant that could be produced without escape of air during the stop phase of the consonant. If this was not possible, intraoral air pressure could not be used as an accurate estimate of subglottal air pressure.

Although aerodynamic estimates of subglottal air pressure are good indicators of the adequacy of respiratory support for speech, this technique requires extensive instrumentation that is not always available clinically. When such instrumentation is unavailable, clinicians may estimate respiratory adequacy with simple devises such as those shown in Figures 9-7 and 9-8. Netsell and Hixon (1978) suggested the use of a manometer with a "leak" tube as an inexpensive means of estimating subglottal air pressure (Figure 9-7). Just as with the aerodynamic transduction equipment described earlier, a velopharyngeal and lip seal is assumed when using a mouth-piece. A full face mask that captures both nasal and oral air flow may be used when either the velopharyngeal or lip seal is inadequate. Using this technique, the client is asked to blow and to maintain a target level of water pressure. Netsell and Hixon give the following clinical rule of thumb, "An individual who can generate and sustain 5 cm H_2O for 5 sec with the 'leak' tube has sufficient pressure capability to meet most speech requirements" (p. 329).

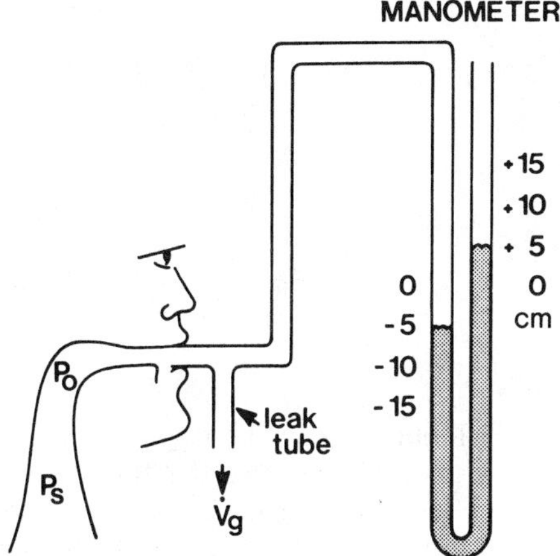

Figure 9-7. A drawing of an individual blowing into a manometer with a "leak" tube and generating 10 cm H_2O (from Netsell & Hixon, 1978).

Hixon, Hawley, and Wilson (1982) suggest an even simpler "homemade" device for determining respiratory driving pressures using a tall (12 cm or more) drinking glass with a straw. After filling the glass with water, the straw is inserted into the water. In Figure 9-8, an individual blowing into the straw would need to generate 10 cm of water pressure in order to initiate the flow of bubbles at the end of the straw.

Many clinicians ask dysarthric individuals to sustain a neutral vowel in order to obtain an indication of respiratory support on a speech-like task. A number of cautions are warranted when using this technique. As was noted earlier, maximum sustained phonation is not a simple task from the standpoint of respiratory control. It reflects phonatory as well as respiratory performance. For example, a speaker with a breathy voice quality due to inefficient laryngeal control will "waste" air with resultant reduction in sustained phonation time. On the other hand, a dysarthric speaker with strained-strangled voice quality may be generating excessive subglottal air pressure in order to initiate phonation. It should also be noted that sustained phonation tasks more accurately reflect maximum respiratory capacity rather than breath support required for a series of breath groups during connected speech. Although most normal individuals can sustain phonation for a longer period of time, a minimum sustained time of 15.0 seconds for adult males and 14.3 seconds for adult females is acceptable (Hirano, Koike, & von Leden, 1968). Remember that the respiratory capabilities of normal individuals are far greater than the respiratory demands for conversational speech. A sustained phonation time of over 15 seconds is unusual in all but the mildest dysarthrias. When speakers are instructed to sustain phonation as long as possible, they usually inhale to lung volume levels much higher than are appropriate for

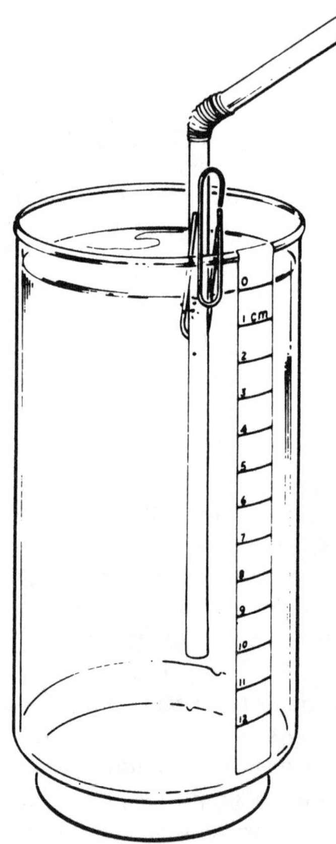

Figure 9-8. A drinking glass with a straw inserted to a depth of 10 cm. This device can be used as an indicator of respiratory driving pressure (from Hixon, Hawley, & Wilson, 1982).

conversational speech. Thus, the dysarthric speaker cannot be expected to produce consecutive breath groups in contextual speech that match in duration the maximal effort seen in sustained phonation. Our approach clinically is not to require maximum phonation, but rather to request that the speaker produce phonation for a relatively brief period of time, four or five seconds. In this way, the task more closely reflects the respiratory demands of connected speech.

Respiratory Movements

APPROACHES TO MEASUREMENT. Observation of the respiratory movements of dysarthric speakers suggests a variety of impairments. Some dysarthric speakers exhibit excessive respiratory movements during speech. In some cases, excessive elevation of the shoulders and expansion of the thorax may be indicative of an effort to compensate for poor abdominal control. In other cases, observations of changes in respiratory shape may reveal paradoxic movements of the thorax and the abdomen. Paradoxing is a maneuver in which the circumference of the thorax is increased during inhalation while the circumference of the abdomen is decreased or vice versa. Because the two movements are, in effect, working at cross purposes, inadequate respiratory support for speech may be the result. In still other cases, dysarthric speakers appear to be attempting to speak at lung volume levels well below those observed for tidal breathing.

Changes in chest wall shape and estimates of lung volume levels can be observed perceptually by placing one hand over the diaphragm and the other on the rib cage. Of course, these perceptual observations are extremely informal and cannot yield precise or objective measures of shape, timing, and respiratory volume. Currently, the most popular devices for objective measurement of respiratory shape are the magnatometer system used by Putnam and Hixon (1984) and described in detail by Hixon and colleagues (1976) and the Respitrace unit described by Hunker and colleagues (1981). Respiratory Inductive Plethysmography (RIP) or Respitrace is a transduction system designed to monitor circumferential size changes in the rib cage and abdomen. The system consists of two coils of insulated wire glued to cotton mesh bands that fit snugly around the speaker's torso (see Figure 9-9). The Respitrace unit electronically sums the individual rib cage and abdominal contributions to obtain a calibrated index of total lung volume change. Results of either the magnatometer system or the Respitrace unit can be displayed in movement-by-time or movement-by-movement (rib-cage-by-abdomen) displays (Abbs, Hunker, & Barlow, 1983; Putnam & Hixon, 1984).

DESCRIPTION OF THE MOVEMENT IMPAIRMENT. Although some dysarthric individuals initiate utterances at lung volume levels similar to normal speakers, many dysarthric individuals with respiratory impairment employ several different patterns that will be reviewed.

Reduced Vital Capacity. Due to reduced vital capacity as compared to normal speakers, some dysarthrics are unable to generate adequate subglottal air pressure amplitudes and durations for functional speech when utterances are initiated at 60 percent of this reduced vital capacity. These individuals may need to routinely initiate utterances at levels greater than 60 percent of vital capacity.

Inconsistent Lung Volume Level. Some dysarthric speakers initiate utterances at the prevailing lung volume level without taking a preparatory breath prior to speech. This pattern is seen in some individuals with head injury. Other individuals initiate utterances at varying lung volume levels. Figure 9-10 illustrates the lung volume levels at which utterances were initiated and terminated by a 28 year old woman with Friedreich's ataxia who was reading a paragraph. This speaker is intelligible, but is producing this passage

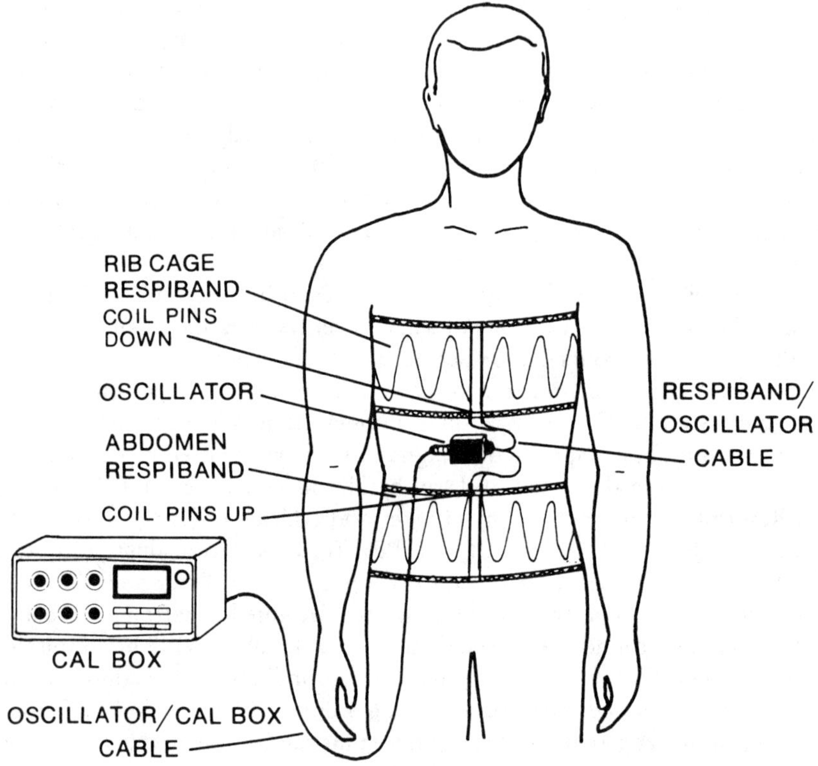

Figure 9-9. A line drawing of the positioning of the rib cage and abdomen Respitrace bands (Ambulatory Monitoring, Inc., Ardsley, New York, 10502).

at a slow rate of 81 wpm. A comparison of this performance with that of the normal speakers in Figure 9-4 suggests many differences. Perhaps the most obvious is the increased number of inhalations produced by the dysarthric speaker. The lung volume level at which she appears to be initiating utterances is generally reduced as compared both to the normal speaker and to her own resting breathing lung volume levels. During speech, this woman does not achieve lung volume levels as high as those she achieves during quiet breathing. The levels at which she inititates utterances are also highly variable. At times she continues to speak at low lung volume levels and fails to return to appropriate levels after inhalation. This is particularly the case with breath group units 11 through 13, where inhalations are insufficient to return the speaker to an appropriate lung volume level. When she fails to return to an appropriate lung volume level, she produces only two or three words before inhaling again.

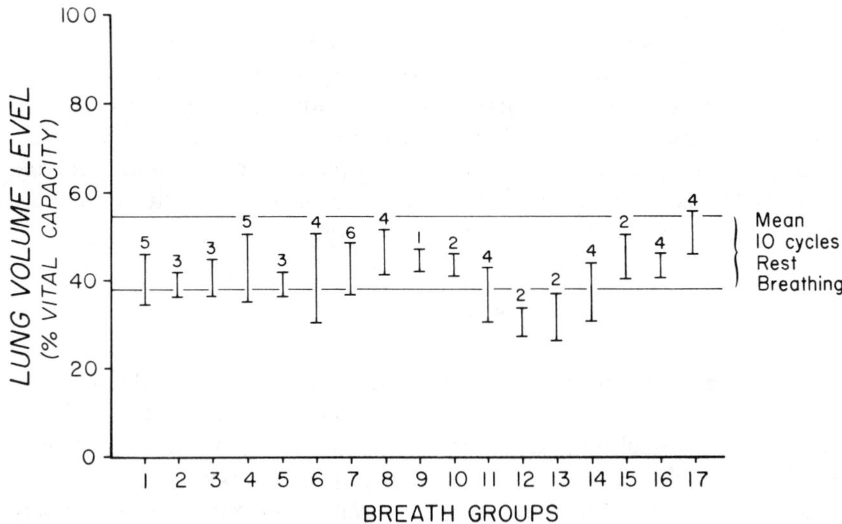

Figure 9-10. Lung volume level produced by an ataxic dysarthric speaker who is reading a portion of the Mount Rainier Paragraph. The range indicates the lung volume levels at which the following breath groups were initiated and terminated: (1) I pointed to the mountain (2) covered with snow, (3) but someone said, (3) "Don't try to show him (4) all that snow. (5) Show Sam some snow." (6) I picked a handful of snow (7) and began (8) to show (9) everyone, (10) but they (11) interrupted and said, (12) "Show Sam (13) some snow." (14) Pretending to be angry, (15) I questioned, (16) "Show Sam some snow? (17) What a ridiculous idea." Also noted as a referent is the range of lung volume level for rest breathing.

Reduced Lung Volume Level. This pattern of lung volume level use has several forms. Many severely dysarthric individuals who are unable to voluntarily modify their rest breathing patterns, and therefore, volume level, initiate inhalation at approximately 60 percent. For those with efficient phonatory and laryngeal systems, this lung volume level range may be adequate for speech. However, many dysarthric individuals need to initiate speech at a lung volume level higher than 60 percent of lung volume level. Other dysarthric individuals will consistently exhale partially before initiating speech. Thus, they inhale to an adequate lung volume level to support speech, but then exhale or allow air wastage before speech is initiated. For some, this pattern may occur because of impairment of laryngeal function, however, for others, the pattern may reflect a maladaptive attempt to compensate for an impairment laryngeal control. Finally, some severely dysarthric individuals are unable to initiate phonation unless they are very low in lung volume level. Then, once phonation is initiated, they have a minimal respiratory reserve for the production of the remainder of the utterance.

Excessive Lung Volume Levels. In an effort to compensate for inefficient phonatory, velopharyngeal, and articulatory function, some dysarthric speakers inhale to excessive lung volume levels prior to the initiation of speech. The resulting high level of subglottal air pressure is associated with excessively loud speech for those who are able to initiate phonation at high lung volume levels. For those who are unable to initiate phonation efficiently at that lung volume level, there may be excessive air wastage.

TREATMENT

The overall treatment goal for respiratory impairments in dysarthria is to achieve a consistent subglottal air pressure level during speech that is produced with minimal fatigue and appropriate breath group lengths. This is usually accomplished by one of a number of general approaches. First, the speaker is taught to compensate for the neuromotor impairment by maximally utilizing their potential respiratory support. Second, the speaker may be involved in an intervention program designed to decrease the extent of neuromotor involvement by using pharmacological therapy or neuromotor training. Third, a prosthetic approach may be used to increase the adequacy of respiratory support for speech. Finally, the impact of the respiratory impairment may be minimized by increasing the efficiency of the laryngeal, velopharyngeal, or oral articulatory valves. The respiratory intervention discussion has been organized in a manner that reflects a sequential approach to the respiratory problems observed in a dysarthric population. The discussion will begin with intervention techniques appropriate for individuals with severe respiratory impairment and proceed through intervention approaches appropriate for the less severely involved.

Establishing Respiratory Support

As in any intervention activity, the clinician is faced with the task of choosing speakers who are candidates for a particular type of treatment program. In an effort to describe speakers for whom basic respiratory patterns for speech must be developed, we have included the following characteristics:

1. The speaker has estimated levels of subglottal air pressure of 3 cm H_20 or less on speech or speech-like tasks
2. The speaker is unable to sustain consistent air pressure (at or above a given level) for two seconds
3. The speaker is unable to generate adequate subglottal air pressure to support phonation
4. The speaker has such limited respiratory support or control for speech that a one-word-at-a-time speech pattern is used during connected speech

Production of Consistent Subglottal Air Pressure

The production of a consistent level of subglottal air pressure is a primary goal of the respiratory function during speech. Netsell and Daniel (1979) reported a biofeedback approach to train a flaccid dysarthric client to sustain air pressures within the range used for speech (5 to 10 cm H_20). At the beginning of treatment their client generated only 2 to 3 cm H_20 for no more than three seconds. They instructed their client to blow into the pressure sensor (a water manometer) as a "leak tube" allowed air to escape at a rate associated with normal phonation (75 to 125 cc/sec). These authors report that their client was able to generate 10 cm H_20 for 10 seconds by the end of the eight 20-minute training sessions.

In our clinical practice, we have modified the simple device described by Hixon and colleagues (1982) by using slightly different materials. We use a plastic bottle with a hole in the cover. A tube is then inserted through the hole and into the water. We have found this approach useful as a training tool, as the plastic materials do not break when dropped, and the cover on the bottle does not allow water to be expelled when excessive air pressures are generated by some ataxic dysarthric speakers.

Another approach to training sustained air pressure generation is to use an air pressure transducer similar to that described in the assessment section. The output from the pressure sensing system is displayed on an oscilloscope for feedback information to the speaker. The target air pressure levels can be set on the oscilloscopic screen using a second cursor. We have used this air pressure feedback approach with head-injured individuals who demonstrate difficulty in maintaining consistent air pressure levels or who produce excessively large air pressure values during speech. Rather than attempt to train them during speech, we have simplified their task by initially training them during nonspeech activities. Generally, training is continued until they are able to sustain intraoral air pressures at approximately 5 cm H_2O for five seconds or until their performance plateaus. Although it is clear that sustaining 5 cm H_20 for 5 seconds is not normal performance, we typically stop training on this task when "5 for 5" target (Netsell & Hixon, 1978) has been achieved. We do this at least in part because our goal is "easy" production rather than maximal production. At times, forced performances encourage the speaker to exhale to excessively low lung volume levels. We do not wish to encourage a habit that may be maladaptive for speech.

In addition to the blowing techniques, another approach to train consistent air pressure generation is to have the client produce sustained vowel sounds. The intensity level of the vowel can be monitored on a VU meter or with an intensity measurement device such as a Visipitch. This task can be used successfully only if laryngeal control is good. It is a more difficult task than the nonspeech tasks described previously. Once respiratory support for sustained phonation can be controlled, we usually attempt to involve the client in tasks that are more speech-like, such as the repetition of syllables. Air pressure can then be monitored with a pressure sensing tube inserted through the corner of the mouth. Vocal intensity can also be monitored using an intensity measurement system.

Finally, clients can be instructed to produce consistent phonation while producing utterances. Utterance lengths are selected so that the speaker is physiologically able to produce the entire utterance in one breath. The air pressure is monitored by constructing the utterances containing many tokens of the phoneme /p/ and sensing the air pressure during those productions as described before. Measurement of vocal intensity during utterances of this type is less effective than aerodynamic measurement, because of the various levels of sound energy associated with different vowel and consonant sounds.

Postural Adjustments

Some dysarthric speakers are unable to develop consistent air pressure values in the seated position. In these situations, postural adjustments and/or prosthetic assistance may be necessary. Posture frequently affects the respiratory support patterns for severely dysarthric individuals. Hardy (1983) reviewed the situation for speakers with cerebral palsy:

> Another procedure that I have frequently seen used is to work with the speaker in a supine position. When the body is upright, gravity pulls the abdominal contents down and thus flattens the diaphragm. In a supine position, those contents will tend to push the diaphragm into the thoracic cavity and thus assist in expiration. There is again, a trade-off, in that inspiratory ability will not be as good since the diaphragm must push against the abdominal contents for inflation of the lungs. (p. 153)

Although Hardy (1964) suggests that there is little difference in the respiratory function of the severely cerebral-palsied individual as a result of static differences in posture, we have observed many dysarthrics, including individuals with head injury, spinal cord injury, and multiple sclerosis, who were able to generate the respiratory support to speak with phonation in the supine and not the seated position. It appears that individuals with greater impairment of the expiratory rather than the inspiratory musculature benefit from posture adjustments. Thus, the "stronger" inspiratory muculature is able to inhale against the added pressure of the abdominal contents and the "weaker" expiratory muscles are benefited by the expiratory forces created by the abdominal contents in the supine position. For the speaker with inspiratory inadequacy, such as ALS or obstructive lung disease, the supine position makes breathing and respiration for speech more difficult. Readers are referred to Putnam and Hixon (1983) for an excellent description of the effect of position on respiratory function in individuals with motoneuron disease.

For speakers who benefit from the postural adjustment, appropriate position can be accomplished by placing the individual in a wheelchair or lawnchair with an adjustable back (Collins, Rosenbek, & Donahue, 1982). Some clients benefit from an adjustment in their posture to provide increased respiratory support for speech during the aspects of the treatment program that focus on phonatory or articulatory proficiency. However, such a speaker might be postured in the seated position while focusing on improving respiratory function. Also, this type of individual should be positioned for maximal respiratory support during times when they are conversing with family, staff, and friends.

Respiratory Prostheses

Two types of respiratory prostheses are utilized to supplement expiratory forces during speech. The abdominal binder (corset) has been used routinely with individuals with spinal cord injury who have intact diaphragmatic innervation but minimal or no innervation of the expiratory musculature. For some individuals with multiple sclerosis and head injury, the abdominal binder provides improved respiratory support for speech. Westlake and Rutherford (1961) suggested the use of abdominal binders for individuals with developmental dysarthria. Hardy (1983), however, does not recommend this procedure for cerebral-palsied speakers. As with postural adjustment, the binder is ineffective and potentially dangerous for the speaker with inspiratory weakness. Because the abdominal binder potentially interferes with inspiration, its use in treatment must involve medical approval and supervision.

A second type of abdominal prosthesis is the expiratory "board" or "paddle" described by Rosenbek and LaPointe (1985). A board is attached to a speaker's wheelchair such that it can be swung into position just anterior to the abdominal musculature. As individuals prepare to speak, they lean forward into the board, thus increasing the expiratory forces. Because individuals can lean back away from the board, this approach does not interfere with inhalation. The efficient use of the board requires some trunkal strength and balance to lean forward and back at the appropriate times without interfering with phonatory or articulatory proficiency. We have found that occasionally the expiratory board is useful; however, usually the speakers who need it most do not have the trunk balance and strength to use it effectively.

Stabilizing the Respiratory Pattern

Even after dysarthric individuals can produce the levels of air pressure necessary for speech, some still manage their respiratory systems very inconsistently. For example, persons with severe dysarthria due to head injury may initiate an utterance at any point in the rest breathing cycle. Some individuals with cerebral palsy may initiate utterances at a variety of lung volume levels; some may be initiated at appropriate levels and others at very inappropriate levels. Dysarthric speakers with several different respiratory patterns are candidates for a respiratory pattern stablization program

1. The speaker initiates phonation at inappropriate lung volume levels that may be either too high or too low
2. The speaker initiates breath groups without taking a preparatory inhalation
3. The speaker initiates breath groups at inconsistent lung volume levels
4. The speaker consistently produces utterances that are excessively loud or quiet
5. The speaker does not terminate a breath group at an appropriate lung volume level, but rather continues to speak until reaching an excessively low lung volume level.

Lung Volume Level

The first step to stablize the respiratory pattern of severe and moderately severe dysarthric speakers is to identify a functional lung volume level range. The range that is selected is an individual judgment, however, normal speakers generally inhale to approximately 60 percent of lung volume level. Hardy (1983) recommends that prior to the production of an utterance, individuals with cerebral palsy inspire to "a relatively high lung-volume level where the relaxation recoil of the respiratory system will assist in generating the needed air pressure in the vocal tract. . ." (p. 154). He recommends this pattern because few individuals with cerebral palsy are able to produce adequate support for speech below the resting respiratory level. Before an optimal inspiratory lung volume level for speech can be determined, the ability of the speaker to check the recoil air pressure generated at high lung volume levels must be assessed. Obviously, there is no reason to have an individual inhale to such high lung volume levels that air pressure cannot be controlled.

For some dysarthric speakers with good control of expiratory musculature, the target inspiratory level for speech may be set at or above 60 percent of lung volume level. For individuals who do not have the ability to inspire to a lung volume level greater than peak tidal volume, the goal is to begin each utterance precisely at that referent level. The lower end of the lung volume level range for speech is also established informally. Usually, speakers are discouraged from exhaling to lung volume levels that elicit abnormal reflexes, result in a change in phonatory quality, or are excessively fatiguing.

The approach for identifying and training a speaker to achieve appropriate lung volume levels for speech depends on the equipment that is available. Water spirometry will assist the clinician in establishing lung volume levels. However, dysarthric individuals often have difficulty speaking into the closed system of a water spirometer during the training activities.

The objective approaches to assess respiratory shape have been very useful in lung volume level training. As mentioned previously, the Respitrace and magnatometers are useful for this type of training, with results displayed on an oscilloscope for feedback purposes. In the past, we have used mercury strain gauges for this type of training. They were more effective than estimating lung volume level visually, but they were much less stable than the Respitrace or the magnatometer approaches. When strain gauges are employed, we found that target levels needed to be adjusted whenever the speaker shifted positions even slightly.

Chest Wall Shape

As was introduced earlier, the respiratory system can be considered an aerodynamic cavity within the chest wall. Hardy (1983) has suggested that there is no "best" respiratory shape pattern for a dysarthric speaker. Generally, we agree, however, there are speakers who have adopted chest wall shape patterns that are extremely fatiguing or maladaptive. In these cases, an attempt is made to teach them a more effective respiratory pattern. For example, a woman with ALS came to our clinic complaining of reduced vocal loudness and fatigue after talking for a period of time. Our evaluation revealed that she was using a paradoxic respiratory pattern. To increase the volume of the thorax, she elevated her shoulders excessively as she increased rib cage circumference. Simultaneous with the increase in rib cage circumference, abdominal circumference decreased. Using a Respitrace system, we trained her to enlarge the circumference of the abdomen or at least stablize the circumference of the abdomen as the rib cage expanded during inhalation. Following two sessions, she learned the new pattern and found that she no longer needed to elevate her shoulders excessively during inhalation. The result was a speech pattern with greater vocal loudness and less fatigue.

Eliminating Abnormal Respiratory Behaviors

The task of eliminating abnormal respiratory behaviors occurs throughout respiratory training. We have included a specific section because some dysarthric speakers have compensated for their motor impairment with behaviors that are now maladaptive. This situation occurs quite frequently with head-injured dysarthric individuals. A case report will illustrate this point. Betty demonstrated a maladaptive respiratory pattern after being injured during a helicopter crash. Early in her recovery, her speech mechanism was so inefficient that she spoke in single syllable utterances and inhaled at the beginning of every syllable. When Betty came to our center, she demonstrated the unusual respiratory pattern of inhaling during or after the first syllable of each utterance, even though she had just inhaled prior to the beginning of the utterance, and her breath groups averaged about four words in length. Evidently, she retained the abnormal respiratory pattern she had adopted earlier in recovery.

Increasing Respiratory Flexibility

The mildly dysarthric speaker usually has accomplished the respiratory goals presented in the previous sections. Usually, the remaining focus of treatment is to increase the flexibility with which the respiratory system is controlled during speech, so that the naturalness of the overall speech pattern can be improved. During this phase of treatment, the stabilized respiratory patterns taught to the severely dysarthric individual may need to be modified. Candidates for this phase of respiratory intervention usually include:

1. Speakers who produce utterances with stereotypic breath group lengths
2. Speakers who never pause without inhaling
3. Speakers who are unable to manage the "quick" inhalation needed to support the short breath group utterance

Adjusting Lung Volume Levels

Normal speakers support their overall speech patterns with subtle adjustments of the respiratory system. For example, in anticipation of loud speech, the normal speaker will inhale to a high lung volume level to take advantage of the greater recoil pressures that will be generated. A similar respiratory maneuver occurs where the speaker anticipates an unusually long breath group. During the production of an extremely long utterance, the normal speaker may pause to inhale and replenish the air supply in the lungs. If the speaker is near the end of the utterance, however, a small inhalation will be taken. If an extensive amount of the utterance remains to be spoken, a larger inhalation will occur. The stabilized breath patterning described earlier for severely dysarthric individuals is simply not subtle enough to support this type of flexible speech performance.

Levels of Training

Training in respiratory flexibility occurs at three levels. Cognitively, the client is taught the general rules that govern respiratory performance during speech. For initial practice, the dysarthric speaker reads paragraphs in which the respiratory patterns have been marked. Next, conversational scripts for two speakers are prepared. The respiratory patterns have been marked in the dysarthric speaker's "lines." Finally, the dysarthric speaker reads aloud or speaks conversationally without the aid of the respiratory pattern markings.

Performance is audio- or video-recorded and discussed. An attempt is made to relate the content of the passage to the interests of the client. The following paragraph was developed for a retired man with parkinsonism. The slashes signal breath group boundaries.

> / For twenty five years / I have been a member / of the Upland Gamebird Club. / For about five years/ I was the president. / We work to preserve habitat / for the birds. / We also lobby the Game Department / for fair hunting seasons. / As you can guess, / that is a matter of opinion. / I have enjoyed the Club / a great deal. / My wife and I travel a lot. / I used to do a lot of speaking, / until the Parkinson's disease / started to affect my voice. / My wife used to complain / that I worked for the Club / and sold insurance on the side.

The following is an example of a dialogue with a dysarthric head-injured young woman named Pat.

David: Hi
Pat: / Hello
David: How are you today?
Pat: / OK / How are you?
David: Fine. Tell me about your weekend pass.
Pat: / It was great. / We went / to the game / on Saturday. / It was / a beautiful day. / My brother / played a good game. / It was good / to be outside / again.
David: Who went with you?
Pat: I went / with Mom and Dad. / Jim's girlfriend / came too.

Maximizing Speech Naturalness

A second goal in increasing the flexibility of respiratory support for the mildly dysarthric speaker is to teach natural stress patterning. A detailed discussion of stress pattern training can be found in Chapter 14. Because the breath group may be the unit of prosody, adequate respiratory control and appropriate phrasing are necessary for natural speech.

Flexibility may also be added to the speech of dysarthric individuals by teaching them to pause without inhalation. Because of the respiratory patterns developed by some dysarthric speakers early in recovery, inhalation occurs at every pause. Thus, they do not produce the momentary pause without inhalations that are so commonly used in speech of nonimpaired individuals to add emphasis. Bellaire, Yorkston, and Beukelman (in press) reported a case study of such a speaker. This young man was taught to increase his speech naturalness by increasing his average breath group length and including momentary pauses in his speech pattern. The training sequence utilized was very similar to that described in the previous section. For a more complete discussion of speech naturalness for dysarthric speakers, see Chapter 14.

REFERENCES

Abbs, J. (1985). Motor impairment difference in orofacial and respiratory speech control with cerebellar disorders: A response to Hixon and Hoit (1984). *Journal of Speech & Hearing Disorders, 50*, 306–312.

Abbs, J., Hunker, C., & Barlow, S. (1983). Differential speech motor subsystem impairments with suprabulbar lesions: Neurophysiological framework and supporting data. In W. Berry (Ed.), *Clinical dysarthria*. Austin, TX: PRO-ED.

Bellaire, K., Yorkston, K.M., & Beukelman, D.R. (1986). Modification of breath patterning to increase naturalness of a mildly dysarthric speaker. *Journal of Communication Disorders*, *19*, 271–280.

Beukelman, D.R., Yorkston, K.M, Dowden, P.A, & Minifie, F.D. (1986, February). *Impact of speaking rate reduction on respiratory patterns of non-impaired and dysarthric speakers*. Paper presented at the third biennal Clinical Dysarthria Conference, Tucson, AZ.

Collins, M., Rosenbek, J., & Donahue, E. (1982). The effects of posture on speech in ataxic dysarthria. *ASHA, 24*, 767.

Darley, F., Aronson, A., & Brown, J. (1975). *Motor speech disorders*. Philadelphia: W. B. Saunders.

Folkins, J.W., & Kuehn, D.P. (1982). Speech production. In N.J. Lass, L.V. McReynolds, J. Northern, & D. Yoder (Eds.), *Speech, language & Hearing: Vol. 1. Normal processes*. Philadelphia: W.B. Saunders.

Hardy, J. (1964). Lung function of athetoid and spastic quadriplegic children. *Develop. Med. Child Neurol., 6*, 378–388.

Hardy, J. (1966). Suggestions for physiological research in dysarthria. *Cortex, 3*, 123–137.

Hardy, J. (1983). *Cerebral palsy*. Englewood Cliffs, NJ: Prentice-Hall.

Hirano, M., Koike, Y., & von Leden, H. (1968). Maximum phonation time and air usage during phonation. *Folia Phoniatrica. 20*, 185.

Hixon, T. (1973) Respiratory function in speech. In F. Minifie, T. Hixon, F. Williams (Eds.), *Normal aspects of speech, hearing, and language* (pp. 73–126). Englewood Cliffs, NJ: Prentice-Hall.

Hixon, T. (1982). Speech breathing kinematics and mechanism interferences therefrom. In S. Grillner, A. Persson, B. Lindbolm, & J. Lubker (Eds.), *Speech motor control*. New York: Pergamon Press.

Hixon, T. (1984). *Parameter-based evaluation of speech breathing functions in dysarthria*. Presentation at the Annual Convention of the Speech-Language-Hearing Association, San Francisco, CA.

Hixon, T., Hawley, J., & Wilson, J. (1982). An around-the-house device for the clinical determination of respiratory driving pressure: A note on making simple even simpler. *Journal of Speech & Hearing Disorders, 47*, 413.

Hixon, T. & Hoit, J. (1984). Differential subsystem impairment, differential motor system impairment, and decomposition of respiratory movement in ataxic dysarthria: A spurious trilogy. *Journal of Speech & Hearing Disorders, 49*, 435–441.

Hixon, T. & Hoit, J. (1985). Reply to Abbs (1985). *Journal of Speech & Hearing Disorders, 50*, 312–317.

Hixon, T.J. (1987). *Respiratory function in speech and song*. San Diego: College-Hill Press.

Hixon, T.J., Mead, J., & Goldman, M. (1976). Dynamics of the chest wall during speech production: Function of the thorax, rib cage, diaphragm, and abdomen. *Journal of Speech & Hearing Research, 19*, 297–356.

Hixon, T.J., Putnam, A., & Sharpe, J. (1983). Speech production with flaccid paralysis of the rib cage, diaphragm, and abdomen. *Journal of Speech & Hearing Disorders, 48*, 315–327.

Hunker, C., Bless, D., & Weismer, G. (1981). Respiratory inductive plethysmography: A clinical technique for assessing respiratory function for speech. Paper presented at the Annual Convention of the American Speech-Language-Hearing Association, Los Angeles, CA.

Kim, R. (1968). The chronic residual respiratory disorder in post-encephalitic parkinsonism. *Journal of Neurology, Neurosurgery, & Psychiatry, 31*, 398–398.

Netsell, R. (1969). Subglottal and intraoral air pressures during the intervocalic contrast of /t/ and /d/. *Phonetica, 20*, 68–73.

Netsell, R. (1973). Speech physiology. In F.D. Minifie, T.J. Hixon, & F. Williams (Eds.), *Normal aspects of speech, hearing, and language* (pp. 211–234). Englewood Cliffs, NJ: Prentice-Hall.

Netsell, R., & Daniel, B. (1979). Dysarthria in adults: Physiologic approach to rehabilitation. *Archives of Physical Medicine & Rehabilitation, 40*, 166–174.

Netsell, R., & Hixon, T.J. (1978). A noninvasive method for clinically estimating subglottal air pressure. *Journal of Speech & Hearing Disorders, 43*, 326–330.

Putnam, A., & Hixon, T.J. (1984). Respiratory kinematics in speakers with motor neuron disease. In M. McNeil, J. Rosenbek, & A. Aronson, (Eds.), *The dysarthrias*. San Diego: College-Hill Press, 1984.

Rosenbek, J.C., & LaPointe, L.L. (1985). The dysarthrias: Description, diagnosis, and treatment. In D.F. Johns (Eds.), *Clinical management of neurogenic communication disorders*. Boston: Little, Brown.

Smitheran, J., & Hixon, T., (1981). A clinical method for estimating laryngeal airway resistance during vowel production. *Journal of Speech & Hearing Research, 46*, 138–146.

Westlake, H., & Rutherford, D. (1961). *Speech Therapy for the Cerebral Palsied*. Chicago: National Society for Crippled Children & Adults, Inc.

Weismer, G. (1985). Speech breathing: Contemporary views and findings. In R. Daniloff (Ed.), *Speech science: Recent advances*. San Diego: College-Hill Press.

APPENDIX TO CHAPTER 9:
Mount Rainier Paragraph

Believe me, my goal is not to perfect your knowledge of nature or any of its attributes, but let's record the story of Sam's first day on the mountain. Unbelievably, this was the first time that he had seen Mount Rainier. It was a perfect day. I didn't know what to show him first. "Show Sam some snow," someone said. I pointed to the mountain covered with snow, but someone said, "Don't try to show him all that snow. Show Sam some snow." I picked a handful of snow and began to show everyone, but they interrupted again and said, "Show Sam some snow." Pretending to be angry, I questioned, "Show Sam some snow? What a ridiculous idea."

CHAPTER 10

Laryngeal Function

Clinical Issues: We were asked to evaluate the "voice" problems of a 23 year old severely dysarthric young man. Prior to evaluation we reviewed his medical records and discovered that he suffered a closed head injury with brain stem contusion one year earlier. Upon admission to the rehabilitation unit three months post onset, the list of medical problems included spastic quadraplegia, swallowing difficulty, anarthria, reduced memory, and cognitive impairment. During the course of inpatient rehabilitation, his physical recovery proceeded gradually. At the time of discharge, he was wheelchair dependent and communicated using a portable typing-based communication augmentation device. Six months after discharge the speech/language pathologist associated with a home health agency referred the patient for a voice evaluation, because she felt that lack of voluntary phonation was limiting the return of his speech. He was beginning to mouth words and to achieve some voicing, according to his parents, "when he wanted to." These episodes of phonation usually occurred when he was lying in bed. When preparing for this evaluation with our student intern, we asked that she be prepared to answer the following questions after completing the evaluation:

- *How do you assess voice production when episodes of voicing occur only once or twice per week?*
- *What factors appear to be contributing to the occasional episodes of voicing?*
- *What is this speaker's level of respiratory function, and how do you decide if respiratory function is adequate to support phonation?*
- *What factors other than respiratory or phonatory control need to be considered when evaluating the voice of severely dysarthric speakers?*
- *What approaches may be appropriate for improving the voice of this individual?*

Phonatory aspects of dysarthria are clinically important for a number of reasons. Phonatory disorders are not only very common among dysarthric speakers but also play an important role in differential diagnosis. Identification of laryngeal signs and symptoms plays a key role in the early differential diagnosis of some progressive disorders such as parkinsonism (Logemann, Fisher, Boshes, & Blonsky, 1978) and myasthenia gravis (Aronson, 1971). With the more severely involved dysarthric speaker, examination of phonatory characteristics may yield important information about the underlying neuropathology. A thorough understanding of the phonatory aspects of dysarthria also is important when planning intervention for speakers at all levels of severity. For the severely involved, inability to produce voice is, at times, the feature that prevents functional speech. Without voluntary phonation, some brain-injured individuals cannot take advantage of their residual articulatory movements. For the somewhat less severely involved, phonatory aspects of speech production warrant attention because imprecise phonatory control prevents some speakers from producing the voiced/voiceless distinctions that are important in speech intelligibility. For the mildly involved dysarthric speaker, phonatory aspects of speech are important contributors to speech naturalness.

NORMAL LARYNGEAL FUNCTION

Neuromotor Function

Production of voice depends on the interaction of the respiratory, phonatory, and resonance components of speech. Although all of these components play a role in the production of the perceptual features of the voice, this chapter will only contain a description of neuromotor aspects of the laryngeal system. A more detailed description of the respiratory requirements for speech is found in Chapter 9 and the resonance system is found in Chapter 11.

The primary vegetative function of the larynx is to protect the airway from entry of foreign material while swallowing. Superimposed on this important vegetative function is voicing. The muscles of the larynx may be divided into two groups: (1) The extrinsic muscles, innervated by cranial nerves V, VII, and XII, are responsible for fixation, elevation, and lowering the position of the larynx. (2) The intrinsic muscles, innervated by the vagus nerve (cranial nerve X), are responsible for the opening and closing of the glottis. Functions of the intrinsic laryngeal musculature include:

- assistance in respiration
- phonation
- protection during swallowing
- assistance in increasing muscular mechanical advantage

Readers are referred to other sources for more comprehensive discussion of normal voice production and neurologic phonatory disorders. (Aronson, 1980; Barlow, Netsell, & Hunker, 1986; Boone, 1977; Prator & Swift, 1984).

Measurement of Laryngeal Function

Generally, we find six parameters to be useful in describing the laryngeal function during speech:

1. Vocal intensity. This is a measure of the level of sound energy produced and is perceptually interpreted as loudness.
2. Fundamental frequency. This reflects the number of vibratory cycles of the vocal folds per second and is perceived as pitch.
3. Vocal quality. This refers to the regularity of the vibratory cycle of the vocal folds and is perceptually described by a variety of terms, including breathiness, roughness, harshness, and hoarseness.
4. Timing of the initiation and cessation of glottal closure for voicing. This aspect of phonation is particularly important in the production of distinctions between voiced and voiceless consonants.
5. Position of the vocal folds on a moment by moment basis. This involves identification of adduction (movement of the vocal folds toward the midline of the laryngeal airway) and abduction (movement of the vocal folds away from the midline) of the laryngeal airway.
6. Aerodynamic resistance of the vocal folds to subglottal air pressure. Laryngeal resistance is the extent to which the larynx offers opposition to the flow of air through it (Smitheran & Hixon, 1981). It is not measured directly but calculated from the ratio of translaryngeal air pressure (the difference between tracheal and pharyngeal pressures) to translaryngeal air flow. Data can also be displayed as subglottal air pressure estimates against laryngeal air flow (Netsell, Lotz, & Shaughnessy, 1984).

Each of these parameters will be described in more detail later in the discussion of assessment of phonatory dysfunction in dysarthria.

Normal phonation requires precise motor control. When weakness, slowness, or incoordination exists in the laryngeal musculature, deviations from normal are heard in the voice. Aronson (1980) describes both normal function and deviation from normal in the following passage:

> The vocal folds must be adducted to the midline and kept there with balanced and bilaterally symmetrical adductor-abductor muscle tonus. Thyroarytenoid and cricothyroid muscle tension must be optimum. Glottal opening and closing has to be precisely timed, the folds adducted at the exact moment for onset of voiced consonants and vowels, and abducted for voiceless. Should they adduct too soon, voiceless sounds would be voiced; too late, voiced sounds would be voiceless. Yet they must not overadduct, for then they would obstruct the exhaled airstream and produce transient changes in voice quality and loudness; should such adduction become extreme, phonation will cease. The extrinsic muscles of the larynx must

be able to elevate and depress the larynx in the neck, otherwise pitch variation will be restricted. On the other hand, if fluctuations are excessive, pitch will change unexpectedly and inappropriately (p. 77.)

LARYNGEAL ASPECTS OF DYSARTHRIA

Because laryngeal signs and symptoms of dysarthria are closely related to the underlying neuropathology, phonatory aspects of the various dysarthrias may be quite distinctive. The following section will contain a description of the laryngeal/phonatory dysfunction observed in the common dysarthrias. The perceptual and physical characteristics of dysphonias associated with dysarthria appear in Table 10-1. Readers should note that there is also a group of neurogenic voice disorders, including paralysis of the vocal folds peripherally below the level of the pharyngeal branch of the Xth nerve, that may not be associated with a generalized dysarthria. These disorders are reviewed in detail elsewhere (Aronson, 1980; Prator & Swift, 1984) and will not be reviewed in this text.

Flaccid Dysarthria

Lesions of the vagus nerve above the level of the pharyngeal nerve branch affects a number of muscles important for speech production, including muscles of the soft palate, pharynx, and the intrinsic laryngeal muscles (Aronson, 1980; Prator & Swift, 1984). These lesions may be either unilateral or bilateral and arise from traumatic injury, vascular disorders, myasthenia gravis, Guillain-Barré syndrome, amyotrophic lateral sclerosis (ALS), and multiple sclerosis (MS). With such lesions, the vocal folds are paralyzed and fixed in the abducted position. Some symptoms of this disorder that are related to impairment in velopharyngeal function include hypernasality, nasal emission, and decreased palatopharyngeal gag. Other symptoms are related to impaired laryngeal function, including breathy voice quality, hoarseness, reduced vocal loudness, low vocal pitch, and a weak or mushy cough. Difficult swallowing, nasal regurgitation, and aspiration of secretion may also be present. Perceptual and physical characteristics of one type of flaccid dysarthria (that associated with myasthenia gravis) appear in Table 10-1.

Spastic Dysarthria

Voice disorders associated with upper motoneuron lesions are found when there is bilateral damage to the cerebral cortex or the corticobulbar fibers. Unilateral cortical or corticobulbar lesions do not typically cause unilateral vocal cord paralysis because of considerable innervation to the laryngeal muscles from the ipsilateral side as well as the contralateral side. This redundancy is thought to have developed because the vegetative function to protect

TABLE 10-1. Laryngeal-Phonatory Characteristics of the Dysarthrias

Flaccid Dysarthria of Myasthenia Gravis

Perceptual: Breathy voice quality; weak intensity; deterioration of phonation during stressful counting or other prolonged speaking activities; reduced sharpness of cough after stressful speaking; can exist in the absence of remaining signs of dysarthria

Physical: In milder cases, vocal folds may appear normal in structure and function despite dysphonia; absence of positive laryngology findings does not exclude presence of milder degree of bilateral adductor weakness of vocal folds; in more severe cases, folds may fail to adduct and abduct completely, bilaterally; bowing may be present

Pseudobulbar (Spastic) Dysarthria

Perceptual: Hoarseness or harshness with a strained-strangled quality; abnormally low pitch; monopitch; loudness is reduced; monoloudness; almost never occurs without accompanying signs of dysarthria; inappropriate crying or laughter may be present

Physical: Vocal folds appear normal in structure; normal to hyperadduction of true and false vocal folds may occur bilaterally

Mixed Dysarthria of Amyotrophic Lateral Sclerosis

Perceptual: Hoarseness or harshness having a strained-strangled quality; "wet" or "gurgly" component; rapid tremor or "flutter" on vowel prolongation; breathy if strong flaccid component; pitch is abnormally low; monopitch; loudness is reduced; monoloudness; inhalatory stridor if severe; reduced sharpness of cough; inappropriate crying or laughter may be present

Physical: Vocal folds appear normal in structure; If major component is spastic, vocal folds appear to adduct normally or may hyperadduct, along with false vocal folds; adduction may be bilaterally symmetric, or one vocal fold may adduct less fully than the other; if there is a major flaccid component, vocal folds may adduct and abduct with less than normal excursions.

Hypokinetic Dysarthria of Parkinsonism

Perceptual: Monopitch; reduced stress; monoloudness; reduced loudness; harsh voice quality; breathy voice quality; note: reduced loudness and breathiness in the absence of other neurologic signs can indicate early parkinsonism

Physical: Vocal folds appear normal in structure; adductor, abductor movements are bilaterally symmetric, but there may be complete closure of vocal folds, accounting for breathy voice quality

Ataxic Dysarthria

Perceptual: Frequently normal; Others have harsh voice quality; monopitch; monoloudness; excess and equal stress on ordinarily unstressed words or syllables; excess loudness; bursts of loudness; coarse voice tremor

Physical: Vocal folds appear normal in structure and function

(continued)

TABLE 10-1 *(continued)*

Hyperkinetic Dysarthria of Chorea

Perceptual: Imtermittently harsh, strained-strangled voice quality; transient breathiness; distorted vowels; monopitch; excess loudness variations; monoloudness; excess, equal stress on ordinarily unstressed words or sylables; reduced stress; sudden forced inspiration/expiration

Physical: Vocal folds appear normal in structure and function

Hyperkinetic Dysarthria of Dystonia

Perceptual: Slow, continous changes in strained-hoarse quality; breathiness; excess loudness variations; voice arrests; monopitch; monoloudness; reduced stress; excess and equal stress on ordinarily unstressed syllables and words

Physical: Vocal folds appear normal in structure and function; however, their physiology has not been studied in detail

Hyperkinetic Dysarthria of Organic (Essential) Tremor

Perceptual: Quavering or intermittent voice arrests during contextual speech; rhythmic tremor and/or voice arrests on vowel prolongation ranging from approximately 5-12 c/sec; note: in severe organic voice tremor, the voice arrests take the form of severe laryngospasm that may be mistaken for the syndrome of spastic (spasmodic) dysphonia; patients with voice arrests may show a smoothing out of these arrests into ordinary tremor when sustaining a vowel at a high pitch level; fluctuating strained-hoarseness along with tremor in more severe cases

Physical: Vocal folds appear normal in structure; on vowel prolongation, adductor-abductor oscillations synchronous with voice tremor can be seen as well as pharyngeal wall movements; tremor movements of larynx can be seen under skin of neck, with the larynx oscillating vertically; voice arrests occur at the maximum laryngeal height of each oscillation

Hyperkinetic Dysarthria of Palatopharyngeaolaryngeal Myoclonus

Perceptual: Momentary voice arrests during contextual speech is severe, but often undetectable; on vowel prolongation, momentary voice arrests occur rhythmically, ranging from 60-240 beats per minute (1 to 4 c/sec), note: because vowel prolongation often is undetectable during contextual speech, it must be documented in all suspected cases

Physical: Vocal folds adduct rhythmically and momentarily on vowel prolongation, synchronously with voice arrests; myoclonic movements of larynx and pharynx can be seen by observing the movements beneath the skin of the neck

Hyperkinetic Dysarthria of Gilles de la Tourette's Syndrome

Perceptual: Involuntary grunting, coughing, throat-clearing, barking, squealing, shrieking, screaming, gurgling, moaning

Physical: Vocal folds appear normal in structure and function

From Aronson, A. (1980). *Clinical voice disorders: An interdisciplinary approach*. New York: Thieme-Stratton Inc.

the airway is critical to survival. The voice quality of individuals with spastic dysarthria typically is called strained-strangled. This voice quality presumably is associated with the hyperadduction of the vocal folds caused by loss of control of inhibitory neurologic signals from the cortex. Smitheran and Hixon (1981) presented the case of an individual with multiple, bilateral cerebrovascular accidents (CVAs) and a marked strained-strangled voice quality. Measures of laryngeal resistance for this speaker were 85 percent higher than the average resistance values of normal males and 53 percent higher than those obtained for the normal subjects with the highest calculated resistance. Harsh voice quality, low pitch, and reduced loudness are also common in spastic dysarthria. The perceptual and physical characterisics of phonation in spastic and mixed spastic-flaccid dysarthria appear in Table 10-1.

Ataxic Dysarthria

Although voice is often normal, especially in milder cases of ataxia, the following symptoms may occur in the more severely involved: hoarse or harsh voice quality, abnormally low pitch, monopitch, monoloudness, inappropriate and imprecise stress patterns, overall excessive loudness, coarse voice tremor. These perceptual characteristics are the result of *dysmetria* (the loss of ability to measure range of movement) and incoordination of the respiratory and laryngeal systems.

Hypokinetic Dysarthria (Parkinsonism)

Damage to the basal ganglia releases inhibition of nerve impulses to the lower motoneuron leading to rigidity and slowness of movement. Several research groups have focused on the phonatory characteristics of hypokinetic dysarthric speakers. Logemann and colleagues (1978) perceptually rated the phonatory and articulatory problems of 200 individuals with Parkinson's disease who represented a range of type and severity. They observed that in the natural progression of parkinsonism, phonatory (laryngeal) symptoms became evident before articulatory symptoms. Further, they reported that 85 percent of their subjects demonstrated phonatory quality disorders as reflected by the symptoms of breathiness, hoarseness, and roughness. Netsell and Rosenbek (1985) have suggested that the laryngeal system can be regarded as a microcosm of the entire speech mechanism. Therefore, the larynx may reflect fine motor central impairment prior to other speech components. Several research groups have confirmed the phonatory symptoms of parkinsonian speakers to be reduced maximal and minimal loudness levels (Boshes, 1966; Canter, 1963) and overall reduced habitual loudness (Boshes, 1966; Canter, 1963; Logemann et al., 1978; Ludlow & Bassich, 1983).

Hyperkinetic Dysarthria

Chorea

Choreic movements are purposeless, quick, jerky, irregular, and unpredictable, and are caused by lesions in the basal ganglia (probably the caudate nucleus). Such movements of the respiratory and laryngeal musculature may produce irregular pitch fluctuations and voice arrests. Other perceptual and physical characteristics of this form of hyperkinetic dysarthria appear in Table 10-1. Forms of chorea include Huntington's chorea (an inherited, degenerative disorder that affects the basal ganglia and the cerebral cortex), and Syndenham's chorea (a self-limiting form of chorea that occurs primarily in children). Choreic movements are also seen in parkinsonian individuals on high doses of levodopa. It is believed that these movements are the result of an imbalance of dopamine and acetylcholine in the striate nucleus. Prognosis for improved phonation with treatment is poor (Prator & Swift, 1984). Phonation improves in cases where the chorea is self-limiting.

Dystonia

Dystonic movements are repetitive, slow, twisting, writhing, and flexing. Phonatory characteristics include uncontrolled adductor and abductor laryngeal spasms that result in strained hoarseness, breathiness, and at times, inhalatory stridor. The dystonias may be either generalized or focal as in tardive dyskinesia, a disorder associated with long-term use of neuroleptic drugs.

Organic (Essential) Voice Tremor

Also known as benign heredofamilial tremor, organic voice tremor may or may not be associated with tremors in other parts of the body. Phonatory characteristics include quavering intonation with rhythmic alterations of vocal pitch and loudness at 5 to 12 cycles per second. Voice arrests with visible, vertical oscillations of the larynx may also be present. Symptomatic voice therapy has not been shown to be effective in reducing the voice tremor (Prator & Swift, 1984).

Palatopharyngeaolaryngeal Myoclonus

Myoclonus is a slow form of tremor resulting in rhythmic movements of the soft palate, pharyngeal walls, laryngeal musculature, eyeballs, diaphragm, and tongue. Aronson (1980) has reported the results of a Mayo Clinic study that suggested a vascular etiology including brainstem or cerebellar infarction, tumor of the cerebellum or fourth ventricle, head trauma producing posterior fossa damage, and degenerative central nervous system (CNS) disease. Site of lesions vary with the following structures being implicated: dentate nucleus, inferior olive, superior cerebellar peduncle, red nucleus, and restiform body. Phonatory signs and symptoms include rhythmic adduction of the vocal folds and gross upward and downward movements of the larynx. The perceptual result is momentary phonatory interruption. Therapy is generally unnecessary because myoclonus usually does not affect contextual speech, but can be observed during sustained phonation or vocal activities such as singing.

Gilles de la Tourette's Syndrome

This syndrome is characterized by multiple tics and involuntary vocalization that includes coprolalia and echolalia (Shapiro, Shapiro, & Wayne, 1973). Treatment with haloperidol usually controls the phonatory symptoms; however, the value of voice therapy is questionable (Prator & Swift, 1984).

Mixed Dysarthrias

Amyotrophic Lateral Sclerosis (Flaccid-Spastic Dysarthria)

ALS is a degenerative disorder of both upper and lower motoneurons. Although in early stages, either flaccid or spastic paralysis may predominate, both types are usually present in later stages. Phonatory characteristics may include those of flaccidity, spasticity, or both. These include breathiness, reduced loudness, audible inhalation, and wet-hoarseness (resulting from accumulation of saliva in the pyriform sinuses and on the vocal folds), and rapid tremor or flutter on vowel prolongation. Carrow, Rivera, Mauldin, and Shamblin (1974) studied the dysarthria of 79 patients and found phonatory impairment prominent with the following features occurring in more than 50 percent of their sample: harsh voice quality, breathy voice quality, voice tremor, and strained-strangled quality.

Multiple Sclerosis (Ataxic-Spastic Dysarthria)

The phonatory characteristics of dysarthria associated with MS vary, depending on the pattern of neurologic involvement. In a study of 168 patients with MS, Darley, Brown, & Goldstein (1972) reported that 41 percent presented an overall speech performance that would be considered abnormal in terms of impact upon the listener. Of those individuals with dysarthria, the two most common symptoms were impaired loudness control and harshness. Also observed were impaired pitch control, inappropriate pitch level, and breathiness.

ASSESSMENT OF LARYNGEAL FUNCTION

As reported earlier, some level of phonatory dysfunction is present in a large percentage of dysarthric speakers. This dysfunction may range in severity from a mild impairment with no associated disability to a disorder so severe that it is a primary factor limiting communication. The assessment of phonatory performance is an integral part of each dysarthria evaluation. Generally, assessment proceeds along the same lines as clinical assessment of other speech components. The first phase involves the documentation of the presence of a phonatory impairment and a perceptual description of its characteristics and severity. This phase essentially serves as a screening process. The second phase of assessment involves an in-depth analysis of phonatory function. Here, a series of questions are posed that are related to the mechanisms underlying the perceptual features of phonation and to various intervention approaches that may potentially benefit the speaker.

Approaches to Measurement

When discussing assessment of voice disorders, Aronson (1980) states, "The trained ear and mind are, at present, the most useful instrument" (p. 182). At the time this book was written, much of the clinical assessment of the presence of phonatory dysfunction of dysarthric speakers was made using perceptual judgments. However, with increasing frequency, the specific characteristics of phonatory dysfunction are being assessed using instrumental measurement techniques. For example, acoustic analysis equipment is becoming more available in the clinical setting. Using this instrumentation, fundamental frequency and relative vocal intensity can be measured. Often, timing relationships (i.e., phonatory versus respiratory timing) may be described more precisely with acoustic analysis and respiratory measures than with perceptual means alone.

A series of perceptual, acoustic, and aerodynamic assessment techniques will be presented in this chapter. Selection of one technique over another for clinical use obviously depends on a number of issues. Perhaps the most important issue is the nature of questions being addressed in the evaluation. Other issues include the importance of the phonatory problems in relation to overall impairment, knowledge and time available to clinician, and equipment at hand.

Researchers are beginning to compare and contrast results of various measurement approaches. For example, Ludlow and Bassich (1983, 1984) studied the relationships between perceptual ratings and acoustic measures of the speech of nonimpaired individuals and those with Parkinson's disease and Shy-Drager syndrome. Shy-Drager syndrome is a progressive neurological disorder whose primary symptom is orthostatic hypotension (dizziness, weakness and disturbances of vision or consciousness upon standing). The underlying neuropathology of this syndrome is different from that of Parkinson's disease. In Shy-Drager syndrome, cell degeneration is found in the cerebellar cortex, substantia nigra, and other basal ganglia, as well as in the spinal ganglion cells (Mumenthaler, 1983). Ludlow and Bassich (1983) identified strengths and weaknesses of perceptual and acoustic approaches in the assessment of this population. For example, they found that either perceptual ratings or acoustic measures were adequate to distinguish the nonimpaired speakers from those with either type of dysarthria and to distinguish one type of dysarthria from another. They also state:

> somewhat different variables were identified as most useful for discriminating between the two types of dysarthria. . . . The acoustic system identified vowel-voicing errors as particularly important for distinguishing between the types of dysarthria, while the perceptual system identified differences in voice quality and overall rate as being particularly important. . . . The perceptual rating system identified three aspects of vocal quality as useful for differentiating between types of dysarthria: breathiness, strain-strangle and wet hoarseness. Neither of the acoustic measures of vocal quality, jitter ratio, or diplophonia ratio were included in the discriminant function for differentiating between the two types of dysarthria. Therefore, the acoustic measures may be more discrete for the analysis of different speech production factors in patients' speech. Further investigation is needed to determine if such is the case. If so, the acoustic system may be more suitable for assessing those aspects that are particularly impaired prior to treatment planning, while the perceptual system may better provide an overall indication of the degree of impairment (Ludlow & Bassich, 1984, p. 140).

In the situation just described, instrumental (in this case acoustic) measurement has permitted an assessment of phonatory timing that is not available using the perceptual approaches alone. Further, the perceptual measures gave an indication of overall voice quality that could not be obtained instrumentally. Thus, it appears when assessing phonatory function in dysarthria, clinicians need to select measurement approaches dependent on the specific aspects of the impairment that are of interest to them.

Identification of Perceptual Signs of Laryngeal Impairment

Generally, the initial phase of the evaluation involves the determination of the presence or absence of a phonatory disorder. For example, when the evaluation is part of an overall neurological assessment to detect the presence of a neurological impairment, slight variation from normal, or at least from previous performance, is important. If no impairment is observed during speech, further assessment of phonatory performance is usually discontinued. If phonatory impairment is confirmed, further description of the phonatory impairment is necessary. The impact of the phonatory impairment on overall disability and handicap must also be assessed.

The assessment of phonatory impairment is usually begun using perceptual measures of loudness, pitch, and quality during production of connected speech. These perceptual observations may be quantified using the seven-point equal-appearing interval scale reported by Darley, Aronson, and Brown (1969 a, b). The specific parameters that relate to phonation include:

Pitch level
Pitch breaks
Monopitch
Voice tremor
Monoloudness
Excessive loudness variation
Loudness decay
Alternating loudness
Harsh voice
Hoarse voice
Breathy voice
Strained-strangled voice
Phrases short

Presence of perceptual changes in these speech dimensions may lead the clinician to ask questions about the mechanisms underlying the impairment and possible intervention approaches. Answers to these questions require the clinician to pursue a more in-depth assessment of phonatory function.

In-depth Assessment of Laryngeal Function

Contribution of Impairments in Other Components

Because dysarthria is typically characterized by impairment in multiple speech components, it is necessary to examine the relationship of phonatory impairment with other aspects of speech production. It is possible that what appears to be an impairment in phonation instead may reflect impairment in respiratory or velopharyngeal performance. For example, poor respiratory support may result in deviations in voice loudness and length of phrase. Answers to the following questions are needed in order to interpret data derived from the assessment of phonatory performance:

- Is the level of subglottal air pressure adequate to support phonatory function?
- How flexible is the respiratory system?
- Can the respiratory system be controlled in a coordinated fashion?
- How efficient is the velopharyngeal valve?
- Is the speaker able to achieve complete velopharyngeal closure?
- Is that closure well-timed in relation to other aspects of speech production?

A detailed discussion of assessment of the respiratory and velopharyngeal components can be found in Chapters 9 and 11, respectively. The following discussion of phonatory function assumes an understanding of respiratory and velopharyngeal function. Once the function of other speech components has been established, then assessment can focus on laryngeal function. A number of aspects of laryngeal-phonatory function are important in the assessment of dysarthric speech. These include efficiency, flexibility, quality, and coordination. Each of these aspects, together with a number of perceptual and instrumental measurement techniques, will be discussed.

Laryngeal Efficiency

Laryngeal efficiency is a term that will be used to describe the adequacy with which the expiratory airstream is valved at the level of the vocal folds. Laryngeal efficiency is compromised when, due to motor impairment, the vocal folds do not adduct properly or when timing of vocal fold closure is not well coordinated. Laryngeal efficiency may be assessed in a number of ways.

PERCEPTUAL CHARACTERISTICS OF THE VOICE. Several perceptual features of the voice may signal laryngeal inefficiency. These qualities may be observed either in connected speech, in sustained phonation tasks, or in both. A breathy voice may indicate air wastage and thus signal inadequate laryngeal closure. On the other hand, a voice with a strained-strangled quality may reflect excessive adduction of the vocal folds. The efficiency of glottal closure may also be assessed by listening to the quality of the cough, a throat-clearing maneuver, or a hard glottal attack. A weak or "mushy" cough may be an indicator of vocal fold weakness.

SUSTAINED PHONATION TIME. Maximum sustained phonation time has been used by some as an indicator of laryngeal efficiency. Prator and Swift (1984) use the following formulas that include measures of vital capacity to predict maximum phonation times for adults.

$$\text{Males: VC/110} \times 0.67 = \text{Maximum Phonation Time}$$
$$\text{Females: VC/100} \times 0.59 = \text{Maximum Phonation Time}$$

Hirano, Koike, and von Leden (1968) indicate a minimum sustained phonation of 15.0 sec for males and 14.3 sec for females. Obviously, performance on this task is not only dependent on the efficiency of glottal closure but also on the level of respiratory support. If the ratio of actual to predicted maximum phonation time falls below .70, a number of dysfunctions may be occurring. For dysarthric individuals one or a number of explanations may pertain:

- Inability to generate sufficient subglottal air pressure
- Inability to control exhalation, or inability to generate a steady, nonexcessive level of subglottal air pressure
- Inability to coordinate exhalation with the initiation of phonation
- Inability to adduct the vocal folds in order to efficiently valve the expiratory airstream
- Hyperadduction of the vocal folds requiring excessive levels of subglottal air pressure in order to produce phonation

Identification of which of these factors is contributing to reduced maximum phonation time can be accomplished in a number of ways. First, the speaker's ability to generate subglottal breath pressure may be evaluated in tasks where laryngeal function is not required. See Chapter 9 for a detailed description of such tasks. Second, speech production tasks with and without voicing can be compared. Sustained /s/ versus /z/ production ratios are one such task. Normal adults are able to sustain /s/ and /z/ for roughly equivalent durations, approximately 20 to 25 sec (Ptacek & Sander, 1963). Thus, the /s/ to /z/ ratio is equal to 1.0. In cases of respiratory insufficiency but efficient laryngeal function, the ratio would continue to be 1.0, however, the maximum durations for both /s/ and /z/ would be shorter than normal. In cases of vocal fold pathology, the /s/ to /z/ ratios often exceed 1.0. Eckel and Boone (1981) report /s/ to /z/ ratios for a group of speakers with vocal pathologies (nodules and polyps). Their results indicated that 95 percent of their individuals had ratios in excess of 1.4. They conclude:

> It would appear that when an additive lesion has developed along the glottal margin, vocal fold approximation is less efficient. This decrement in efficiency appears to result in a decrease in glottal resistance, increasing airflow and resulting in shortened phonation time (p. 149)

Unfortunately, data regarding /s/ to /z/ ratios for dysarthric individuals with various laryngeal neuropathologies have not been reported in the research literature.

MEASURES AND ESTIMATES OF AIR FLOW DURING PHONATION. Laryngeal efficiency may also be assessed by measuring or estimating the rate of air flow during sustained phonation. Instrumentation required for the measurement of air flow rate includes a pneumotachometer (a device that senses the volume velocity of air flow through a face mask), a microphone, and a recording device. With the microphone and face mask in place, speakers are asked to sustain a vowel for several seconds at a comfortable pitch and intensity level. Mean flow rates are computed by dividing volume exhalation during phonation by time. For males, mean flow rates average 115 ml/sec and for females they average 100 ml/sec (Yanagihara, Koike, & von Leden, 1966). Because of the possibility of inconsistent laryngeal control by dysarthric speakers, average measures of air flow may not accurately reflect the status of laryngeal function (Netsell et al., 1984).

When a pneumotachometer is not available, an estimate of air flow can be calculated using a measure called the phonation quotient (Prator & Swift, 1984). This measure has been shown to correlate well with mean flow rates (Hirano et al., 1968; Yanagihara & Koike, 1967; Yanagihara et al., 1966; Yanagihara & von Leden, 1967). The phonation quotient is calculated by dividing the vital capacity by the maximum phonation time. Normative data suggest a phonation quotient of 145 ml/sec for males and 137 ml/sec for females. Data outside the following ranges are considered abnormal (Hirano et al., (1968):

Males: 69—307 ml/sec
Females: 78—241 ml/sec

ESTIMATES OF LARYNGEAL RESISTANCE. The extent to which the larynx offers opposition to the flow of air through it is known as laryngeal resistance. Although it cannot be measured directly, Smitheran and Hixon (1981) described an approach to estimate the aerodyanmic impedance of the laryngeal structures. Briefly, the level of subglottal air pressure for vowels is estimated from intraoral air pressure levels of voiceless consonants adjacent to the vowel in question. The volume velocity of airflow through the glottis during vowel production is measured. Using the formula (laryngeal airway resistance = translaryngeal pressure / translaryngeal flow) an estimate of laryngeal resistance is calculated. This measure provides information about the resistance to airflow through the larynx. The authors have reported that persons with harsh voices have resistance levels that are considerably higher than those with normal voices and persons with breathy voices have lower levels of resistance. Netsell, and colleagues (1984) have reported a different way of displaying laryngeal resistance in air pressure by air flow plots. One limitation of this procedure with dysarthric persons is that the measure does not necessarily reflect the stiffness of the vocal folds. In a severely spastic individual, the folds may be very stiff and yet because of vocal fold position, produce a breathy voice quality. Also, the measurement technique assumes a complete velopharyngeal and bilabial seal during the production of the voiceless stop /p/. This level of performance is not always present in dysarthric speakers.

MOVEMENT MEASURES. Movement of the vocal folds in dysarthric speakers has been routinely observed through indirect laryngoscopy. This technique is useful when evaluating for vocal fold paralysis. However, the rapid movement of the vocal folds does not permit cycle-by-cycle evaluation of the vocal folds using this technique. During recent years, the use of a fiberscope, a stroboscopic light source, and video-recording equipment shows promise for visualizing and measuring vocal fold movement in dysarthric speakers.

Fiberscopic technology is becoming available in many medical clinics that specialize in laryngeal or velopharyngeal function. This technology permits observation of laryngeal movement, and taken together with perceptual and aerodynamic measures, can provide important information regarding laryngeal dysfunction. D'Antonio, Lotz, Chait, & Netsell (in press).

Electroglottography is another technique that shows promise in the laryngeal assessment of vocal fold movement of dysarthric speakers. Electroglottography estimates the degree of contact between the vocal folds using an electric impedance approach. Electroglottography is described in detail in Davis (1981). Electroglottography has not yet received widespread use as a research or clinical measurement tool in the dysarthria field.

Vocal Flexibility

Aronson refers to vocal flexibility as "variations in pitch and loudness that aid in the expression of emphasis, meaning, or subtleties indicating the feelings of the individual" (1980, p. 6). This aspect of voice can be assessed perceptually by judging parameters of pitch variation, loudness, and quality. Typically, habitual performance may be compared to maximum performance by asking the speaker to perform structured tasks designed to heighten flexiblity. Examples of such tasks are the emphatic stress patterning tasks described in more detail in Chapter 14. Vocal flexibility can also be measured acoustically with parameters related to fundamental frequency such as range of fundamental frequency within an utterance, range of peak fundamental frequencies of each syllable within an utterance, or slope of the fundamental frequency contour. Lack of vocal flexibility is a characteristic of certain types of dysarthria, including the hypokinetic dysarthria seen in Parkinson's disease.

Vocal Quality

Voice quality is a complex perceptual phenomenon relating to vocal fold periodicity and glottal and vocal tract resonance (including the respiratory system). Aronson (1980) classified neurogenic voice disorders according to consistency or variability of vocal production. For example, there is a group of relative constant neurologic voice disorders where the quality deviation is relatively constant. This group includes the phonatory properties of flaccid, spastic, and hypokinetic dysarthria. Another group of phonatory disorders is characterized by arrhythmical fluctuations. Ataxic, choreic, and dystonic dysphonias fall into this group. Rhythmically fluctuating dysphonias include those associated with tremor, including palatopharyngeaolaryngeal myoclonus and organic (essential) voice tremor. Paroxysmal neurologic dysphonia is evidenced where voice quality is altered relatively infrequently by sudden bursts. Gilles de la Tourette's syndrome is included in this group.

Coordination

Laryngeal coordination refers to the timing of laryngeal activity with other aspects of speech production. Timing of respiratory and phonatory efforts are particularly important in dysarthria. This type of coordination can be assessed in several ways. For example, the speaker can be asked to produce in rapid succession the series of vowels /i-i-i-i-i/. This task may be difficult for many dysarthric individuals, especially those with respiratory or laryngeal coordination problems. It requires not only rapid initiation and cessation of vocal fold vibration, but also a steady respiratory drive. In severe impairment, evidence of such incoordination is visually apparent during connected speech. At other times, observations of respiratory—laryngeal incoordination require instrumental measurement. Acoustic measurement has permitted assessment of phonatory timing that is not available using only the perceptual approach. For example, measures of the latency between the initiation of phonation following the beginning of the expiratory phase of respiration may be obtained using aerodynamic techniques. Some dysarthric individuals waste their air supply by exhaling a portion of their lung volume before initiating phonation.

Still another example of phonatory incoordination can be seen in the production of voicing distinctions. Some dysarthric individuals are unable to produce perceptually different voiced versus voiceless cognate pairs. Often, this is a consequence of poorly controlled and timed phonation. Although this type of voicing problem can certainly be identified perceptually, acoustic analysis is often helpful in examining the details of this problem. Durational measures of the timing of phonation cessation and reinitiation during the production of a voiceless consonant sound can be made.

TREATMENT

This discussion of treatment of laryngeal dysfunction is organized according to severity. Thus, we will begin with a description of the development of voluntary phonation in the severely involved speaker. Development of the respiratory/laryngeal control needed for phonation is often the first step in intervention. Once phonation has been established, efforts can be turned to the management of other aspects of speech production, such as improving velopharyngeal function and oral articulation. Techniques to increase vocal loudness and improve vocal quality and coordination will also be presented. Readers should note that, with the possible exception of focusing on improved vocal quality in mild dysarthria, laryngeal function is rarely treated in isolation from other aspects of speech production. For example, management of respiratory and laryngeal function are often closely related in the severely dysarthric individual. Likewise, oral articulation and laryngeal function are closely related when attempting to improve the production of voiced/voiceless sound distinctions.

Treating the Aphonic Individual

Evaluating Reflexive Phonation

Some severely dysarthric individuals are unable to produce phonation voluntarily. The speakers described in the following section generally exhibit reduced respiratory support, velopharyngeal incompetency, and bilateral vocal fold weakness that prevents them from forcibly adducting the vocal folds. Common etiologies include closed head injury with brain stem contusion and brain stem CVA. With both of these etiologies, there is a sudden onset followed by a gradual course of recovery that may extend over years.

With these individuals, the various nonspeech reflex patterns that might be associated with phonation are inventoried, including laughing, coughing, sighing, and expressions of pain or discomfort. When phonation occurs, note is taken not only of the type of activity (i.e., laughing) but also the speaker's position (supine, prone, or sitting). When respiratory drive is weak, the speakers' efforts are supplemented with abdominal pressing to increase the subglottal air pressure being generated. Family members and attendant staff are encouraged to keep a diary of the times when phonation occurs, thus carefully documenting situations that produce successful phonation including stimulus, body position, assistance provided, and associated activity such as response to pain or discomfort. An example of such a phonation diary appears in Table 10-2. A review of this table suggests a gradual change over a four month period. Voicing was initially present only in response to discomfort, phonation then became consistent in the supine position, and finally, phonation became consistent and voluntary when the speaker was seated.

Developing Voluntary Phonation

The transition from reflexive to voluntary phonation varies from individual to individual. For some, the transition is almost immediate; for others, the transition takes months or years. Our first approach is usually to have individuals attempt to produce a reflexive behavior on a repetitive basis. Next, we ask them to produce the phonation voluntarily. Commonly, these speakers are simultaneously participating in a program designed to increase their ability to generate subglottal air pressure. During phonatory practice sessions, we position the individual for maximal generation of subglottal air pressure when attempting phonation. Many persons are positioned supine with an abdominal press to increase subglottal air pressure. Rarely is initial phonatory initiation produced in the upright or seated position.

TABLE 10-2. An Example of a Phonation Diary Completed by the Family of a Severely Dysarthric 23 year old Individual with a Closed Head Injury

NAME: Tom Matthews
RECORDER: Ellen Matthews

INSTRUCTION: Remember to include information about date, voicing behavior, consistency, position, stimulus, and whether or not the speaker could continue to produce voicing.

Make an entry at least once a week. Pick a particular day each week, if that will help you be consistent.

1/15/85	no voicing today, supine or prone, with verbal instruction
1/22/85	no voicing this week in any position, with verbal instruction
1/29/85	voice in response to an uncomfortable transfer from bed to wheelchair
2/05/85	sound occurred when choking on saliva no voluntary voicing supine or prone, with verbal instruction
2/12/85	cough and choking sound supine when swallowing saliva no voluntary sound in any position with verbal instruction
2/19/85	same
2/26/85	same
3/05/85	same
3/12/85	same
3/19/85	voice during laughing, both prone & supine, but not seated, still voice when coughing and choking occasionally
3/26/85	same
4/02/85	same
4/09/85	same
4/16/85	same, maybe voluntary sound supine with verbal instruction and while pushing stomach
4/23/85	occasional voluntary sound when supine with verbal instructions and abdominal push no voluntary sound in seated position
4/30/85	sound 50% of time in supine with abdominal push, sound occasionally without abdominal push, occasional sound in seated position with abdominal push
5/07/85	consistent voluntary sound in prone and supine, sound 30% of time in seated position with abdominal push
5/14/85	consistent sound in seated position, voice is almost a whisper
5/21/85	voice stronger every day, especially after a coughing spell

Because the goal of this phase of intervention is more forcible vocal fold adduction, traditional pushing exercises such as those described by Prator and Swift (1984) may be used. These exercises typically involve forceful muscular activity such as lifting, pulling, or pushing. Pushing the hand, arms, or legs against resistance may elicit reflexive glottal closure for those who are unable to achieve it under other circumstances. Because severely dysarthric individuals may have arm and leg weakness, the anatomic site used and the specific pushing activity will vary from speaker to speaker. Some individuals push against the arm rests or lap tray of the wheelchair, others push against overhead slings mounted to hospital beds or wheelchairs (see Figure 10-1).

Once severely dysarthric speakers are able to consistently initiate phonation voluntarily, they are asked to attempt to shape the oral cavity to produce a number of different vowel sounds and to initiate phonation when assuming various articulatory postures. Once they have demonstrated the ability to do

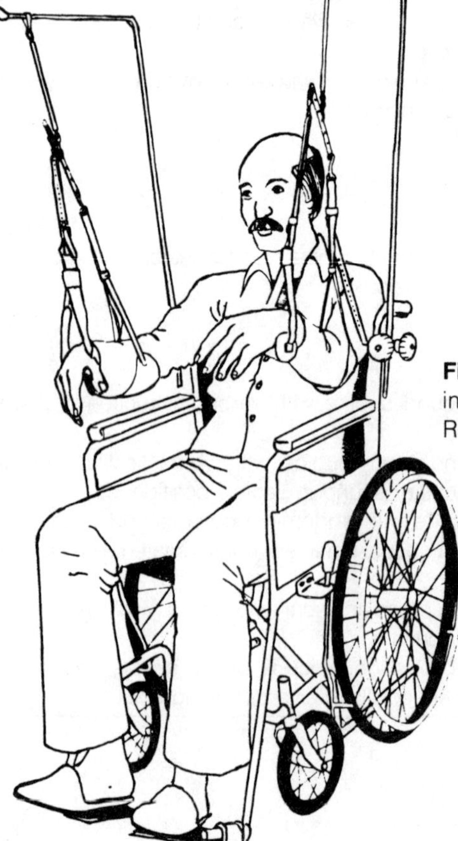

Figure 10-1. Overhead slings for increasing speaking effort (From Rosenbek, 1984).

this, they are introduced to vowel intelligibility drills similiar to those discussed in Chapter 12.

Case Presentation

Sam was 72 years old when he suffered an extensive brain stem stroke. He was admitted to the rehabilitation unit one month post onset. At that time, he was anarthric and was communicating with a yes/no eye blink system. He had severely compromised respiratory support, bilateral vocal fold paralysis, severe reduced swallow reflex, no observable velopharyngeal movement, and some weak bilabial movement. After an augmentative communication approach had been established using a head-mounted light pointer and an alphabet board, focus of attention turned to speech production. Goals for the first hospitalization included increasing respiratory support for speech, increasing ability to produce spontaneous phonation in the supine position, and increasing ability to produce understandable vowels. At the time of his hospital discharge at eight months post onset, he was able to consistently initiate voluntary phonation in the supine position. Although he was able to produce two or three syllables per utterance when lying down, he was not able to vocalize voice when seated.

Five months after his discharge from the first hospitalization, he was readmitted for management of an unrelated medical problem. When we evaluated him at the beginning of the second hospitalization, we found that he had made some small but important gains. He and his wife reported that speech had become sufficiently understandable so that the communication augmentation system was no longer needed when he was lying down. However, he was still unable to initiate phonation in the seated position. This lack of phonation was beginning to pose more and more of a problem because he wished to spend the majority of his day seated in the wheelchair. Our goal during the second hospitalization was to develop phonation in the seated position. As is frequently the case, both respiratory and phonatory impairments were implicated in Sam's lack of phonation.

Evaluation of respiratory function revealed that although his ability to generate adequate levels of subglottal air pressure was severely compromised in both positions, it was considerably worse in the seated than in the supine position. Observations of respiratory movements were made using the Respitrace unit. See Chapter 9 for a more detailed discussion of this instrument. This examination indicated that resting breathing was accomplished almost exclusively with abdominal movements. Rib cage movements appeared to contribute only minimally during rest breathing.

Several pushing techniques were explored in an effort to increase the frequency of voicing in the seated position. Most of these were unsuccessful. First, Sam did not have the trunk control to push a respiratory paddle such as the one that appears in Figure 10-2. Likewise, he did not have sufficient arm strength to push against his own abdomen when attempting to initiate

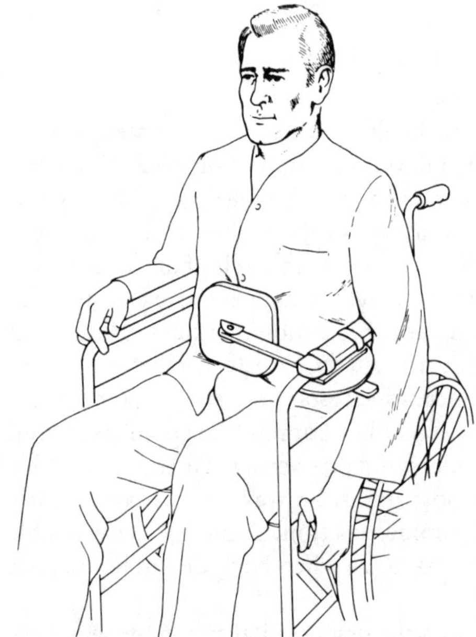

Figure 10-2. A respiratory paddle (from Rosenbek, 1984).

phonation. Only one technique appeared to be associated with consistent production of phonation. This technique involved both pushing and an attempt to initiate phonation at maximum lung volume. Sam was asked to extend his legs and arms and, at the same time, to move his shoulders back. When performing this maneuver, Sam was displacing his rib cage and presumably initiating phonation at a higher lung volume level than when relying on his abdominal movements alone. Further, the generalized pushing movement appeared to increase Sam's tone. This may have been responsible for better adduction of the vocal folds. Sam quickly learned to use this technique during conversational speech, and began to use it consistently and successfully in day-to-day communication. Although more effort was required to speak when seated, Sam considered this part of his "training routine." Once voluntary phonation was established, we began to consider techniques to manage the incompetent velopharyngeal mechanism. These efforts are described in Chapter 11.

Increasing Loudness

Behavioral Training

Respiratory support and control are critical aspects in determining voice loudness. The respiratory capabilities of dysarthric individuals who are not sufficiently loud should be examined carefully. Behavioral training for loudness may involve training the speaker to generate greater levels of subglottal air pressure or to initiate phonation at appropriate lung volume levels or at appropriate times in the respiratory cycle. These and other techniques are discussed in detail in Chapter 9.

Prosthetic Management

In cases where speakers are unable to change their respiratory pattern, loudness may be enhanced by portable amplification systems. Figure 10-3 illustrates one such amplifier. The system is small enough to be carried in a pocket or purse, and a microphone small enough to be mounted on eyeglasses or behind the ear may be used. We have found that such amplifiers are successful for some parkinsonian speakers. The amplifiers appear to be much more effective when quiet phonation is present than when the speaker produces only a whisper.

The speech amplifier just described is considered a prosthetic device and one would not expect continued improved performance without the device. Rubow and Swift (1985) described a microcomputer-based wearable device designed to improve the loudness of parkinsonian speakers. Briefly, the device performs the following functions:

- It samples intensity of voiced segments from a throat microphone
- It discriminates speech from background noise

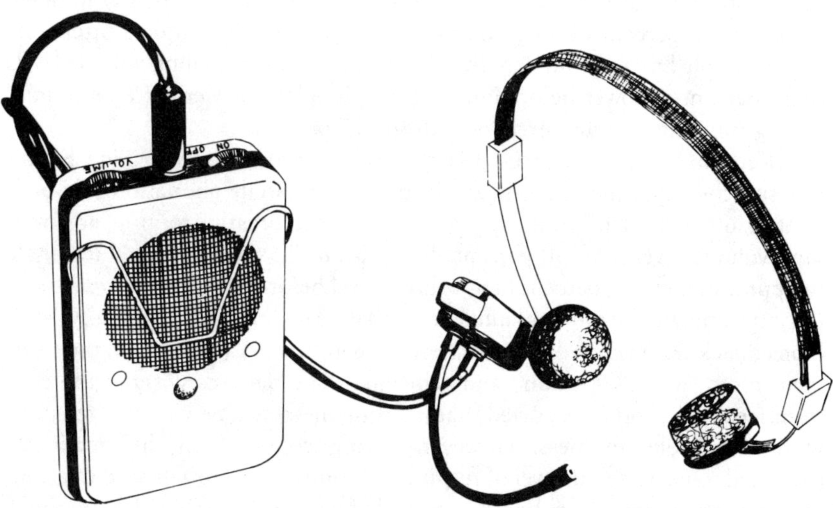

Figure 10-3. A portable, battery-operated voice amplifier (Cooper-Rand).

- It determines if the vocal intensity is below a defined threshold
- It delivers appropriate auditory feedback to the patient
- It collects and stores time-coded data on performance
- It transfers those data to a host computer for analysis

These authors report the successful use of such a device in aiding the transfer of training with a 67 year old man with mild to moderate Parkinson's disease.

Case Presentation

Ken was diagnosed with Parkinson's disease 10 years before he was referred to our clinic. He was the supervisor of a custom tool shop in a local industry. He found that he was unable to speak loudly enough to be heard in the noisy environment, so for at least a year, he had invited all of his employees into his office to communicate with them. In Ken's opinion, his method of staff communication was inadequate, because it did not allow him to discuss problems and solutions in the shop where the work was being done. The problem that brought Ken to us was his increasing inability to communicate effectively at management team meetings. He was concerned that he was losing his ability to represent his area well.

A brief conversation revealed the presence of a voice impairment. Ken's voice was characteristic of many people with Parkinson's disease. His voice was breathy and vocal intensity was low, however, phonation was consistently present. A more complete assessment revealed that Ken's estimated subglottal air pressure during speech averaged between 2 and 3 cm of water pressure. His respiratory pattern was unusual in several ways. He frequently initiated speech at 40 percent of lung volume level or lower. To complete utterances of reasonable breath group lengths, he frequently spoke to lung volume levels of 20 percent or lower before inhaling. His inhalations were often minimal, raising his lung volume levels only 10 or 15 percent.

Ken was involved in a trial of respiratory treatment described in Chapter 9. Using the Respitrace unit, he was instructed to.initiate phonation at appoximately 60 percent of vital capacity and end the breath group at no lower lung volume level than 30 percent. In addition, he was instructed to inhale to approximately 60 percent lung volume level before each breath group, and thus to eliminate the minimal inhalations that he had ultilized habitually. With biofeedback, Ken achieved those objectives with remarkable ease. In the treatment room, he was speaking and achieving the objectives without the constant feedback, and he reported that in group meetings, he was able to speak with acceptable loudness. However, during conversation, he frequently neglected to exercise the level of respiratory control that he achieved in group meetings or in treatment. Ken was provided with a portable voice amplifier and a boom microphone mounted on his glasses for communication in the shop. Depending on the progression of his disease, the portable amplification system may become a regularly worn prosthesis.

Improving Voice Quality

Rough, hoarse, harsh, or breathy voice are frequent characteristics of dysarthric speech. Often, these symptoms are not treated. For severely involved speakers, other aspects of speech production may be more critical to the improvement of speech intelligibility. For mildly involved speakers, the presence of a slight phonatory impairment may not be an important handicap. When voice quality impairment is present and it is felt to contribute to overall disability and handicap, intervention may be warranted.

When voice quality disorders are associated with hyperadduction of the vocal folds, traditional voice therapy techniques designed to reduce laryngeal hyperadduction and increase airflow through the glottis may be appropriate. For a review of these treatment techniques see Prator and Swift (1984).

Smitheran and Hixon (1981) report intervention with a 57 year old man who had had multiple bilateral CVAs. Among the characteristics of his mixed dysarthria was a markedly strained-strangled voice quality. Estimates of laryngeal airway resistance suggested excessive laryngeal obstruction of airway with a resistance score 85 percent higher than those of normal individuals. It was assumed these high resistance values were associated with the probable spastic component of his laryngeal problem. Voice quality was judged to be perceptually better when the speaker was asked to perform under one of the following conditions: to raise his fundamental frequency, to rotate his head backward, or to initiate his utterance from a high lung volume level. These perceptual changes also were associated with decreases in laryngeal airway resistance. Smitheran and Hixon state: "It was assumed that this improvement was related to passive abduction of the vocal folds brought about by the tracheal tug associated with a lower diaphragm position at a high lung volume level" (p. 145).

Improving Laryngeal Coordination

Respiratory—Laryngeal Timing

Appropriate laryngeal timing usually involves two issues for dysarthric speakers. One is the prompt initiation of phonation at the beginning of the exhalation phase of respiration for speech. Prompt initiation of phonation reduces air wastage and fatigue during speech. We have found respiratory biofeedback using the Respitrace unit particularly helpful in training this aspect of phonatory timing. With a respiratory signal displayed on one channel of a scope and a raw acoustic waveform or intensity contour from an intensity analysis system, such as the Visipitch (Kay Elemetrics Corp., Pine Brook, NJ, 07058-9797), on the second channel of a storage scope, the respiratory-phonatory timing patterns can be "captured" and presented to the speaker as biofeedback.

Voiced—Voiceless Distinctions

A second aspect of phonatory timing is voice onset and cessation during the production of voiceless consonants in vowel environments. Many dysarthric individuals have extreme difficulty producing perceptually different voiced/voiceless cognate pairs. Because the phonatory timing requirement for this task is so demanding, we have successfully taught some individuals to exaggerate other aspects of the voiced/voiceless distinction. For example, some speakers may produce the distinction by aspirating final unvoiced plosives and producing final voiceless plosived without aspiration. Rosenbek and LaPointe (1985) have listed some other differences that may suggest useful training techniques. For example, voiced plosives are usually accompanied by greater intraoral breath pressure and airflow than their voiceless counterparts. Vowel duration before voiceless productions is typically longer than before unvoiced productions. We typically train dysarthric individuals to produce voiced/ voiceless distinctions within the framework of the intelligibility drill (see Chapter 12). Briefly, when voicing contrasts such as "cap" and "cab" are present, a listener naive to the target utterance is asked to transcribe the utterance produced by the speaker. The speaker is informed of the perceived message as an indication of whether or not the target distinction was adequately produced.

REFERENCES

Aronson, A. (1980). *Clinical voice disorders: An interdisciplinary approach.* New York: Thieme-Stratton, Inc.

Aronson, A.E. (1971). Early motor unit disease masquerading as psychogenic breathy dysphonia: A clinical care presentation. *Journal of Speech & Hearing Disorders, 36*, 116–124.

Barlow, S.M., Netsell, R., & Hunker, C.J. (1986). Phonatary disorders associated with CNS lesions. In *Otolaryngology—Head and neck surgery.* St. Louis: C.V. Mosley.

Boone, D. (1977). *The voice and voice therapy* (2nd ed.). Englewood Cliffs, NJ: Prentice-Hall.

Boshes, B. (1966). Voice changes in parkinsonism. *J. Neurosurg, 24*, 286–288.

Canter, G. (1965). Speech characteristics of patients with parkinsons disease II: Physiological support for speech. *Journal of Speech & Hearing Disorders, 30*, 44–49.

Carrow, E., Rivera, V., Mauldin, M., & Shamblin, L. (1974). Deviant speech characteristics in motor neuron disease. *Arch. Otolaryngeaol, 100*, 212.

D'Antonio, L., Lotz, W., Chrit, D., & Netsell, R. (in press). Perceptual-physiologic approach to evaluation and treatment of dysphonia. *Annuals of Otology, Rhinology & Laryngology.*

Darley, F., Aronson, A., & Brown, J. (1969b). Clusters of deviant speech dimensions in the dysarthrias. *Journal of Speech & Hearing Research, 12*, 462–496.

Darley, F., Aronson, A., & Brown, J. (1975). *Motor speech disorders.* Philadelphia:

W.B. Saunders Company.

Darley, F., Brown, J.R., & Goldstein, N.P. (1972). Dysarthria in multiple sclerosis. *Journal of Speech & Hearing Research, 15*, 229–245.

Davis, S.B. (1981). Acoustic characteristics of normal and pathological voices. *ASHA Reports: Number 11*, 97–115.

Eckel, F.C., & Boone, D.R. (1981). The S/Z ratio as an indicator of laryngeal pathology. *Journal of Speech & Hearing Disorders, 46*, 147–149.

Hirano, M., Koike, Y., & von Leden, H. (1968). Maximum phonation time and air usage during phonation. *Folia Phoniatrica, 20*, 185–201.

Logemann, J.A., Fisher, H.B., Boshes, B., & Blonsky, E.R. (1978). Frequency and concurrence of vocal tract dysfunctions in the speech of a large sample of parkinson patients. *Journal of Speech & Hearing Disorders, 42*, 47–57.

Ludlow, C., & Bassich, C. (1983). The results of acoustic and perceptual assessment of two types of dysarthria. In W. Berry (Ed.), *Clinical dysarthria*. Austin, TX: PRO-ED.

Ludlow, C., & Bassich, C. (1984). Relationships between perceptual ratings and acoustic measures of hypokinetic speech. In M. McNeil, J. Rosenbek, & A. Aronson (Eds.), *The dysarthrias*. San Diego: College-Hill Press.

Mumenthaler, M. (1983). *Neurology: A textbook for physicians and students with 185 self-testing questions*. New York: Thieme-Stratton.

Netsell, R., Lotz, W., & Shaughnessy, A.L. (1984). Laryngeal aerodynamics associated with selected voice disorders. *American Journal of Otolaryngology, 5*, 397–403.

Netsell, R., & Rosenbek, J.C. (1985). Treating the dysarthrias. In *Speech and language evaluation in neurology: Adult Disorders*, New York: Grune & Stratton.

Prator, R.J., & Swift, R.W. (1984). *Manual of voice therapy*. Boston: Little, Brown & Company.

Ptacek, P.H., & Sander, E.K. (1963). Maximum duration of phonation. *Journal of Speech & Hearing Research, 28*:171.

Rosenbeck J.C. (1984). Selected alternatives to articulation training for the dysarthric adult. In H. Winitz (Ed.), *Treating articulation disorders: For clinicians by clinicians*. Austin, TX: PRO-ED.

Rosenbek, J.C., & LaPointe, L.L. (1985). The dysarthrias: Description, diagnosis, and treatment. In D.F. Johns (Ed.), *Clinical management of neurogenic communicative disorders*. Boston: Little, Brown, & Co.

Rubow, R., & Swift, E. (1985). A microcomputer-based wearable biofeedback device to improve transfer of treatment in parkinsonian dysarthria. *Journal of Speech & Hearing Disorders, 50*, 178–185.

Shapiro, A.K., Shapiro, E., & Wayne, H.L. (1973). The symptomatology and diagnosis of Gilles de la Tourette's syndrome. *J. Clild Psychiat., 12*, 702–723.

Smitheran, J., & Hixon, T., (1981). A clinical method for estimating laryngeal airway resistance during vowel production. *Journal of Speech & Hearing Disorders, 46*, 138–146.

Yanagihara, N., & Koike, Y. (1967). The regulation of sustained phonation. *Folia Phoniatrica, 19*, 1.

Yanagihara, N., Koike, Y., & von Leden, H. (1966). Phonation and respiration: Function study in normal subjects. *Folia Phoniatrica, 18*, 323.

Yanagihara, N., & von Leden, H. (1967). Respiration and phonation: The functional examination of laryngeal disease. *Folia Phoniatrica, 19*, 153.

CHAPTER 11

Velopharyngeal Function

Clinical Issues: Two speech/language pathology students were observing through a one-way mirror as a speech pathologist was evaluating a severely dysarthric speaker with multiple speech component impairment including profound velopharyngeal dysfunction. The students were questioning whether or not management of the velopharyngeal component would have any effect, considering how severely impaired the speaker appeared to be. As they discussed management options for velopharyngeal dysfunction, behavioral exercises, palatal obturators, and surgical management were included. It was clear that their information on managing velopharyngeal dysfunction was based entirely on their cleft palatal coursework. In the discussion that followed, the students raised several important questions:

- *How do velopharyngeal management options differ for dysarthric speakers as compared to speakers with cleft palate?*
- *When multiple speech components are impaired, where should intervention begin?*
- *Who is a candidate for a palatal lift?*
- *Can dysarthric speakers with velopharyngeal incompetence be managed successfully with behavioral methods alone?*

Velopharyngeal dysfunction is frequently, but not universally, associated with dysarthria. Although incidence of velopharyngeal dysfunction is unavailable for most populations of dysarthric speakers, Hardy, Rembolt, Spriestersbach, and Jaypathy (1961) reported that 39 percent of children with cerebral palsy have velopharyngeal closure problems that are considered important to their speech problems. Perceptual evidence of hypernasality and nasal emission have been reported to occur in many types of dysarthria, including flaccid, mixed (amyotrophic lateral sclerosis), spastic, ataxic, and hyperkinetic dysarthria of chorea (Darley, 1984). This suggests that velopharyngeal dysfunction occurs not only in those individuals with lower motoneuron damage affecting innervation of the soft palate, but also in individuals with other underlying neuropathologies, including cortical and cerebellar damage.

Despite the fact that velopharyngeal dysfunction does not occur in all dysarthric speakers, an understanding of the velopharyngeal mechanism, its disorders, and its management is extremely important clinically. Case reports of interventions ranging from prosthetic management to behavioral training and surgery suggest that the velopharyngeal mechanism can be managed successfully in selected individuals. There are more case reports of successful interventions in the area of velopharyngeal dysfunction than any other specific aspect of dysarthria. These interventions will be described in detail later in this chapter. Although it is encouraging to read reports of successful intervention, a review of the literature also suggests that there is no single best approach to velopharyngeal management. Rather, because velopharyngeal dysfunction in dysarthria may vary widely in its characteristics, interventions must also be tailored to the specifics of the dysfunction. Thus, the clinician not only must be able to verify whether or not there is a velopharyngeal problem, but also must be able to carefully describe the extent and consistency of the deficit before an appropriate intervention can be recommended.

Velopharyngeal dysfunction of dysarthric speakers is of critical interest to the clinician because it tends to exaggerate the impairment of other speech mechanism components. For example, a speaker with an impaired respiratory system may perform adequately to produce functional speech if the laryngeal, velopharyngeal, and oral articulatory valves are functioning efficiently. However, in the presence of velopharyngeal dysfunction, the speaker may not be able to achieve adequate respiratory drive for speech. Velopharyngeal dysfunction distorts the production of vowel and consonant sounds even though they may be produced with accurate oral articulatory gestures. In the presence of velopharyngeal dysfunction, vowels will be perceived as hypernasal and many consonants will be perceived as imprecise.

VELOPHARYNGEAL FUNCTION DURING SPEECH

Normal Speakers

The Mechanism

The velopharyngeal mechanism consists of the soft palate and that portion of the pharynx that approximates the soft palate. The velopharyngeal mechanism functions to separate or couple the nasal cavity with the oropharyngeal cavity. The soft palate is a richly innervated structure. The levator veli palatini, uvula, and superior pharyngeal constrictor muscles are dually innervated by the facial nerve and branches of the pharyngeal plexus derived from the glossopharyngeal and vagus nerves (Nishio, Matsuya, Machida, & Miyazaki, 1976). Studies conducted on rhesus monkeys suggest that the movements observed on stimulation of the vagus or glossopharyngeal nerve were similar to those observed in swallowing in humans whereas stimulation to the facial nerve resulted in velopharyngeal movement similar to that observed in human phonation (Nishio, Matsuya, Ibuki, & Miyazaki, 1976). Thus, the motor nerves innervating the velopharynx may be responsible for different types of movements.

A number of different patterns of velopharyngeal closure occur in both normal and disordered populations. Using multiview videofluoroscopy, Croft, Shprintzen, and Rakoff (1981) classified large groups of normal and cleft palate individuals into the following valving categories:

1. Coronal: The velum approximates to the posterior pharyngeal wall which remains immobile. The lateral pharyngeal walls move medially to approximate the lateral edges of the velum. The major component of velopharyngeal valving occurs in the anteroposterior direction. This pattern occurred in 55 percent of normal individuals and 45 percent of disordered individuals.

2. Sagittal: There is marked movement of the lateral pharyngeal walls occurring posterior to the velum which moves posteriorly only slightly, approximating to the anterior edge of the abutted lateral walls. This pattern occurred in 16 percent of normal and 11 percent of disordered individuals.

3. Circular: There is an equal amount of movement in the velum and lateral pharyngeal walls, creating a circular closure pattern. This pattern occurred in 10 percent of normal individuals and 20 percent of disordered individuals.

4. Circular with Passavant's ridge: As in the circular pattern, there is equal contribution to closure of the velum and lateral walls, but there is also anterior movement in the posterior pharyngeal wall (Passavant's ridge), resulting in a truly sphincteric closure pattern. This pattern occurred in 19 percent of normal individuals and 24 percent of disordered individuals.

Maue-Dickson (1977) presents an excellent review of the anatomy and physiology of the velopharyngeal mechanism.

The Speaking Task

The role of the velopharyngeal mechanism for normal speakers varies depending upon the speaking task. During the production of nonnasal consonant sounds, the velopharyngeal mechanism can be viewed as an aerodynamic valve that usually is completely sealed to prevent the escape of air from the oral cavity through the nasal cavity (Thompson & Hixon, 1979; Warren, 1975; Warren & DuBois, 1964). For most speakers, the velopharyngeal seal is complete during some aspects of "pressure consonant" production, although the pattern and duration of closure varies from speaker to speaker. However, a small number of normal speakers demonstrate very small velopharyngeal openings during the production of nonnasal consonants.

During the production of nasal consonants, the velopharyngeal mechanism is opened to allow the coupling of the oral-pharyngeal and nasal cavities to form the primary acoustic resonator for these sounds. The oral cavity is the occluded side branch resonator (Shoup, Lass, & Kuehn, 1982). This resonance pattern yields the acoustic patterns that are associated with hypernasal speech: low first formant, high sampling of formants, and high density of formants that is associated with nasal consonants.

During vowel production, the status of the velopharyngeal mechanism is influenced by the velopharyngeal requirements of the adjacent consonants. Some nasalization of the vowels is common. In fact, the complete closure of the velopharyngeal mechanism results in denasality, which is judged to be abnormal. However, excessive nasality during vowel production is also judged as abnormal.

Dysarthric Speakers

Velopharyngeal function in dysarthric speakers has not been studied as thoroughly as it has in normal or cleft palate speakers, and case reports of dysarthric individuals suggest different patterns of dysfunction. Neurological deficits seen in dysarthria result in slowness, weakness, and incoordination of palatal movements. In contrast to the speaker with a cleft palate, the dysarthric speaker has adequate palatal tissue to achieve velopharyngeal closure. Clinical experience suggests dysarthric speakers vary considerably in terms of severity and pattern of velopharyngeal dysfunction. Some individuals demonstrate essentially normal function without hypernasality, nasal emission, or abnormal movement patterns on radiographic examination. Others exhibit consistent dysfunction with little evidence of closure of the velopharyngeal port during rest breathing or speech. However, a third group exhibit somewhat less consistent patterns. Netsell (1969a) utilized an aerodynamic approach to measurement of velopharyngeal function in cerebral-palsied dysarthric speakers. He reported several types of velopharyngeal dysfunction in dysarthric speakers:

1. Gradual Closing—The speaker opens the velopharyngeal orifice at the beginning of an utterance, but it gradually closes as speech continues
2. Anticipatory Opening—The speaker opens the velopharyngeal orifice in anticipation of an upcoming nasalized sound

3. Retention Opening—The speaker slowly closes the velopharynx after the production of a nasalized sound, but not until nasal emission has occurred during subsequent sound production
4. Premature Opening—The speaker opens the velopharynx during the production of a "pressure consonant" allowing nasal emission of air during a portion of the consonant production

Hardy (1983) reviewed the patterns of velopharyngeal dysfunction he has observed in speakers with cerebral palsy. In addition to many of the patterns described by Netsell, Hardy indicated that velopharyngeal closure may be associated with vowel height: "There may be closure in association with high back vowels and proximal consonants, but not for high front vowels and neutral vowels and consonants adjacent to such vowels." Hardy also suggested that velopharyngeal function might be affected by speaking rate: "There may be more competence at rapid than at slow speaking rates or vice versa." In addition, he observed that patterns of velopharyngeal closure may be compounded by head position.

The important relationship between velopharyngeal function and other aspects of speech production in dysarthria has been frequently suggested, but has remained largely unstudied. One exception was a report Netsell (1969b) in which he studied changes in oropharyngeal cavity size of cerebral-palsied children as a function of whether or not a velopharyngeal prosthesis was in place. Results indicated a decrease in oropharyngeal cavity size with the prosthesis. Netsell states:

> some dysarthric speakers routinely use an abnormally large oropharyngeal cavity size during certain vowel productions, and that use of such an opening is a compensatory effort to offset excessive velopharyngeal opening. (p. 649)

The implication is that the velopharyngeal component of speech must be considered in relationship to other aspects of speech production. Not only may velopharyngeal incompetence exaggerate impairment in other speech components, but such incompetence may bring about maladaptative compensatory adjustments in other aspects of speech.

ASSESSMENT OF VELOPHARYNGEAL FUNCTION

During the assessment of a dysarthric speaker, the clinician usually attempts to address several questions:

- Is there evidence of velopharyngeal dysfunction in this speaker?
- What is the extent and pattern of the dysfunction?
- Does the velopharyngeal dysfunction influence other aspects of speech performance?
- What options are available to improve velopharyngeal function for this speaker?

As in the evaluation of other aspects of dysarthria, a number of approaches to measurement are available, including perceptual and instrumental techniques. The specific measurement approach depends on the nature of the clinical question. The general question, "Is there a velopharyngeal problem?" can best be answered perceptually as the clinician listens to the speech and identifies the presence or absence of those features that are typically associated with velopharyngeal dysfunction. However, after the clinician has confirmed the presence of a problem and is seeking information regarding the extent and pattern of the dysfunction, approaches other than perceptual ones are appropriate.

Perceptual Adequacy

The first phase of assessment is the confirmation of the presence of a velopharyngeal dysfunction. The adequacy of velopharyngeal function during speech is often perceptually assessed. Ratings of hypernasality, occurrence of nasal emission, and patterns of articulatory errors can be employed as indicators of adequacy of velopharyngeal function. Each of these features will be discussed.

Hypernasality

The term *hypernasality* refers to the perception of excessive nasality. In the field of dysarthria, it has traditionally been assessed by rating samples of connected speech on the seven-point equal-appearing interval scale used by Darley, Aronson, and Brown (1975). Presence of hypernasality may also be identified clinically by alternate pinching of the nostrils while the speaker is producing a sustained vowel (Moser, 1942). A fluttering vowel quality signals the presence of hypernasality. Sustained phonation is a speech-like task and may not reflect the degree of hypernasality in contextual speech.

The use of perceptual ratings of hypernasality are associated with a number of limitations, one of which is judge reliability. Kuehn (1982) states:

> One of the main disadvantages is that perceptual measures, specifically listener judgments, are difficult to calibrate. Perceptual judgments depend on training and experience, among other factors, and different listeners may not agree as to the severity of a particular problem. (p. 505)

Mild to moderate hypernasality is an aspect of some dialectic patterns of normal speakers. In this case, hypernasality is not associated with velopharyngeal dysfunction. Perceptual judgments of hypernasality may be influenced by factors unrelated to velopharyngeal function. Moll (1968) grouped these factors into the following categories for individuals with cleft lip and palate: phonetic aspects, pitch level, loudness level, and articulatory proficiency. Although unconfirmed in the research literature, the same factors may affect judgments of hypernasality in dysarthric speakers. Hypernasality ratings are no doubt influenced to some extent by the severity of the articulatory deficit of dysarthric speakers. Judges tend to inflate hypernasality ratings for speakers with extensive articulation errors. Hypernasality ratings may also be affected by loudness level. If respiratory drive and therefore, loudness levels, are reduced, the extent of hypernasality may be underestimated. However, if loudness is excessive, hypernasality may be exaggerated.

The problems associated with perceptual ratings of hypernasality has led researchers to seek objective or instrumental means of measurement. To date, no substitute for perceptual ratings of hypernasality has been developed. Kuehn (1982) states:

> Although resonance is an acoustic phenomenon with underlying structural correlates, there are no existing explicit standards for normal resonance patterns in either the acoustic or the anatomic/physiologic domain and there are not likely to be any in the near future. (p. 505)

Nasal Emission

The term *nasal emission* refers to air flow through the nose during production of nonnasal consonants. Nasal emission may appropriately be considered an articulatory rather than a resonance problem. However, both nasal emission and hypernasality may be a consequence of velopharyngeal incompetence, although the two features may exist independently (Peterson-Falzone, 1982). A speaker may exhibit moderate hypernasality without audible nasal emission, or inconsistent nasal emission with hypernasality. The presence of nasal emission is frequently associated with velopharyngeal dysfunction. Because nasal emission during production of the nasal consonants is not associated with normal speech, the perceptual identification of this feature is usually taken as an indication of dysfunction. However, inability to perceptually detect nasal emission should not be taken as an indication of adequate velopharyngeal function. If the nasal emission is minimal, it may not be audible and can be detected only by instrumentation that measures airflow. If a speaker is unable to impound air pressure in the oral cavity due to severely reduced respiratory drive or inability to achieve a constriction or obstruction of airflow in the oral cavity, only a minimal amount of air will escape through the nasal cavity, regardless of the degree of velopharyngeal dysfunction.

Articulatory Error Patterns

Velopharyngeal incompetence results in inability to generate sufficient intraoral air pressure to produce certain consonants, particularly the plosives, fricatives, and affricates. Evaluation of the pattern of consonant articulation errors with particular emphasis on the pressure sounds has long been used in the field of cleft palate research (Morris, Spriestersbach, & Darley, 1961; Prins & Bloomer, 1968; Van Demark et al., 1985).

Analysis of articulatory patterns may indicate the presence of velopharyngeal dysfunction. Most obvious of the articulatory patterns is the nasalization of voiced consonants such as /b/, /d/, and /g/. Because of the effect of neuromotor impairment on the overall articulation performance of the dysarthric speaker, determining the contribution of the velopharyngeal dysfunction to the specific articulatory pattern may be somewhat more difficult to determine in the dysarthric than in the cleft palate speaker. In an effort to deal with this issue, Yorkston, Honsinger, Mitsuda, and Beukelman (1986) investigated the articulatory performance of two groups of dysarthric speakers, those who were determined through aerodynamic studies not to achieve velopharyngeal closure and those who, at least occasionally, achieved velopharyngeal closure. Analysis of their results revealed that in those speakers who achieve some velopharyngeal closure, the percentage of nasal sounds that were correctly produced was very similar to the percentage of "pressure consonants" that were correctly produced. However, for the group of dysarthric subjects who did not achieve complete velopharyngeal closure, the percentage of nasal and glide sounds correctly produced was much greater than the percentage of pressure consonants correctly produced.

Figure 11-1 contains a scattergraph of attempted versus perceived consonants produced by an individual with velopharyngeal incompetence in addition to other impairments in the respiratory, phonatory, and oral articulatory components of speech. The scattergraph is typical of those obtained from velopharyngeally incompetent speakers. Examination of the figure suggests that the judge is misidentifying many of the pressure consonants as nasals. Overall scores for consonant production indicate that the judge is able to identify 17 percent of the consonant productions correctly. Further analysis reveals a marked difference between accuracy of the nasal/glide category (45 percent accurate) as compared to pressure consonants (7 percent accurate).

Patterns of Velopharyngeal Dysfunction

After the presence of velopharyngeal dysfunction has been identified, an attempt is often made to describe the pattern of dysfunction. The velopharyngeal port cannot be directly viewed during connected speech. Further, precise inferences about the size of the velopharyngeal port and the timing of closure in relation to other aspects of speech production cannot be made solely on the basis of perceptual judgments. Therefore, a number of instrumental measurement techniques are typically used to supplement perceptual judgment and to give a more detailed description of the pattern of the dysfunction. The following discussion will be restricted to those techniques that are routinely employed clinically when evaluating dysarthric speakers. Kuehn (1982) gives an excellent review of approaches to assessment

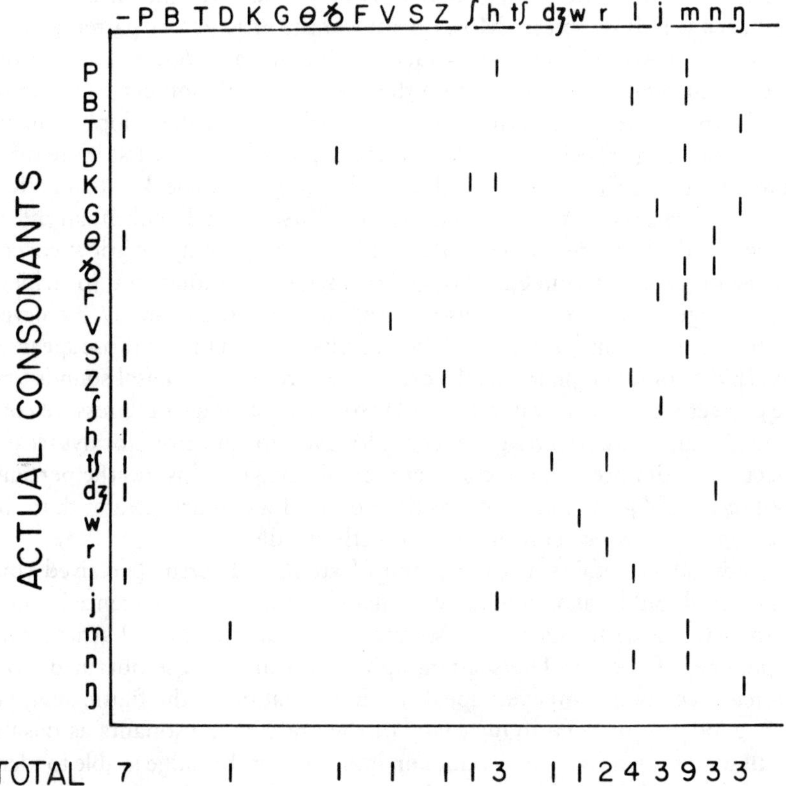

Figure 11-1. Scattergraph plot of actual versus perceived consonants produced by a speaker with severe dysarthria and velopharyngeal incompetence.

of resonance disorders, including acoustic analysis and those techniques that assess resonance by comparing nasal and oral sound pressure levels.

Aerodynamic Measures

Because the velopharyngeal port is one of the most important valves that interrupts the breath stream during the production of speech sounds, measurement of oral air pressure and volume velocity of air flow across the port are useful indicators of velopharyngeal function. Aerodynamic techniques do not provide a direct measure of velopharyngeal movement, rather they are used to make estimates of velopharyngeal resistance and/or area of the velopharyngeal orifice.

EQUIPMENT. The basic components for aerodynamic measurement include an air flow meter, an air pressure transducer, and a microphone (Kuehn, 1982; Netsell, 1969a; Warren, 1975). The pneumotachograph is the most frequently used type of air flow meter. Use of this device requires that the speaker wear a nose mask that traps nasally emitted air. Measurement of air flow is based on the detection of pressure difference across the wire screen of the pneumotachograph. Air flow rate measures alone are not a good index of velopharyngeal adequacy because these measures are affected by such factors as nasal or oral cavity resistance and intraoral air pressure. Therefore, intraoral air pressure measures are obtained simultaneously with those of nasal airflow. This is accomplished by placing a small, flexible polyethylene tube on the tongue, oriented perpendicular to the flow of air in the oropharynx. Pressures are sensed within this tube and are converted to electrical voltage by a transducer. The simultaneously obtained measures of nasal air flow rates and intraoral air pressure may be used in standard equations to calculate velopharyngeal orifice area, nasal airway resistance, and oral cavity constriction size (Warren & Dubois, 1964; Warren & Ryon, 1967).

SPEECH SAMPLE. Netsell (1969a) suggested the use of a speech sample that varied both speaking rate and the phonetic context of speech. A review of Table 11-1 reveals the list of utterances produced includes voiceless and voiced plosive and nasal consonant productions accompanied by a neutral vowel. Utterances are produced at conversational levels of pitch and loudness.

TABLE 11-1.
A List of Utterances Produced During Aerodynamic Measurement Procedures

	Utterance	**Rate**
Rate Variation:	/tʌ/	1, 2, 4, and 5/sec
	/dʌ/	1, 2, 4, and 5/sec
	/nʌ/	1, 2, 4, and 5/sec
Phonetic Context Variation:		
	/ʌtʌdʌ/	Conversational
	/ʌdʌtʌ/	Conversational
	/ʌndʌntʌn/	Conversational
	/ʌntʌndʌn/	Conversational
	/ʌtʌnʌ/	Conversational
	/ʌdʌnʌ/	Conversational
	/ʌnʌtʌ/	Conversational
	/ʌnʌdʌ/	Conversational

From Netsell, R. (1969a). Evaluation of velopharyngeal function in dysarthria. *Journal of Speech & Hearing Disorders, 34,* 113.

INTERPRETING THE RESULTS. Figure 11-2 contains results of simultaneous recording of nasal air flow and intraoral air pressure for a normal speaker who is repeating the utterance /apapapa/. For ease of interpretation, an audio signal is also displayed. Examination of this figure reveals that no nasal emission is present during any of the stop phases of the voiceless plosive /p/. Further, the speaker is consistently achieving intraoral air pressures of approximately 7 cm H_20.

In contrast to the measurements obtained from a normal speaker, the measurements represented in Figure 11-3 are from a dysarthric speaker. This figure illustrates the audio signal, nasal air flow, and intraoral air pressure as the speaker is repeating the sentence "Buy a pie" two times. Note that consistent nasal emission occurs simultaneously with the build up of intraoral air pressure during the stop phase of the plosive sounds. Further, increases in intraoral air pressure are associated with proportional increases in the level of nasal air flow.

LIMITATIONS OF THE TECHNIQUE. Although aerodynamic measures allow the clinician to make precise inferences about the extent and timing of velopharyngeal closure, the technique has certain limitations. In order to interpret the results, the speaker must be able to achieve either tongue tip to alveolar ridge contact for /tʌ/ or bilabial contact for /pʌ/. If the speaker is unable to achieve an air tight seal, accurate measures of intraoral air pressure cannot be obtained.

Radiographic Techniques

In addition to aerodynamic measures of velopharyngeal dysfunction, radiographic techniques have been utilized extensively with cleft palate speakers and also with dysarthric speakers. Rather than relying on inference about

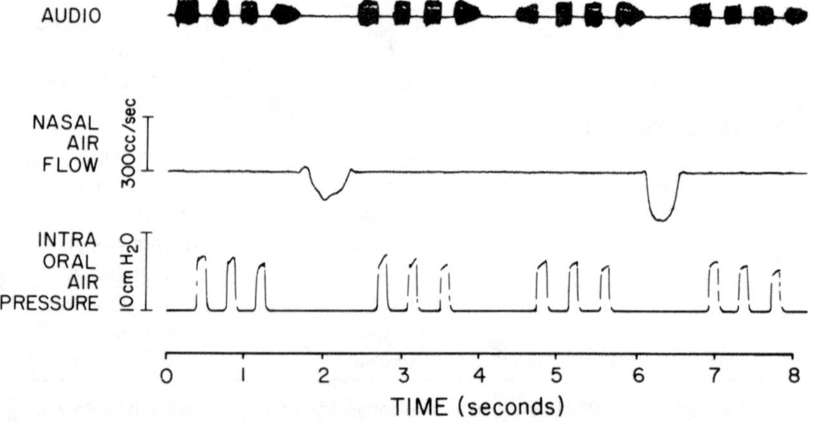

Figure 11-2. Illustration of the speech signal (audio), nasal airflow rate, and intraoral air pressure from a normal speaker repeating the utterance /apapapa/ four times.

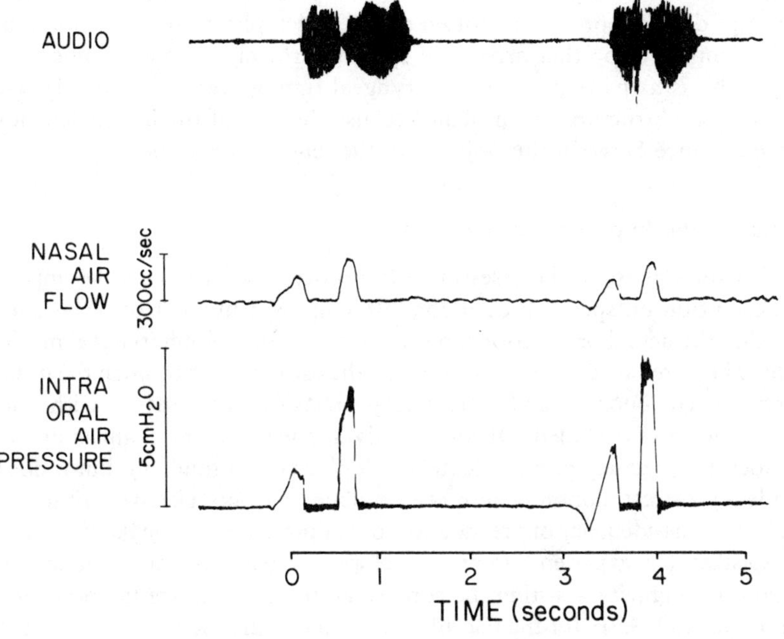

Figure 11-3. Illustration of the speech signal (audio), nasal airflow rate, and intraoral air pressure from a dysarthric speaker repeating the sentence "Buy a pie" two times.

movement from perceptual observation, these techniques allow for the examination of movements in speech structures typically hidden from view. Cineradiographic or videofluoroscopic approaches have been used extensively to evaluate velopharyngeal function in cleft palate speakers. Kuehn (1982) presents a review of these procedures. In the dysarthria field, radiographic procedures have been used somewhat more sparingly. Typically, radiographic procedures are not utilized as a routine part of our examination of an individual with dysarthria. Radiographic procedures are frequently employed by some in the palatal lift fitting process.

Direct Visualization

Fiberoptic equipment allows the direct visual observation of structures without radiation exposure. To assess velopharyngeal function, the flexible shaft of the fiberscope is inserted through the nares and nasal cavity until the soft palate and pharyngeal wall movement can be observed (Miyazaki, Matsuya, & Yamaoka, 1975). Reports of the usefulness of this technique are beginning to appear in the literature (D'Antonio, Chart, Lotz, & Netsell, 1986; Ibuki, Karnell, & Morris, 1983; Karnell, Ibuki, Morris, & Van Demark, 1983). This technique also allows the movement of the structures to be viewed. However, several features have limited its use: (1) Many dysarthric patients are unable to tolerate the presence of the fiberscope in the nasal cavity. (2) The fiberscope does not provide a written record of velopharyngeal function that can be compared to other aspects of speech performance on a moment by moment basis as patterns of velopharyngeal timing are measured. (3) Size estimates of a structure are difficult because the size of the image depends on the distance between the object and the lens of the scope.

Estimating the Impact of Intervention

The final phase of the assessment is a process of estimating the impact of intervention on speech production. We employ a number of techniques to modify the actual or functional performance of the velopharyngeal mechanism. The nares are occluded to eliminate the escape of air through the nasal cavity. Speech loudness and articulatory precision are assessed with and without the nares occluded. Of course, valving the speech mechanism in this way does not precisely mimic adequate velopharyngeal function, but it does provide a gross estimation of improved function, if one selectively observes such features as adequacy of pressure consonant production. The flaccid dysarthric speaker may experience improved velopharyngeal function in the supine position with gravity assisting the soft palate to approximate the posterior pharyngeal wall. Also, for the flaccid speaker, a dental mirror can be inserted into the oral cavity and the soft palate elevated into the position approximating the pharyngeal wall. Change in vowel quality may be noted as the velopharyngeal port is occluded. Finally, we instruct the client to speak at a variety of rates, in an attempt to determine the impact of speaking rate on velopharyngeal function.

TREATMENT OF VELOPHARYNGEAL DYSFUNCTION

The decision whether or not to focus the intervention on improvement of velopharyngeal function is dependent on several factors. The overall neurological stability of the speaker is considered. If a speaker is improving rapidly, the decision not to intervene directly to improve velopharyngeal function is frequently made. Likewise, if a speaker is deteriorating rapidly, intervention with the velopharyngeal mechanism may not be considered. Thus, intervention is usually selected for persons with relatively stable conditions.

Velopharyngeal dysfunction has important consequences for speech production. In fact, Hardy (1983) suggests that it "is likely to be more dehabilitating than inefficiency of oral structures" (p. 88). At times, the velopharyngeal dysfunction is so severe that intervention to improve other aspects of speech performance will probably be ineffective, if velopharyngeal function is not properly managed (Netsell & Daniel, 1979). For example, respiratory function may be severely compromised in the dysarthric speaker. When this occurs in conjunction with an open velopharyngeal port, air will follow the path of least resistance and escape through the nose rather than the oral cavity. As long as air pressure escapes through the nasal cavity, improvement in respiratory drive will not result in an increase in intraoral air pressure during the production of consonant sounds. Also, in some speakers with severe flaccid dysarthria, the soft palate is draped on the posterior aspects of the tongue. Because the palate is not elevated during speech efforts, the speaker radiates all sound energy into the nasal cavity through the velopharyngeal port and none through the oral cavity. Without some intervention to improve function of the velopharyngeal mechanism, efforts to improve articulation will be ineffective.

For other dysarthric speakers, velopharyngeal dysfunction will not be so severely affected by the neuromotor impairment. In these cases, the speech/language pathologist may take several different courses of action. If the speaker has an improving dysarthria, the decision to focus intervention on other aspects of the disorder may be taken while monitoring changes in velopharyngeal dysfunction. This is especially true in cases of brain injury, in which overall changes in motor control are occurring. At other times, the dysarthria is stable with a history of unchanging patterns of velopharyngeal dysfunction, and the decision to focus intervention on the velopharyngeal mechanism is initiated.

Behavioral Methods

Behavioral approaches for the management of velopharyngeal dysfunction in dysarthric speakers appear to be as controversial as they are in managing cleft palate speakers. Noll (1982) suggests that there are similarities in management of those dysarthric and cleft palate speakers. If the speaker is unable to achieve closure, either because of lack of tissue or neuromotor deficits, behavioral intervention may not be appropriate. Noll states:

> the only way to modify the problem is to improve the apposition of the soft palate with the pharyngeal walls, regardless of whether it is due to a structural deficiency of the palatal mechanism (as in cleft patients) or to a neuromuscular dysfunction of the soft palatal (as in some dysarthric patients). If the structural defect is of such a degree that there is insufficient anatomic tissue to accomplish velopharyngeal closure whatsoever, then no amount of speech therapy will result in significantly altering the problem of excessive nasality. By the same token, if there is severe neuromuscular involvement such that the patient cannot possibly accomplish closure, then a program of speech therapy is undoubtedly futile. (p. 566)

With the caution that the following approaches are likely to succeed only with those speakers with mild velopharyngeal dysfunction who are able to achieve adequate closure, a number of behavioral approaches can be found in the literature (Ruscello, 1982). Froeschels (1943) and Froeschels, Kastein, and Weiss (1955) suggest a pushing technique for speakers with velar paralysis. Their rationale is that voluntary contraction of one group of muscles will overflow onto other groups. Daly and Johnson (1974) reported successful training of three mentally retarded individuals with excessive nasality using an instrumental system known as TONAR (The Oral Nasal Acoustic Ratio [Fletcher, 1970]). However, some suggest that such direct exercises are ineffective because speech and nonspeech velopharyngeal closure involve different underlying mechanisms (Moll, 1974) and no evidence exists that increasing soft palate strength improves speech performance (Shelton, Hahn, & Morris, 1968).

At times, it is appropriate to treat mild velopharyngeal dysfunction simply as an articulatory problem. Many of the techniques reported in Chapter 12 may be employed to improve the production of nasal as well as nonnasal consonants. Rate control may also have an impact on velopharyngeal performance. A reduction in velopharyngeally associated symptoms (hypernasality) was reported in selected ataxic dysarthric subjects when their speaking rate was reduced (Yorkston & Beukelman, 1981). Because these ataxic speakers spoke at an excessively rapid rate, they may have been unable to achieve articulatory targets and the velopharyngeal movements for closure were not accomplished. However, when speaking rates were reduced with the resultant increase in speech intelligibility, articulatory targets were achieved by oral and velopharyngeal structures and hypernasality was within the normal range.

Prosthetic Methods

The Palatal Lift

When dysarthric speakers are unable to achieve velopharyngeal closure by voluntarily modifying their speech pattern, better function can be accomplished by prosthetically managing the dysfunction with a palatal lift, a rigid acrylic appliance fabricated by a prosthodontist. The palatal lift consists of a retentive portion covering the hard palate and fastening to the maxillary teeth by means of wires and a lift portion that extends along the oral surface of the soft palate. At times, orthodontic bands or acrylic ridges are added to selected teeth to improve the retention capability of the palatal portion of the lift. The lifting action of the device is illustrated in Figure 11-4.

The palatal lift is usually constructed in a series of steps:

1. The speaker's teeth are checked and needed restoration is completed
2. Orthodontic bands or acrylic ridges are secured to selected teeth (optional)
3. An oral cavity desensitization program is begun for those speakers with hyperactive gag reflexes (Daniel, 1982)
4. A mold of the maxillary arch is taken
5. A dental retainer (the palatal portion) of the lift is fabricated with a wire loop extending posteriorly as an anchor for the posterior portion
6. The posterior portion of the lift is shaped using temperature-sensitive wax. The wax is shaped when warm and becomes firm when cool. The lift is adjusted using the wax until an optimal fit is achieved

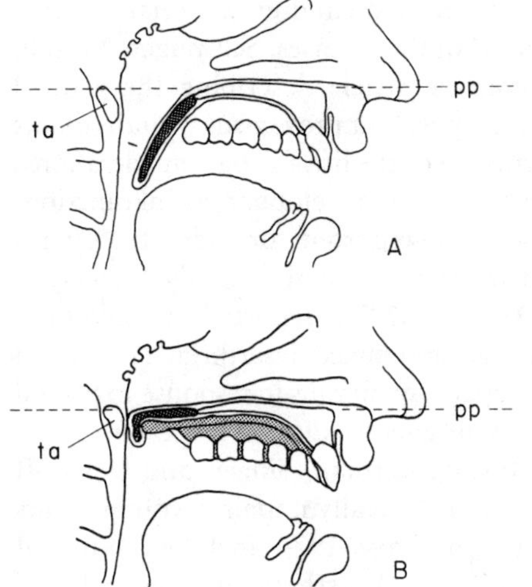

Figure 11-4. A line drawing representation of a neurologically involved speaker with velopharyngeal incompetence. Illustrated are views without (A) and with (B) the palatal lift (pp, palatal plane; ta, median tubercle of the atlas) (From Gonzalez & Aronson, 1970).

7. The posterior portion of the lift is cast in acrylic and polished
8. Further adjustments are made by removing or adding acrylic to the lift

For individuals with minimal tolerance of objects in their mouth, the palatal lift may be fitted in several stages, with the patient wearing the partially completed lift for several days or weeks to adjust to it, before the next adjustment is made.

An alternative palatal lift design was reported by Aten, McDonald, Simpson, and Gutierrez (1984), who described their intervention with 16 moderately to severely dysarthric patients. The purpose of their research was to evaluate the efficacy of a specifically designed palatal lift in treating patients with a wide variety of neurological conditions. The traditional lift was modified so that the lift portion was attached to the body of the maxillary retainer with wire connectors instead of traditional solid acrylic material. This design allowed the lift to be adjusted by bending the wires to achieve the desired height and anterior-posterior dimensions. The authors report that palatal lifts were demonstrated to reduce hypernasal resonance in all patients but one.

Historical Review

The use of the palatal lift prosthesis to manage velopharyngeal dysfunction has a relatively long history. The prosthetic approach to palatal dysfunction in dysarthria was initiated nearly 30 years ago by Gibbons and Bloomer (1958), who introduced the procedure when they developed a lift for an individual with palatal paralysis due to bulbospinal poliomyelitis. Lang (1967) and Kipfmueller and Lang (1972) presented a detailed description of palatal lift fitting and construction. Hardy, Netsell, Schweiger, and Morris (1969) reported on their efforts to fit 11 cerebral-palsied children with palatal lifts, and reported successful intervention in 10 of the 11 cases. Schweiger, Netsell, and Sommerfield (1970) wrote a summary article describing the general methods of prosthetic management and speech improvement in individuals with dysarthria. They reviewed construction of the lift, fitting considerations, and radiographic and aerodynamic measurement of velopharyngeal function. Successful palatal lift fitting has also been reported for individuals with velopharyngeal dysfunction of unknown etiology (Lawshe, Hardy, Schweiger, & Van Allen, 1971). Gonzalez and Aronson (1970) reported on successful fitting of 19 individuals with flaccid, spastic, and mixed dysarthria. They noted reductions in hypernasality and nasal emission symptoms in response to palatal lift fitting. However, some patients with progressive disease lost their speech gains over time following palatal lift fitting. Kerman, Singer, and Davidoff (1973) constructed palatal lifts for two neurologically impaired young adults with severe dysarthria. Fletcher, Sooudi, and Frost (1974) included results of four dysarthric speakers in their report of prosthetic management of "nasalance" in speech. They reported improvement for all four subjects, but the most severe of the degenerative subjects (familial spastic paraplegia) responded less satisfactorily to the prosthesis than did her less-involved sister.

Guidelines for Candidacy

The candidacy requirements for palatal lifts appear to differ from center to center. Generally, the following guidelines cover the major considerations (Gonzalez & Aronson, 1970; Netsell & Rosenthal, 1985; Rosenbek & La Pointe, 1985).

SEVERITY OF THE DYSFUNCTION. A palatal lift should be considered for speakers who demonstrate consistent inability to achieve velopharyngeal closure. For such individuals, behavior intervention, in the absence of spontaneous recovery, is usually ineffective. For individuals who are able to achieve closure during some, but not all, speech attempts, palatal lift intervention is less clear-cut. If the disorder is mild, behavioral intervention may be useful. Typically, a brief period of trial intervention can indicate whether or not the behavioral approach is likely to succeed.

IMPAIRMENT IN OTHER SPEECH COMPONENTS. Palatal lifts are most likely to succeed immediately with those individuals who exhibit a relatively isolated velopharyngeal impairment. Unfortunately, for most dysarthric speakers, velopharyngeal impairment is most frequently accompanied by respiratory, phonatory, and oral articulatory impairment. Although speakers with severe articulatory or respiratory disorders may be considered for palatal lift fitting, clinicians should not expect more from the lift than the speaker's symptom complex will allow (Rosenbek & LaPointe, 1985). When multiple speech components are involved, palatal lift fitting must be followed by a traditional program of respiratory or articulatory training. For the severely involved speaker, managing the velopharyngeal mechanism may serve to improve the efficiency of the respiratory system and to allow for progress in the modification of oral articulation. At our center, we do not require good oral articulation and respiratory function before proceeding with palatal lift fitting for stable or gradually recovering speakers. However, we do not typically recommend palatal lifts for individuals who are unable to achieve voluntary phonation because of a severely compromised respiratory system.

COOPERATION. Lack of motivation and failure to cooperate are frequently cited as contraindications for palatal lift fitting (Gonzalez & Aronson, 1970; Dworkin & Johns, 1980). We do not consider palatal lifts for severely brain-injured speakers who are still easily agitated, unable to tolerate minimal amounts of discomfort, or unable to understand the purpose of the intervention.

PALATAL SPASTICITY. Speakers with extremely spastic palates may be difficult to fit with a palatal lift. The result of spasticity is a stiff soft palate that may not tolerate elevation and may make retention more difficult.

COURSE OF THE DISORDER. When considering a palatal lift for a speaker with a degenerative disease, consider the natural course of the disease and realize the benefits of the lift may be of short duration. Be particularly conservative when the speaker's articulation capability is deteriorating rapidly. Unlike individuals with a stable or recovery course, we typically require good oral articulation before proceeding with palatal lift fitting for speakers with rapidly degenerating disorders.

SWALLOWING DIFFICULTIES. If a speaker has difficulty swallowing secretions without aspiration, the presence of a palatal lift will reduce swallowing efficiency to some extent in these individuals. Typically, the flow of saliva is increased during the phase in which the speaker is accommodating to the lift. This period is typically a brief one.

DENTURES. Edentulous persons are considered difficult to fit with palatal lifts by some centers, whereas other centers report considerable success with this group of speakers. Ill-fitting dentures are particularly problematic when combined with a spastic soft palate.

Documenting the Effects of the Lift

Frequently, the goals of palatal lift intervention involve a number of different issues:

1. Velopharyngeal closure during the production of the "pressure consonants" of speech
2. Velopharyngeal opening during the nasal sounds of speech
3. Painless, efficient, comfortable swallow of secretions, food, and drink
4. Ability to breathe through the nose during rest breathing
5. Improvement in overall speech function in terms of improved intelligibility, normalized nasality, elimination or reduction in nasal emission, improved precision of consonant production, and more efficient valving of the breath stream during speech

Successful achievement of these goals can be documented in a variety of ways. Nearly all of the measures used to assess velopharyngeal function may also be used to document the effects of palate lift fitting. Perhaps the most direct means of documenting the impact of a palatal lift is aerodynamically. The relationship between rate of nasal air flow and intraoral air pressure generation can be seen in Figure 11-5. This figure contains measures obtained from a speaker with severe dysarthria as a result of closed head injury. This speaker was six months post onset when first evaluated. Aerodynamic measures were again obtained at nine months post onset. On both occasions, the speaker was unable to generate more than 1.5 cm H_20 intraorally. These low intraoral air pressures were produced in the presence of high nasal air flow rate, thus indicating velopharyngeal incompetence. Further, these

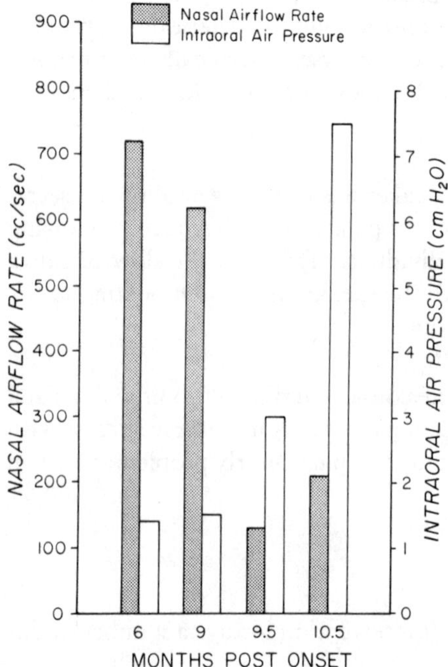

Figure 11-5. Measures of nasal airflow rate and intraoral air pressure produced during the stop phase of voiceless plosives by a severely dysarthric speaker. Measures at 9.5 and 10.5 months post onset were obtained while the speaker wore a palatal lift.

measures obtained three months apart indicated essentially no change over time. The initial fitting of the palatal lift was completed at 9.5 months post onset. Measures obtained at that time indicated that with the lift in place, the speaker was able to generate as high as 3 cm H_20 in the presence of airflow rates approximately one third of those obtained without the lift. Aerodynamic measures were obtained once again at 10.5 months post onset. At that time, the speaker was able to generate 7.5 cm H_20 during the stop phase of voiceless plosives.

Still another useful technique for measuring palatal lift effect is the examination of articulatory error patterns for speakers with and without the lift in place. Figure 11-6 illustrates data obtained during the first three months post fitting of a palatal lift for a severely dysarthric individual. The palatal lift was initially fitted at 23 months post onset (MPO) of closed head injury. An inventory of perceived articulatory adequacy was obtained using a task in which judges without knowledge of the target attempted to identify the phoneme produced (Yorkston, Dowden, Beukelman, & Traynor, 1986). Immediately following fitting at 23 MPO, results suggested a marked improvement in nonnasal consonant production. Judges identified only five percent of these sounds when the speaker was not wearing the lift as compared to 45 percent when the lift was in place. However, accuracy of production of nasal consonants was reduced markedly when the lift was first introduced.

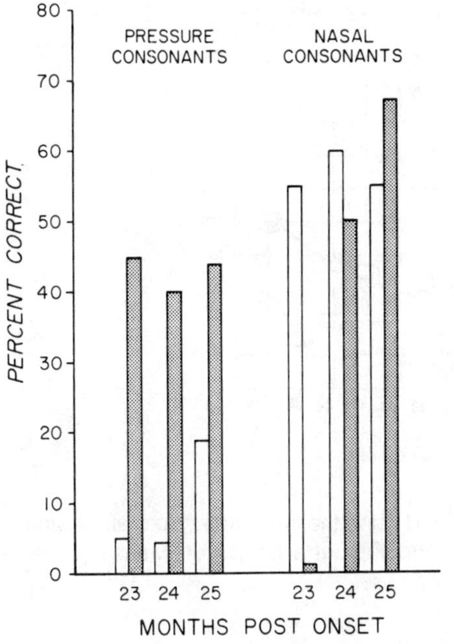

Figure 11-6. Measures of perceived articulatory adequacy for pressure and nasal consonants obtained from a dysarthric speaker with and without a palatal lift. Measures were obtained at 23 months post onset (initial fitting) and at 24 & 25 months post onset.

Over the course of the next two months, performance with and without the lift was monitored. Results indicated that adequacy of nonnasal consonant production remained relatively stable. However, production of nasal consonants with the lift in place consistently improved to the point where performance on these sounds with the lift in place was better than without the lift. This case illustrates the point made by many clinicians (Kerman, Singer, & Davidoff, 1973; LaVelle & Hardy, 1979; Shaughnessy, Netsell, & Farrage, 1983) that optimum speech results come only after a period of accommodation and, in this case, speech training.

Improvement in the overall adequacy of speech intelligibility is perhaps the best means of assessing the functional changes brought about by the palatal lift. Figure 11-7 contains longitudinal speech intelligibility data (from Yorkston, Beukelman, & Traynor, 1984) for the closed-head-injured speaker just described. The graph plots single word intelligibility, with and without the palatal lift, during the period of time from 23 to 30 MPO. Examination of the figure suggests that the speaker consistently demonstrated a 15 to 20 percent increase in single word speech intelligibility when wearing the lift. Although some improvement is noted over the course of time without the lift, the speaker continued to benefit from the lift.

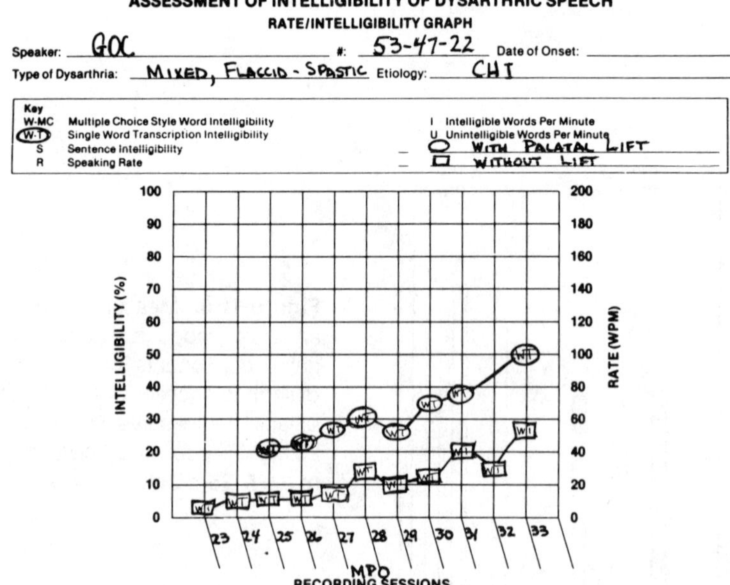

Figure 11-7. Single word intelligibility (judged using the transcription format) obtained from a severely dysarthric speaker with and without a palatal lift. Measures were obtained from 23 through 33 months post onset.

Still another potential impact of palatal lift fitting is the suggestion made by some (Dworkin & Johns, 1980; Lang & Kipfmueller, 1969; Mazaheri & Mazaheri, 1976) that placement of the lift stimulates or facilitates development of lateral and posterior wall movements in some speakers. Lateral movement may contribute in an important way to the success of the outcome. With an optimal fitting lift, velopharyngeal contact is made in the anteroposterior dimension, but lateral airways are left in order to maintain nasal breathing and nasal sound production. Schwieger, Netsell, and Sommerfeld (1970) report that many dysarthric speakers with well-fitted lifts are able to close off the velopharyngeal orifice completely during speech duration. Presumably, this is accomplished with lateral wall movements.

Difficult Populations to Serve with Palatal Lifts

EDENTULOUS SPEAKERS. Through the years, attempts have been made to fit edentulous speakers with palatal lifts. Rosenbek & LaPointe (1985) reported that their clinical group had attempted to fit five edentulous, flaccid dysarthric patients with palatal lifts, but that only one was successful. The others were unable to retain the prosthesis. Aten, McDonald, Simpson, and Gutierrez (1984) reported fitting palatal lifts for 16 patients, 9 of whom wore dentures. They concluded that for 15 of the 16 speakers, the palatal lifts were effective in reducing hypernasality. One subject with ataxic dysarthria was judged to be more nasal with than without the lift. The authors wrote, "Denture seals were maintained and retention was not a major problem" (p. 240).

VERY YOUNG CHILDREN. Shaughnessy, Netsell, and Farrage (1983) reported the successful palatal lift fitting of a four year old boy with severe dysarthria. They summarized an intervention program that involved a variety of treatment approaches, including the palatal lift. Although this four year old boy appears to be the youngest child with palatal lift fitting thus far reported in the literature, Holley, Hamby, and Taylor (1973) report the successful palatal lift fitting of a seven year old boy with a "lifelong history of grossly nasal speech" of unknown etiology. This boy's pre-fitting hypernasality was "greatly reduced" and "speech intelligibility was improved."

CHANGING NEUROLOGICAL STATUS. The need to adjust palatal lifts to meet the requirements of the changing client has been a long-standing problem. At times, prosthodonists become frustrated with the repeated visits needed to achieve a properly fitting lift. Then, as the neurological status of the individual changes, further adjustment often is needed.

PERSONS WITH DIFFICULTY ADJUSTING TO THE PROSTHESES. Patients who have difficulty adjusting to the presence of a palatal lift are managed quite differently, depending on the philosophy of the intervention team. There is no research supporting one approach over the others. Daniel (1982) suggested that there are individuals who have difficulty adjusting to a palatal lift, including persons with spasticity of the soft palate, hypersensitivity to touch, and hyperactive gag reflexes. For those individuals, Daniel suggested a palatal desensitization program prior to palatal lift fitting. In the program, someone other than the patient applies pressure in a rubbing motion on the alveolar ridge of the patient with a cot placed on the index finger. Gradually, the hard palate is stimulated at the midline farther and farther posteriorly. When the patient feels the urge to gag, he or she is instructed to utter a sound and the posterior progression of the stimulating finger is stopped and lateral movements begun. After 30 seconds of lateral massage, a 15 second rest period is provided. The stimulation pattern then begins again. Daniel suggested that exercises should be completed for five minutes, four times per day, seven days per week, and that desensitization, if it is going to occur, usually takes two or three weeks.

Hardy (1983) and colleagues have adopted an approach in which the completed palatal lift is inserted without a desensitization program. Although the adaptation process may be difficult, the gag reflex is gradually inhibited. In our clinical practice, we have taken a moderate position on this issue. For individuals, especially those with head injury who have difficulty tolerating discomfort, we initiate a program of desensitization during the tooth brushing routine. This familiarizes the patient with another person stimulating their oral area. In addition, during the initial insertions of the palatal lift, we have the individual wear the lift for very brief periods of time (often five to ten seconds). During each subsequent insertion, the duration is doubled. With two or three insertions per day, the duration of palatal lift wearing soon reaches several hours.

Follow-up Approaches

After the palatal lift is optimally fitted, a follow-up program should be initiated to meet several needs. First, the fit of the lift should be checked, especially during the first months of use. Some early users bend the wires that attach the dental portion of the lift to the teeth, and the lift does not fit properly. Second, although the lift users may be somewhat uncomfortable initially, they should no longer experience pain after they adapt to the lift. If pain or discomfort persists, the lift probably will need to be modified slightly. Third, the condition of the tissues of the soft palate should be checked to ensure that the fit of the lift is appropriate. For severely involved speakers with impairment in multiple speech components, follow-up to palatal lift fitting takes the form of speech treatment. Typically, this treatment focuses on attempting to achieve increased respiratory support and on increasing the precision of pressure consonant production. Finally, long-term follow-up is necessary, especially with speakers gradually recovering from closed head injury or stroke, because for many, the palatal lift is a temporary device worn until adequate velopharyngeal function returns. It is essential to follow these individuals so that return of function can be adequately monitored.

Surgical Methods

At the time this book was written, surgical procedures were being used very infrequently with dysarthric speakers. Noll (1982) summarizes his review of surgical management of velopharyngeal dysfunction in dysarthria by saying:

> It would appear from a review of the published reports that any form of surgical treatment of the velopharyngeal system for dysarthric patients is less than totally successful. It is true that some authors report good results with their patients. However, other studies indicate that some postoperative hypernasality or impaired speech persists. At any rate, this form of management certainly does not seem to be as successful with patients who have an impaired velopharyngeal mechanism due to neuromotor problems as it is with those patients who have structural deficits. (pp. 561–562)

Teflon Injections

Teflon injections have been reported by Lewy, Cole, and Wepman (1965), who injected Teflon and glycerin mixture into the area of Passavant's line in patients with neurogenically based dysfunction. They reported improved speech as a result. Bluestone, Musgrave, McWilliams, and Crozier (1968) injected Teflon into the nasopharynxes of 12 individuals with velopharyngeal incompetence. They excluded from their sample any persons with poorly defined or erratic levator action.

Pharyngeal Flap

Hardy, Rembolt, Spriestersbach, and Jaypathy (1961) reported their experience with pharyngeal flaps for three cerebral-palsied children. Two children, both over 10 years of age, showed good speech gains. The child under 10 years of age was able to attain intraoral air pressure following surgery. However, Hardy (1983) wrote that the results of the pharyngeal flap program proved disappointing and that the palatal lift prosthesis proved to be a viable alternative.

Crikelair, Kastein, and Cosman (1970) reported successful inferiorly based pharyngeal flap surgery for an individual two years post onset of closed head injury. Their patient had previously undergone a period of "voice therapy" without success. A "marked" improvement was noted although a "slight residual dysarthria" persisted. Johns (1985) reported a case study of a patient with dysarthria following a gunshot wound to the left frontal region of the brain as well as the left shoulder and left mandible. He demonstrated severe mixed dysarthria. A superiorly based pharyngeal flap surgery was performed. From perceptual and acoustic analysis, Johns concluded "improved post-operative velopharyngeal closure correlated with perceptual judgments of clarity, improved intelligibility, and decreased nasality" (p. 168)

A number of approaches to management of velopharyngeal dysfunction in dysarthria have been described in this chapter. In addition to eliminating, as reducing such features as nasal emission and excessive hypernasality, effective management of this component is often necessary before effective treatment of oral articulation problems can be carried out. The following chapter will describe assessment and intervention for this aspect of dysarthria.

REFERENCES

Aten, J., McDonald, A., Simpson, M., & Gutierrez, R. (1984). Efficacy of modified palatal lifts for improved resonance. In M. McNeil, J. Rosenbek, & A. Aronson (Eds.), *The dysarthrias: Physiology, acoustics, perception, management.* San Diego: College-Hill Press.

Bluestone, C., Musgrave, R., McWilliams, B., & Crozier, P. (1968). Teflon injection pharyngoplast. *Cleft Palate Journal*, *5*, 19–22.

Crikelair, G.F., Kastein, S., & Cosman, B. (1970). Pharyngeal flap for post-traumatic palatal paralysis. *Plastic & Reconstructive Surgery*, *45*, 182–185.

Croft, C.B., Shprintzen, R.J., & Rakoff, S.J. (1981). Patterns of velopharyngeal valving in normal and cleft palate subjects: A multi-view videofluoroscopic and nasendoscopic study. *Laryngoscope*, *91*, 265–271.

Daly, D.A., & Johnson, H.P. (1974). Instrumental modification of hypernasal voice quality in retarded children: Case Reports. *Journal of Speech & Hearing Disorders*, *39*, 500–507.

Daniel, B. (1982). A soft palate desensitization procedure for patients requiring palatal lift prostheses. *Journal of Prosthetic Dentistry*, *48*, 565–566.

D'Antonio, L., Chait, D., Lotz, W., & Netsell, R. (1986). Pediatric videonasoendoscopy for speech and voice evaluation. *Otolaryngol Head Neck Surg.*, *94*, 578–83.

Darley, F.L. (1984). Perceptual analysis of dysarthria. In J. Rosenbek (Ed.), *Seminars in speech and language*, *5*, 267–278.

Darley, F.L., Aronson, A.E., & Brown, J.R. (1975). *Motor speech disorders.* Philadelphia: WB Saunders.

Dworkin, J.P., & Johns, D.F. (1980). Management of velopharyngeal incompetence in dysarthria: A historical review. *Clinical Otolaryngology*, *5*, 61–74.

Fletcher, S.G. (1970). Theory and instrumentation for quantitative measurement of nasality. *Cleft Palate Journal*, *7*, 601–609.

Fletcher, S., Sooudi, I., & Frost, S. (1974). Quantitative and graphic analysis of prosthetic treatment for "nasalance" in speech. *Journal of Prosthetic Dentistry*, *32*, 284–291.

Froeschels, E. (1943). A contribution to pathology and therapy of dysarthria due to certain cerebral lesions. *Journal of Speech Disorders*, *8*, 301–321.

Froeschels, E., Kastein, S., & Weiss, D.A. (1955). A method of therapy for paralytic conditions of the mechanisms of phonation, respiration, and glutination. *Journal of Speech & Hearing Disorder*, *20*, 365–370.

Gibbons, P., & Bloomer, H.H. (1958). The palatal lift: A supportive-type prosthetic speech aid. *Journal of Prosthetic Dentistry*, *8*, 363–369.

Gonzalez, J., & Aronson, A. (1970). Palatal lift prosthesis for treatment of anatomic and neurologic palatopharyngeal insufficiency. *Cleft Palate Journal*, *7*, 91–104.

Hardy, J., *Cerebral palsy.* Englewood Cliffs, NJ: Prentice-Hall.

Hardy, J., Netsell, R., Schweiger, J., & Morris, H. (1969). Management of velopharyngeal dysfunction in cerebral palsy. *Journal of Speech & Hearing Disorders*, *34*, 123–137.

Hardy, J., Rembolt, R., Spriestersbach, D., & Jaypathy, B. (1961). Surgical management of palatal paresis and speech problems in cerebral palsy: A preliminary report. *Journal of Speech & Hearing Disorders*, *26*, 320–325.

Holley, L., Hamby, G., & Taylor, P. (1973). Palatal lift for velopharyngeal incompetence. *Journal of Dentistry for Children*, 43–46.

Ibuki, K., Karnell, M.P., & Morris, H. (1983). Reliability of the nasopharyngeal fiberscope (NPF) for assessing velopharyngeal function. *Cleft Palate Journal*, *20*, 97–104.

Johns, D. (Ed.) (1985). *Clinical management of neurogenic communication disorders.* Boston: Little Brown.

Karnell, M.P., Ibuki, K., Morris, H.L., & Van Demark, D.R. (1985). Reliability of the nasopharyngeal fiberscope (NPF) for assessing velopharyngeal function: Analysis by judgment. *Cleft Palate Journal*, *20*, 199–208.

Kerman, P., Singer, L., & Davidoff, A. (1973). Palatal lift and speech therapy for velopharyngeal incompetence. *Archives of Physical Medicine and Rehabilitation*, *54*, 271–276.

Kipfmueller, L., & Lang, B. (1972) Treating velopharyngeal inadequacies with a palatal lift prosthesis. *Journal of Prosthetic Dentistry*, *27*, 63–72.

Kuehn, D.P. (1982). Assessment of resonance disorders. In N. Lass, L. McReynolds, J. Northern, & D. Yoder (Eds.), *Speech, language and hearing: Vol. III. Pathologies of speech and language.* Philadelphia: WB Saunders.

Lang, B. (1967). Modification of the palatal lift speech aid. *Journal of Prosthetic Dentistry*, *17*, 620–626.

Lang, B., & Kipfmueller, L. (1969). Treating velopharyngeal inadequacy with the palatal lift concept. *Plastic and Reconstructive Surgery*, *43*, 467–480.

LaVelle, W.E., & Hardy, J.C. (1979). Palatal lift prostheses for treatment of palatopharyngeal incompetence. *Journal of Prosthetic Dentistry*, *42*, 308–315.

Lawshe, B., Hardy, J., Schweiger, J., & Van Allen, M. (1971). Management of a patient with velopharyngeal incompetency of undetermined origin: A clinical report. *Journal of Speech & Hearing Disorders*, *36*, 547–551.

Lewy, R., Cole, R., & Wepman, J. (1965). Teflon injection in the correction of velopharyngeal insufficiency. *Annuals of Otology, Rhinology, & Laryngology*, *78*, 874.

Maue-Dickson, W. (1977). State of the art report: Section II. Anatomy and physiology. *Cleft Palate Journal*, *14*, 270–287.

Mazaheri, M., & Mazaheri, E.H. (1976). Prosthodontic aspects of palatal elevation and palatopharyngeal stimulation. *Journal of Prosthetic Dentistry*, *35(3)*, 319–326.

Miyazaki, T., Matsuya, T., & Yamaoka, M. (1975). Fiberscopic methods for assessment of velopharyngeal closure during various activities. *Cleft Palate Journal*, *12*, 107–114.

Moll, K.L. (1968). Speech characteristics of individuals with cleft lip and palate. In D.C. Spriestersbach, & D. Sherman (Eds.), *Cleft palate and communication*. New York: Academic Press.

Morris, H., Spriestersbach, D., & Darley, F. (1961). An articulation test for assessing competency of velopharyngeal closure. *Journal of Speech & Hearing Research*, *4*, 48.

Moser, H.M. (1942). Diagnostic and clinical procedures in rhinolalia. *Journal of Speech & Hearing Disorders*, *7*, 1–4.

Netsell, R. (1969a). Evaluation of velopharyngeal function in dysarthria. *Journal of Speech & Hearing Disorders*, *34*, 113.

Netsell, R. (1969b). Changes in oropharyngeal cavity size of dysarthric children. *Journal of Speech & Hearing Research*, *12*, 646–649.

Netsell, R., & Daniel, B. (1979). Dysarthria in adults: Physiologic approach to rehabilitation. *Archives of Physical Medicine & Rehabilitation*, *60*, 502–508.

Netsell, R., & Rosenbek, J.C. (1985). Treating the dysarthrias. In *Speech and Language Evaluation in Neurology: Adult Disorders*. New York: Grune & Stratton, Inc.

Nishio, J., Matsuya, T., Ibuki, K., & Miyazaki, T. (1976). Roles of the facial, glossopharyngeal and vagus nerves in velopharyngeal movement. *Cleft Palate Journal*, *13*, 201–214.

Nishio. J., Matsuya, T., Machida, J., & Miyazaki, T. (1976). The motor nerve supply of the velopharyngeal muscles. *Cleft Palate Journal*, *13*, 20–30.

Noll, J.D. (1982). Remediation of impaired resonance among patients with neuropathologies of speech. In N. Lass, L. McReynolds, J. Northern, & D. Yoder (Eds.), *Speech language and hearing: Vol. III: Pathologies of speech and language.* Philadelphia: WB Saunders.

Peterson-Falzone, S.J. (1982). Resonance disorders in structural defects. In N. Lass, L. McReynolds, J. Northern, & D. Yoder (Eds.), *Speech, language and hearing: Vol. III: Pathologies of speech and language.* Philadelphia: WB Saunders.

Prins, D., & Bloomer, H.H. (1968). Consonant intelligibility: A procedure for evaluating speech in oral cleft subjects. *Journal of Speech & Hearing Research*, *11*, 128–137.

Rosenbek, J.C., & LaPointe, L.L. (1985). The dysarthrias: Description, diagnosis, and treatment. In D.F. Johns (Ed.), *Clinical management of neurogenic communicative disorders*. Boston: Little Brown.

Ruscello, D. (1982). A selected review of palatal training procedures. *Cleft Palate Journal*, *19*, 181–194.

Schweiger, J., Netsell, R., & Sommerfield, R. (1970). Prosthetic management and speech improvements in individuals with dysarthria of the palate. *Journal of the American Dental Association*, *80*, 1340.

Shaugnessy, A., Netsell, R., & Farrage, J. (1983). Treatment of a four year old with palatal lift prosthesis. In W. Berry (Ed.), *Clinical dysarthria*. Austin, TX: PRO-ED.

Shelton, R.L., Hahn, E., & Morris, H.L. (1968). Diagnosis and therapy. In D.C. Spreistersbach & D. Sherman (Eds.), *Cleft palate and communication*. New York: Academic Press.

Shoup, J., Lass, N., & Kuehn, D. (1982). Acoustics of speech. In N. Lass, L.

McReynold, J. Northern, & D. Yoder (Eds.), *Speech, language, and Hearing.* Philadelphia: W.B. Saunders.

Thompson, A.E., & Hixon, T.J. (1979). Nasal air flow during normal speech production. *Cleft Palate Journal, 16,* 412–420.

Van Demark, D., Bzoch, K., Daly, D., Fletcher, S., McWilliams, B.J., Pannbacker, M., & Weinberg, B. (1985). Methods of assessing speech in relation to velopharyngeal function. *Cleft Palate Journal, 22,* 281–285.

Warren, D.W. (1975). The determination of velopharyngeal competence by aerodynamic and acoustic techniques. *Clinical Plastic Surgery, 2,* 299–304.

Warren, D.W., & DuBois, A.R. (1964). A pressure-flow technique for measuring velopharyngeal orifice area during continuous speech. *Cleft Palate Journal, 1,* 52.

Warren, D.W., & Ryon, W.E. (1967). Oral port constriction, nasal resistance, and respiratory aspects of of cleft speech: An analog study. *Cleft Palate Journal, 4,* 3X.

Yorkston, K.M., & Beukelman, D.R. (1981). Ataxic dysarthria: Treatment sequences based on intelligibility and prosodic considerations. *Journal of Speech & Hearing Disorders, 46,* 398–404.

Yorkston, K.M., Beukelman, D.R., & Traynor, C.D. (1984). *Computerized assessment of intelligibility of dysarthric speech.* Austin, TX: PRO-ED.

Yorkston, K.M., Dowden, P., Beukelman, D.R., & Traynor, C.D. (1986, February). *A phoneme identification task as a measure of perceived articulatory accuracy.* Paper presented at the third biennial Clinical Dysarthria Conference, Tucson, AZ.

Yorkston, K.M., Honsinger, M., Mitsuda, P., & Beukelman, D.R. (1986). Perceived articulatory adequacy in two groups of brain-injured dysarthric speakers. *ASHA.*

CHAPTER 12

Oral Articulation

Clinical Issues: In preparation for their internships with us, students are given a reading list designed to familiarize them with the nature and management of disorders frequently occurring in our clinical practice. Often this reading list is the students' first exposure to management of dysarthric speakers. At times, students who are more familiar with management of developmental articulation disorders than adult motor speech disorders are confused by the dysarthria literature. For example, as they read the research reports of Darley, Aronson, and Brown (1975), students find that the speech dimension of imprecise consonants is consistently listed among the most deviant dimensions across all of the dysarthrias. Yet, despite the apparent frequency of occurrence of articulatory impairment, they will also read the following statement representing a current philosophy of management: "Indeed, traditional articulation treatment alone is seldom salutary for the dysarthric talker even if the impairment involves only his tongue, lips, or jaw." (Rosenbek, 1984, p. 250)

- *How can the apparent prevalence of articulation impairment in dysarthria be reconciled with the lack of clinical focus on oral articulation in intervention programs?*
- *How does the management of articulatory impairment in dysarthria differ from the management of developmental articulation disorders?*
- *How is oral articulation influenced by other speech components such as respiration, phonation, and the velopharyngeal system?*
- *How is the articulatory impairment of dysarthric speakers managed clinically?*

A PERSPECTIVE ON ARTICULATION IN DYSARTHRIA

Broadly defined, articulation is considered the movement of speech structures employed in producing the sounds of speech. However, this chapter will only focus on the movements of the tongue, lips, and jaw that shape the oral resonance cavity during production of vowels and the movements that constrict or obstruct the voiced or voiceless airstream during consonant production. Rosenbek (1984) advocates viewing dysarthria as more than an articulatory disorder and its treatment as more than articulatory training. Fully aware of potential problems, the relatively narrow view of the articulatory process selected for this chapter was dictated by convenience rather than by a belief that treatment should focus only on oral articulation in isolation from other aspects of speech production.

The oral articulatory component of speech provides an excellent illustration of the interdependencies among various speech components. For example, Hardy (1967) presented the case of a 24 year old individual who, at the time of evaluation, was two years post brain injury with cerebral concussion-contusion, right hemiparesis, and probable brain stem injury. His unintelligible speech was characterized by an extremely rapid rate with an initial "explosive" burst followed by rapidly diminishing loudness. Cinefluorographic films revealed "gross immobility of the tongue and velum" at habitual rates. However, an increase in the extent of lingual and palatal movement was noted at reduced speaking rates. Hardy offered a possible explanation for the severely impaired movements of the oral articulators. He suggested that the patient "attempts to compensate for his speech physiological problems during recovery from the severe neurological damage by completing an utterance 'before he ran out of air'." Hardy further stated that the patient's inappropriate speaking rate worked against his compensatory efforts. This case illustrates an instance where severely restricted movements of the oral articulators may not have been the direct result of damage to the neuromotor control of these structures. Rather, those severely restricted movements may have been the consequence of a poorly controlled respiratory system and the attempt to compensate for that impairment.

The interdependence of the oral articulators and other speech components can also be illustrated with an example related to phonation. The perceptual distinction between voiced and voiceless cognate pairs is based on precise laryngeal timing as well as subtle adjustments in the duration of oral articulatory gestures. Voiced versus voiceless distinctions are often difficult for a dysarthric speaker to achieve, perhaps because of the complex timing and coordination required between a number of speech components. Imprecise production of speech sounds is not simply an oral articulatory phenomenon, but is the result of laryngeal, velopharyngeal, and oral articulatory impairments. Respiratory and phonatory examples have been provided to illustrate that the management of oral articulation must be considered only in the context of other aspects of speech. Often the sequence of treatment requires focus on training other components first, or on prosthetic management of other components, before training of oral articulation can be expected to result in perceptually acceptable productions.

DESCRIPTIVE STUDIES

An understanding of the nature and variety of articulation disorders seen in dysarthria is essential for planning appropriate treatment. No other dysarthric speech component has received as much study. However, a review of the literature quickly indicates that research investigations vary widely in terms of the approaches to measurement, subjects, and tasks speakers are asked to perform. We have prepared a series of tables to summarize the pertinent features of selected studies. Although a number of these studies examine aspects of motor speech disorders other than articulation, discussion will focus on the results as they pertain to the oral articulation components of the lips, tongue, and jaw.

Perhaps the best way of understanding the implications of this literature is to follow the progression from the benchmark studies of large clinical populations carried out at the Mayo Clinic in the late 1960s (summarized in 1975 by Darley et al.) through the research contributions from the University of Wisconsin over the past 15 years. By considering the study of articulation in this way, it becomes apparent that measurement approaches have changed during this 15 year period of research. New approaches to measurement have broadened our understanding of the nature of articulatory impairment in several forms of dysarthria.

Perceptual Studies

Darley and colleagues (1975), in their introduction to *Motor speech disorders*, indicated that historically informal observation of motor speech disorders led to a series of "quaint and colorful" (p. 7) descriptive terms, including "slurred," "forced," "labored," "drawling," or "jerky." The limited usefulness of such terms is obvious. First, they overlook the fact that motor speech can be disordered in a number of different ways, depending on the site of neurological damage. These differences, resulting from varying underlying pathophysiologies, are important for differential diagnosis. Second, these descriptive phrases do not reflect the impairment of the various speech components. An understanding of the contribution and relative impairment of each speech component is critical for the appropriate planning of intervention. Finally, the descriptive phrases give the clinician no direct way of evaluating the severity of a disorder and thus provide no useful way of monitoring change over time or the effects of treatment.

Spurred at least in part by their dissatisfaction with informal observation and descriptive phrases, Darley and colleagues undertook a classical series of studies which are reviewed in Chapter 3. These studies remain the most comprehensive description of the various dysarthrias (Table 12-1). Among other findings, their results indicated that imprecise consonant articulation ranked as the most perceptually deviant speech dimension in five of the seven groups studied. Only in bulbar palsy was hypernasality ranked higher than articulation and in parkinsonism were the prosodic features of monopitch, reduced stress, and monoloudness ranked higher than articulation. In speakers with cerebellar lesions and ataxic dysarthria, three of the four most deviant dimensions were related to articulation. They were imprecise consonants, irregular articulatory breakdown, and distorted vowels. Thus, for the majority of the dysarthric speakers studied by the Mayo group, articulatory disorders played a key role in the perceptual characteristics of the disorder and, coupled with certain other aspects of motor speech, produced the distinctive perceptual characteristics of that disorder.

The work of Darley and colleagues was important for the breadth and depth of the disorders studied and for the quantification of symptoms in order to identify the most deviant dimensions of speech within and across diagnostic categories. Their comparative ranking system places the deviant articulatory features in perspective in relation to other aspects of motor speech. Thus, articulatory impairments, although seen as important, and perhaps a characteristic feature of dysarthria, are not viewed in isolation from other respiratory, phonatory, resonance, and prosodic features of the disorder.

The rating scales used by Darley and colleagues gave information only about the general severity of the articulatory impairment, but did not provide detailed information about the pattern of articulatory deficits in the various dysarthrias. A more detailed examination of articulatory performance in dysarthria was also carried out by the Mayo group. Johns and Darley (1970) reported measures of articulatory performance for a group of 10 dysarthric speakers with a variety of etiologies. Although the primary interest of Johns and Darley was the study of articulation in apraxia, data from a group of normal speakers and a group of dysarthric individuals served as a point of comparison. These data provide some interesting insights into the nature of articulatory patterns in dysarthria. Subjects produced a series of single-syllable real and nonsense words under a number of stimulus (auditory, visual, and auditory-visual presentation) and response conditions. They also produced a series of words of increasing length (e.g., "thick," "thicker," "thickening"). Phonemes were transcribed using broad IPA and errors were categorized as omissions, substitutions, distortions, additions, repetitions, and prolongations. Results indicated that the dysarthric group did not differ from the apraxic group in terms of the number of errors or phonemes that the speakers failed to produce. However, the groups differed significantly in terms of the types of errors they made. Sixty-five percent of the errors made by dysarthric speakers were distortions, as compared to 10 percent of the errors made by apraxic speakers. Less

TABLE 12-1.
Perceptual Studies

Subjects:	Tasks:	Measures:	Results:
Darley, Aronson, & Brown (1975)			
30 Ss with bulbar palsy	Connected speech (paragraph reading; in some cases conversation or sentence imitation)	Perceptual ratings of 38 speech dimensions	(1) 28 of 30 had consonant imprecision (mean scaled score = 2.91) (2) Most prominent characteristic was hypernasality
30 Ss with pseudobulbar palsy	"	"	(1) All had consonant imprecision (mean scales score = 3.9) (2) 17 of 30 had vowel distortion (1.77) (3) Imprecise consonant, distorted vowels, & hypernasality formed a distinctive cluster of articulatory/resonance features
30 Ss with cerebellar lesions	"	"	(1) 28 of 30 had imprecision of consonants (3.19) (2) 25 had vowel distortions (2.14) (3) 28 had irregular articulatory breakdowns (2.59)
32 parkinsonian Ss	"	"	(1) all had consonant imprecision (3.59) (2) Prosodic changes were more pronounced than articulatory ones
30 Ss with chorea	"	"	(1) 27 of 30 had imprecise consonants (2.93) (2) 27 had distorted vowels (2.13)
30 dystonic Ss	"	"	(1) All had imprecise consonants (3.32) (2) 24 of 30 had distorted vowels (2.4) (3) 24 of 30 had irregular articulatory breakdowns (2.28)
30 Ss with ALS	"	"	(1) Distortion of vowels, slow rate, shortness of phrase, & imprecision of consonant (4.39) were more deviant in ALS than in any other neurologic disease studied

(*continued*)

TABLE 12-1 (continued)

Subjects:	Tasks:	Measures:	Results:
Darley, Brown, & Goldstein (1972)			
168 Ss with MS	Connected speech DDK rates	5-point rating scale	(1) 59% had normal speech (2) 46% had defective articulation
Logemann & Fisher (1981)			
200 parkinsonian Ss	Fisher-Logemann Test of Articulation Competence (Sentence Version)	IPA Transcription of misarticulations	(1) Classes most affected were stop-plosive, affricates & fricatives (2) Suggest inadequate tongue elevation to achieve complete closure on stop-plosives & affricates, & close constriction of the airway in lingual fricatives
Logemann, Fisher, Boshes, & Blonsky (1978)			
200 parkinsonian Ss	11 sentences from Fisher-Logemann Test of Articulation Competence	Judgments of presence or absence of misarticulations	(1) 45% had articulatory disorders (compared to 89% with laryngeal disorders) (2) Those consonants requiring greatest constriction are most affected
Platt, Andrews, Young, and Quinn (1980)			
32 spastic cerebral palsied male adults 18 athetoid cerebral palsied male adults	Syllable repetition 50 single words Grandfather passage	Diadokokinetic rates IPA transcription of words Orthographic transcription of words Estimates of intelligibility	(1) Higher phoneme transcription scores than intelligibility scores (2) Scores on all speech measures were higher for spastic than for athetoid (3) Phonemic features: anterior lingual place inaccuracy; reduced precision of fricative manner; inability to achieve extreme position in vowel articulation
Platt, Andrews, & Howie (1980)			
32 spastic cerebral palsied male adults 18 athetoid cerebral palsied male adults	29 CVC words	IPA transcription with diacritical marks	(1) Within manner errors more frequent than between manner errors (2) Difference between severely disabled & less disabled was one of degree rather than quality

than 10 percent of the errors made by dysarthric speakers were substitutions, in contrast to 50 percent for the apraxic group. Johns and Darley suggested that "consistency of production" characterized dysarthric performance. Thus, if a phoneme were misarticulated in spontaneous speech, it would usually be misarticulated in reading and imitative conditions, and, if a phoneme were distorted in one position, it would usually be distorted in another.

Other research groups have also carried out detailed articulatory inventories of selected dysarthric speakers. Such investigations, relying on perceptual measures, lend themslves to large group studies such as those carried out with parkinsonian speakers at Northwestern University by Logemann and her colleagues (Logemann & Fisher, 1981; Logemann, Fisher, Boshes, & Blonsky, 1978). Two hundred parkinsonian speakers were recorded as they read the sentence version of the Fisher-Logemann Test of Articulation Competence (Fisher & Logemann, 1971). Judges identified the presence or absence of articulatory errors. Forty-five percent of the parkinsonian speakers exhibited disorders of articulation. This is in contrast to 89 percent who exhibited laryngeal disorders. Logemann and Fisher (1981) reported the results of an articulatory error analysis on this sample. Like Johns and Darley (1970), they found a "remarkably consistent" pattern in their dysarthric speakers. For example, when a particular phoneme was misarticulated by these parkinsonian speakers, essentially all speakers produced the same error pattern. This analysis led the authors to suggest an "articulatory undershoot" characterized by inadequate tongue elevation to achieve complete closure on stop plosives and affricates, and inadequate constriction of the airway in lingual fricatives.

Still another group utilizing perceptual techniques studied the relationship between articulation and certain other aspects of motor speech production. Platt and his colleagues (Platt, Andrews, & Howie, 1980; Platt, Andrews, Young, & Quinn, 1980) obtained measures of diadokokinetic rates and articulation (percent of selected phonemes correctly transcribed) from a group of spastic and a group of athetoid cerebral-palsied males. Single words were orthographically transcribed for intelligibility and prose reading samples were also rated for intelligibility. They found that scores from IPA transcription of phoneme accuracy obtained from trained judges were higher than intelligibility scores obtained from naive listeners. Further, they found that mean scores on all of the speech measures for the spastic group were higher than for the athetoid group. An analysis of the articulatory error pattern (Platt, Andrews, & Howie, 1980) indicated that the spastic group did not differ from the athetoid group and that differences between severely and less severely disabled individuals were of degree rather than quality. Furthermore, although the articulation scores of this group of cerebral-palsied adults were higher than those for a group of children reported earlier by Bryne (1959), the profiles of the two groups across place and manner features are strikingly similiar. Thus, despite the fact that the dysarthric groups studied obviously had differing underlying pathophysiologies, perceptual measures of articulatory error patterns did not differentiate the groups. Articulatory inventories are useful in providing global measures of articulatory adequacy. However, they may not provide information related to the movement abnormalities or the underlying causes of those abnormalities.

Acoustic Studies

Thus far, studies have been reported that rely largely on perceptual measures. In these studies, judges listened to samples of connected speech and rated the adequacy of what they heard. Weismer (1984 a, b) took a somewhat different approach to the measure of articulation in dysarthria. He used acoustic signal analysis because those signals "sit in the middle of the communication process," thus potentially providing more information than other signals such as muscle contraction or perceptual judgments (Table 12-2). He studied selected speech samples from a small number of dysarthric individuals and made detailed inferences about motor production from the acoustic characteristics. Weismer (1984a) provided a tutorial in which he illustrated the use of acoustic spectrography to make physiological inferences and to better understand the perceptual characteristics of dysarthria. He cautioned the reader not to believe that spectrographic records always reflect articulatory events in a straightforward way. He further cautioned that perceptual phenomenon are complexly related to various characteristics of the speech waveform. This relationship is not completely understood.

Ansel (1985) and Ansel & Kent (1986) reported the results of a study in which they sought to identify the specific acoustic features that would predict speech intelligibility in a group of adult cerebral-palsied males. The following contrasts were studied: syllable-initial voicing; syllable-final voicing; stop-nasal; fricative-affricate; front-back, high-low, and tense-lax vowel. The acoustic factors of vowel duration and F1 and F2 formant locations and noise duration were found to be major predictors of speech intelligibility scores. Thus, the physiological parameters of temporal control and tongue position appeared to influence speech intelligibility.

Studies of Movement

Quantification of articulatory adequacy has been the goal of the perceptual and acoustic analyses presented thus far. However, caution must be exercised when making inferences about articulatory movement and underlying pathophysiology from these perceptual and acoustic measures. Other investigators study the articulatory disorders in dysarthria by focusing on movement abnormalities (Table 12-3). Their rationale for this approach to measurement is straightforward. Since dysarthria is basically a movement disorder, then one needs to understand the movement abnormalities in order to understand the disorder.

TABLE 12-2.
Acoustic Studies

Subjects:	Tasks:	Measures:	Results:
Ansel (1985) Ansel and Kent (1986)			
16 Adult cerebral palsied males	CVC words	Spectrographic & perceptual analysis	Vowel duration & F1 and F2 format locations; fricative-affricate rise time & noise duration were major predictors of intelligibility
Weismer (1984a)			
1 parkinsonian male 1 spastic cerebral palsied male 1 normal male	Spontaneous speech	Spectrographic analysis	(1) Pk S tended to omit constricted part of consonants (2) In Spastic S, vowel distortion was associated with aberrant formant transition: imprecise consonants with weak intensity & aberrant spectrum of fricatives:
Weismer (1984b)			
8 parkinsonian speakers 5 young adults 8 geriatric adults	Sentence repetition at conversational & rapid rates	Spectrographic analysis	(1) Spirantization most frequent in Pk group (2) Voicing into stop closure occurred frequently in geriatric & Pk group (3) Pk group had segmental & phrase level durations slightly shorter than geriatric group

Measurement of oral articulatory movements has become increasingly more sophisticated since the early studies of Hixon and Hardy (1964), who measured diadokokinetic movement rates of the oral articulators during speech and nonspeech tasks. Kent and Netsell (1975) used cineradiographic as well as spectrographic analysis to study the speech of a woman with ataxic dysarthria. They found “conspicuous abnormalities in speaking rate, stress patterns, articulatory placements of both vowels and consonants, velocities of articulator movements, and fundamental frequency contours” (p. 115). Later, Kent and Netsell (1978) studied movements of five athetoid cerebral-palsied individuals using cinefluorographic tracings of vocal tract shapes during speech samples.

TABLE 12-3.
Movement Studies

Subjects:	Tasks:	Measures:	Results:
Hirose, Kiritani, Ushijima, & Sawashima (1978)			
1 ataxic male 1 female with ALS 1 normal male	Syllable repetition	EMG Pellet tracking using X-ray microbeam	(1) For ataxic S, difficult initiating purposeful movements & inconsistency of articulatory movements (2) For ALS S, decrease in range & velocity of movement (3) For slowed normal, no decrease in velocity but increase in closure duration
Hixon & Hardy (1964)			
25 spastic cerebral palsied children 25 athetoid cerebral palsied children	Samples of connected speech Repetition of CVs Repetition of nonspeech movements	Ratings of speech defectiveness Rates of speech & nonspeech movements	Nonspeech activities are not as highly related to speech defectiveness as were rates of speech movement
Kent & Netsell (1975)			
1 female with cerebellar lesion & ataxic dysarthria	Isolation & sustained vowels Sentence repetition	Cineradiography spectrography	Abnormalities in articulatory placement of vowel & consonants & in velocities of articulatory movements
Kent & Netsell (1978)			
5 athetoid cerebral palsied Ss	Vowels Nonsense syllables Short sentences	Cinefluorographic tracing of vocal tract shapes	(1) Large range of jaw movement (2) Inappropriate tongue positioning (3) Intermittent v/p closure & instability of velar elevation (4) Prolonged transition times
Kent, Netsell, & Bauer (1975)			
4 dysarthric adults 4 normal speakers	Speech sounds Short sentence	Cineradiographic measurement of fleshpoint displacement	Abnormalities in range, rate & direction of speech movements
McClean, Beukelman, & Yorkston (1986)			
10 normal & 6 dysarthric adults (parkinsonian & ataxic)	Visuomotor tracking	Cross correlation between target and cursor	Dysarthric performance reduced compared to normal: wide range of tracking performance; generally consistent with overall level of speech performance

Their findings supplemented the earlier work of Kent, Netsell, and Bauer (1975). Specifically, Kent and Netsell found large ranges of jaw movements, inappropriate tongue positioning, abnormalities in the timing and range of velopharyngeal movement, and prolonged articulatory transition times.

Hirose, Kiritani, Ushijima, and Sawashima (1978) studied the articulatory movements of the lip and jaw using a pellet tracking technique with an X-ray microbeam system. In selected cases, EMG data were also available. Their subjects included a speaker with cerebellar degeneration and ataxic dysarthria, a speaker with bulbar-type ALS, and a normal speaker who performed at normal and slowed speaking rates. Results indicated that the articulatory movement patterns of their subjects were each quite different. Specifically, the articulatory movements of the ataxic speaker was characterized by inconsistency in both range and velocity, whereas the maximum velocity was not much less than that of the normal speaker. For the ALS speaker, results indicated a reduced range of articulatory movement and reduction in the rate of speech. However, the "slowness" of the ALS speaker was found to be different from that produced by a normal speaker who was asked to repeat syllables slowly. The movement pattern of the slowed normal speaker was characterized not by a reduction in the velocity of the lip but instead by a prolonged closure period.

A visuomotor tracking task was used to assess the nonspeech performance of normal and dysarthric subjects (McClean, Beukelman, & Yorkston, 1986). Among other speech components, lower lip and jaw movements were transduced and displayed on an oscilloscopic screen. Subjects were asked to track a visual target moving at low frequency. The dysarthric subjects exhibited a wide range of tracking performance. All dysarthric subjects showed reduced performance as compared with normal subjects. Dysarthric performance was generally consistent with overall levels of speech performance and levels of neurological impairment.

Barlow and Abbs (1986) studied fine force and movement control in groups of normal and cerebral-palsied individuals. Subjects were asked to make movements of their upper lip, lower lip, tongue, and jaw "as rapidly and accurately as possible." They found that quantitative physiologic measures of force and movement control were highly related to impairment in speech intelligibility.

Studies of Muscle Function

Perhaps even more basic than the studies of articulator movement during connected speech are those studies completed in speech physiology laboratories that seek to understand the basis of the movement problems (Table 12-4). Results of these studies carry important implications for selection of appropriate approaches to treatment. A better understanding of the basis of movement problems in the various dysarthrias should ultimately lead to a series of specific treatments based on the nature of the neuropathologies.

TABLE 12-4.
Studies of Muscle Control

Subjects:	Tasks:	Measures:	Results:
Barlow & Abbs (1983)			
1 parkinsonian speaker 1 spastic dysarthric speaker 1 normal speaker	Matching target force levels with tongue, lips, & jaw	Comparison of applied to target force over time	Variable results depending on the level of target force & subsystem
Barlow & Abbs (1984)			
6 adult spastic males 3 normal adults	Matching target force levels with tongue, lips, & jaw	Comparison of applied to target force over time Comparison of instability & force	Disproportionate degrees of motor impairment at finer levels of force control
Dworlin, Aronson & Mulder (1980)			
19 adults with ALS 125 normal adults	Tongue movement Syllable repetition Grandfather passage	Anterior & lateral tongue force Diadokokinetic rates Judgments of articulatory defectiveness	(1) Dysarthric tongue force lower than normal (2) Lateral less than anterior (3) High correlation between tongue force & articulatory deficit (4) High negative correlation between syllable rates & severity of artic. deficit
Hunker, Abbs, & Barlow (1982)			
4 parkinsonian males 4 normal males	Application of known force to lips Single sentence utterance	Labial stiffness Labial speech movements EMG	Labial rigidity correlated with decrements in range of lip movement EMG results suggest a causal relationship between rigidity & hypokinesia
Neilson & O'Dwyer (1984)			
5 athetoid cerebral palsied adult males 5 normal speakers	Single stimulus sentences recited 50 times	EMG Speech intensity waveforms	Athetoid Ss produced syllables slower & with greater variability than normals Abnormal voluntary activity was the cause
Netsell, Daniel, & Celesia (1975)			
22 parkinsonian speakers	Syllable repetition Short sentences	EMG Oral & nasal air pressure Acoustic signal	Acceleration & weakness found May be associated with reduced range of movement in absence of rigidity

O'Dwyer, Neilson, Guitar, Quinn, and Andrews (1983) doubted that weakness or pathological imbalance in the orofacial and mandibular muscles contributed to movement disorders in their cerebral-palsied population. Rather, they suggested that "the motor deficit in cerebral palsy is considered to reflect an inappropriate set of motor commands for achieving a desired sensory goal" (p. 169). By asking groups of normal and athetoid cerebral-palsied speakers to repeatedly produce a single sentence and by examining the reproducible and variable components, Neilson and O'Dwyer (1984) were able to conclude that abnormal voluntary activity, rather than variable involuntary activity, was the primary cause of the movement disorders of athetoid dysarthria.

Other researchers examined weakness and its relationship to the speech disorders of individuals with ALS. Dworkin, Aronson, and Mulder (1980) studied the anterior and lateral tongue force and syllable repetition rates in groups of normal and dysarthric individuals with ALS. They compared these measures in dysarthric individuals with judgments of articulatory defectiveness. They found that maximal tongue forces for the ALS groups were significantly lower than normal. High correlations were found between measures of tongue force and the extent of articulatory deficit.

Several groups of researchers have studied the underlying control deficits in parkinsonism. Netsell, Daniel, and Celesia (1975) obtained muscle action potentials from the orbicularis oris superior along with nasal and oral air pressure from 22 parkinsonian patients during a speech task. Their illustrative examples indicate that weakness in the control signals, rigidity, or the acceleration phenomenon could be the neuromuscular basis for this reduced range of movement, and that various combinations of these three conditions are present in many parkinsonian individuals. In another study of parkinsonian subjects, Hunker, Abbs, and Barlow (1982) measured labial rigidity by applying known forces to the lips and observing the displacement for four parkinsonian and four normal speakers. Hypokinesia during speech was assessed using a head-mounted lip and jaw movement transduction system. They found differences in rigidity were consistently correlated with decrements in the range of lip movement. The authors provided EMG information that indicated a causal relationship between rigidity and hypokinesia. Thus, there appear to be different reasons for movement disorders even within a single diagnostic group.

Barlow and Abbs (1983) presented data that suggested that motor control deficits may vary within one speaker from one speech component to another. They found that the ability of their subjects to achieve and maintain target levels of force differed among the lingual, labial, and mandibular systems. They also presented evidence suggesting that their parkinsonian speakers had a similiar pattern of poor mandibular control for speech as well as nonspeech activities. They discouraged reliance on global measures such as aerodynamic, acoustic, and perceptual observations when attempting to understand how the speech components function in dysarthria. They suggested that global measures do not allow for the understanding of the contribution of various components to the overall impairment. Further, they suggested such an understanding is necessary if treatment is to focus on the most important problems.

Clinical Questions to the Researcher

In closing this discussion of research focusing on the physiology of oral articulation of dysarthric speakers, we will present questions that appear to be critically important for the clinical management of dysarthria. Answers to these questions will come only after careful investigation using the technology and the skills of the speech physiologists. The first question is, "Are motor control deficits seen in dysarthric speakers as unique as they appear to be in the case presentations that appear in the literature, or have the researchers selected particularly interesting subjects?" The answer to this question will come when studies of large groups of dysarthric individuals are completed. These studies will not only allow the clinician to compare and constrast the motor control impairment of the various dysarthrias, but will also allow the clinician to see individual differences within a group of dysarthric speakers as well as differences between speech components within a single individual.

Another clinically important question that only recently has been addressed (Barlow & Abbs, 1986) is, "What is the relationship between movement abnormalities and perceptual measures of articulatory adequacy?" We know that the relationship is not a simple one. Studies are needed to examine simultaneous measures of neural activity, movement, aerodynamics, and acoustics and compare these measures to perceptual aspects of articulation. Our final question, particularly relevant to the clinical management of dysarthria, is, "How is the motor control impairment in dysarthria affected by frequently employed treatment strategies?" Speech physiologists quite understandably have begun their studies of dysarthric speech by examining habitual speech patterns or nonspeech tasks and comparing them with the productions of normal speakers. However, clinicians are equally interested in the effects that common treatment strategies may have on articulatory movements. For example:

- What is the effect of reduced speech rate on the articulatory movements of ataxic or parkinsonian speakers?
- What is the effect of a general biofeedback program that focuses on reduction of muscle tone on the articulatory movements of athetoid cerebral-palsied individuals?
- What is the effect of prosthetically compensating for a defective velopharyngeal mechanism on the articulatory movements of brain-injured individuals?

Answers to these and many other questions are needed before our clinical management programs can specifically address and treat motor control problems.

CLINICAL APPLICATIONS OF ARTICULATION MEASURES

The previous review of research literature is intended to provide a description of the articulatory impairment of dysarthric speakers. From this review, it is apparent that a number of different measurement techniques are available to the researcher. Each of these techniques provides its own type of information. In the following section, we will review measures of articulatory performance available to the clinician and will discuss interpretation of the information obtained from each of these measures. For a more general discussion of approaches to assessment, see Chapter 7.

Perceptual Rating of Speech Component Performance

The first level of clinical assessment involves obtaining an overall assessment of the adequacy of articulatory performance and comparing that to ratings of other components of speech performance. General questions are asked by the clinician in this portion of the evaluation. These include:

Is there an oral articulatory impairment?
If so, how severe is it?
How does the severity of the articulatory impairment compare to the respiratory, phonatory, or velopharyngeal impairment?

Thus, the first measures obtained are global ones in which we confirm the presence of an articulatory impairment and rank its severity in relation to other components of performance. This step is important for treatment planning because it allows one to sequence treatment tasks and deal first with those aspects of the problem that have the most potential for changing the overall adequacy of speech. In many cases, this means beginning with treatment that focuses on aspects of speech other than articulation.

Estimation of the relative contribution of the oral articulatory impairment to overall communication disability typically is based on informal assessment and relies heavily on subjective clinical judgment. By selecting various sounds and sound combinations, the clinician can sample movements of the lips (by asking the speaker to repeat /papapa/), the tongue tip (/tatata/), the tongue back (/kakaka/), and a combination (/pataka/). Movement rates for single structures can be compared and contrasted with one another and with combinations of sounds. These simple tasks can also be performed with and without voicing to estimate the contribution of inadequate respiratory and phonatory control to articulatory movement impairments. Typically, a dysarthric individual with inadequate respiratory support will perform much more poorly when attempting to speak a series of syllables than when simply "mouthing" the syllables. When this is the case, the clinician may choose to work on increasing respiratory and laryngeal control before focusing on articulatory movements in treatment.

Simple alternating movement tasks also may be used to estimate the contribution of various articulatory components to the overall articulatory adequacy. For example, asking a speaker to repeat the bilabial consonant-vowel combination /papapa/, with and without a bite block, may give an indication of the contribution of abnormal jaw movement to articulatory impairment. See Netsell (1985) for a more detailed interpretation of bite block use. In addition to overall diadokokinetic movement rates, the clinician may also make judgments about the range of excursion of the movements and the variability of the movement rates.

Clinically, tasks used for assessment of articulatory movement are, for the most part, perceptually judged. The clinician initially confirms the existence of an articulatory impairment and estimates its severity in relation to other components of speech production. As is apparent, we have not included acoustic, aerodynamic, radiographic, or movement transduction in the list of clinical approaches for assessment of articulation in dysarthria. Although these measures have been used in research, they have not found their way into routine clinical practice. This probably has occurred because the necessary instrumentation to make these measurements is only now routinely becoming clinically available.

Articulation Inventories

Administration of traditional articulation inventories (e.g., The Fisher-Logemann Test of Articulatory Competence [1971]) or less formal word lists that sample all of the speech sounds (e.g., those used by Johns & Darley, 1970; or Platt, Andrews, Young & Quinn, 1980) appear not to have been accepted as a routine part of clinical assessment of dysarthric speakers. However, measures of perceived articulatory adequacy have a place in dysarthria management because the information obtained from them may provide answers to specific questions. For selected individuals, information about articulatory performance would allow the clinician to document the impact of intervention. For example, consider the severely involved flaccid dysarthric speaker. Treatment may have focused on lip strengthening exercises in order to achieve bilabial closure. An articulation inventory would allow the monitoring of changes in the perceived adequacy of bilabial sounds. Or, consider the severely involved individual for whom a palatal lift has been fitted. An articulation inventory would allow the comparison of articulatory adequacy with and without the lift. Use of an articulation inventory to make decisions regarding palatal lift management is discussed in Chapter 11. Finally, consider the severely dysarthric individual recovering from brain injury for whom treatment has focused on inclusion of final consonants. An articulation inventory would allow for the monitoring of change in final consonant production and for comparison of that change with changes in nontreated sounds. In short, articulation inventories may provide answers to specific questions, usually involving the performance of severely dysarthric speakers. To date, there are no reports in the literature on the performance of dysarthric speakers on structured articulation inventories as compared to free speech sampling techniques.

In our opinion, there are a number of reasons why articulation inventories have not enjoyed widespread clinical use in dysarthria. First, traditional articulation inventories often require judges to transcribe speech samples using IPA and a number of modifiers for such features as dentalization, lip rounding, and tongue position. This type of transcription is based on the assumption that a speaker's articulatory movements can be inferred from a judge's perception of the speech end product. Speech physiologists have repeatedly cautioned against making such inferences. Second, distortions rather than substitutions, omissions, or other error categories predominate in dysarthria. Traditional articulation inventories, in which the target phoneme is known to the judge, often fail to adequately make the critically important distinction between a phoneme that is distorted but recognizable and one that is distorted but no longer within phoneme boundaries. Finally, in traditional articulation inventories, judges who know the target phoneme may overestimate the accuracy of productions as compared to listeners who are naive to the phoneme targets.

In order to circumvent some of these measurement problems, we routinely use a Phoneme Identification Task (Yorkston, Dowden, Beukelman, & Traynor, 1986) to obtain a measure of perceived articulatory adequacy. Speakers are recorded as they produce a series of single words or sentences containing 57 target phonemes (22 prevocalic consonants, 19 postvocalic consonants, and 16 vowels and diphthongs). Judges view a word frame such as "ma-" and are asked to identify the missing phoneme. All frames are selected so that a variety of real-word options are possible. For example, possible words for the frame "ma-" include "mass," "mat," "mad," "mack," "map," "mash," "match," and so forth. In addition to attempting to identify the phoneme, judges score each attempt according to the following distortion scale:

3—Correct, undistorted phoneme
2—Correct but distorted (judges are confident that they have identified the correct phoneme, but the production is distorted)
1—Guess (the phoneme is so distorted that the judge's response is a guess)
0—No basis for a guess

In order to illustrate how the results of the Phoneme Identification Task can be used to make clinical decisions, the case of an 18 year old brain-injured individual will be presented. Table 12-5 contains a chronology of some important events in Brian's recovery. To summarize briefly, Brian began making some voluntary verbal responses 3.5 months post onset (MPO). One month later (4.5 MPO), his speech was characterized by his primary speech clinician as unintelligible, grossly hypernasal, and produced with little oral articulatory movement. Spontaneous speech was marked by short utterances. Although initial portions of utterances were adequately loud, the patient frequently appeared to "run out of air," finishing the utterance without phonation.

TABLE 12-5.
Chronology of Brian's recovery

MONTHS POST ONSET	
1.5	Began arousing from coma
3.0	Vocalized to discomfort No yes/no responses
3.5	Used an alphabet board Some verbal responses
4.5	Palatal lift first considered First recording of Phoneme Identification Task
4.6	Training focused on achieving lip closure
5.0	Second recording of Phoneme Identification Task Aerodynamic assessment of velopharyngeal function
5.5	Third recording of Phoneme Identification Task
6.0	Spasticity medications increased Increased swallowing difficulties noted Fourth recording of Phoneme Identification Task
6.5	Fifth recording of Phoneme Identification Task
7.5	Sentence intelligibility reached 97% at a speaking rate of 67 wpm

At approximately 4.5 MPO, Brian's primary clinician consulted us regarding the possibility of evaluating him for palatal lift fitting. A Phoneme Identification Task was recorded and judged. Results of this and other subsequent recordings appear in Figure 12-1. This figure contains the perceived adequacy of three consonant groups: (1) labials & bilabials, (2) stops, fricatives, & affricates, and (3) nasals & others. Results of the first recording indicate severely impaired performance with a mean score across consonants of approximately 20 percent correct. Both labial-bilabial and stop-fricative-affricate categories were only 10 percent correct. Aerodynamic measures of velopharyngeal performance could not be obtained at that time because of the patient's inability to achieve lip closure. See Chapter 11 for a detailed description of these measurement techniques. It was recommended that treatment focus on attempts to achieve bilabial closure during speech production.

After a two week interval, his clinician indicated that she felt he could achieve sufficient lip closure to be tested aerodynamically. During this testing, Brian demonstrated the ability to consistently achieve lip closure and to produce air pressure in the oral cavity during the stop phase of the /p/ at 10 cm of water pressure or more. This supported the observation that Brian had adequate respiratory control to support speech. However, he demonstrated nasal

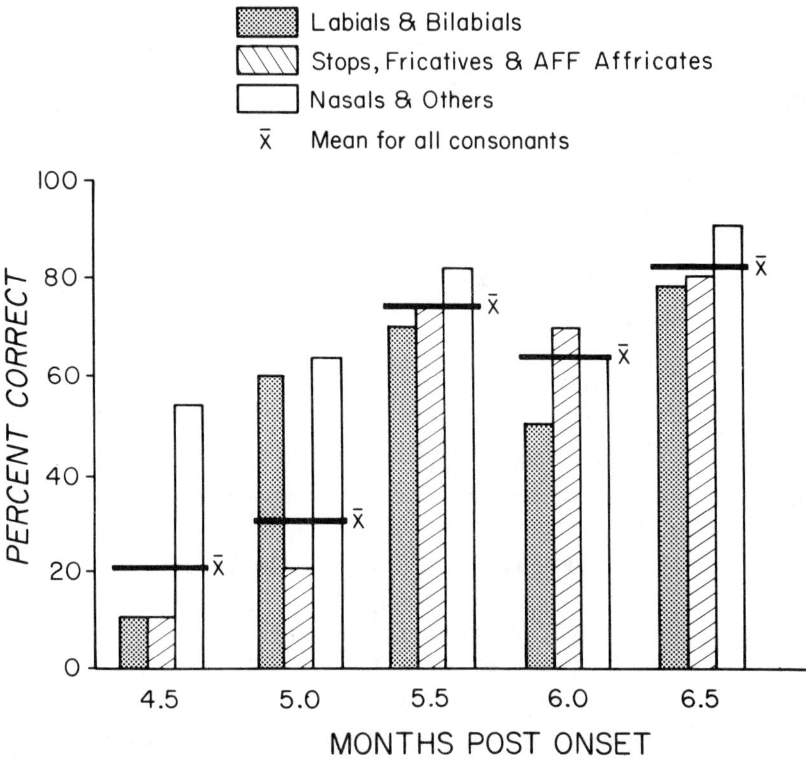

Figure 12-1. Results of the Phoneme Identification Task for Brian from 4.5 months post onset to 6.5 months post onset.

flow of air each time he attempted to impound intraoral air pressure during speech. This suggested that his velopharyngeal mechanism was not functioning adequately. A visual examination of the soft palate revealed some movement during sustained phonation. The Phoneme Identification Task was recorded again at the time of the aerodynamic evaluation. Results of this recording at 5.0 MPO indicated that the labial-bilabial group of consonants had improved to 60 percent accurate. Thus, the clinician's intervention appeared to have had the desired effect. Because of the improvement that had been observed over a two week period of time, the decision was made to delay palatal lift fitting and monitor closely the changing performance. The third recording of the Phoneme Identification Task along with aerodynamic measures were obtained two weeks later at 5.5 MPO. Results indicated that Brian was now achieving adequate velopharyngeal closure, at least at times, during connected speech. Perceived accuracy of stop, affricate, and fricative consonants was now over 70 percent.

Close examination of Figure 12-1 suggests that performance at 6.0 MPO was decreased as compared to the testing done two weeks earlier. This decrease in articulatory performance was coincident with an increase in Brian's antispasticity medications. Subjectively, Brain's clinician also observed increased drooling and swallowing difficulties. She reported the measures of articulatory performance as evidence of undesirable drug effects, and dosages of medications were lowered. This case illustrates the usefulness of articulation inventories for providing answers to specific questions related to intervention with severely impaired dysarthric individuals.

TREATMENT

The treatment of articulatory disorders in dysarthria may take on many forms. For purposes of this discussion, procedures will be reviewed under two general headings. The first set of techniques contains those that attempt to normalize function by reducing the impairment. Included in this category are those procedures that employ medical management, biofeedback training, or strengthening exercises in order to restore muscle function as nearly as possible to normal. The second set of techniques contains those that are compensatory. These techniques utilize behavioral training or prosthetic management in an effect to help dysarthric speakers compensate for their motor impairment. The selection of specific techniques and their sequencing in relation to other training tasks is dependent on a number of factors, including the underlying neuropathology of the articulatory system deficit and the severity of articulatory impairment in relation to other components of the speech mechanism. In presenting the following techniques, an attempt will be made to provide a framework for deciding for whom a technique is appropriate and when it should be applied.

Normalizing Function

More often than not in dysarthria treatment, intervention programs involve compensatory adjustments rather than attempts to achieve normalcy. With this caution in mind, some approaches will be reviewed that are designed to normalize the muscular function in dysarthria. These are the articulatory techniques that come to mind first when the clinician asks if anything can be done to reduce the physiologic impairment.

Normalizing function or reducing the overall impairment may occur in a number of ways. Many disorders resulting in dysarthria are characterized by a natural course of spontaneous recovery or reduction of the impairment. For example, Guillain-Barré syndrome typically involves a course of rapid recovery following the acute paralytic phase. Strokes typically involve a sudden onset, followed by a slow course of natural recovery that may last months and even years. Multiple sclerosis may be characterized by periods of exacerbations and remissions. In other disorders that cause dysarthria, the impairment may be reduced by medical management. For example, the rigidity seen in parkinsonism may be reduced by medication and the impairment seen in Wilson's disease is typically managed with diet and medication.

The techniques described in the following section involve attempts to reduce the impairment, thus normalizing function, through training. This training is typically carried out in the presence of a natural course that is either stable or improving and typically involves some form of biofeedback. Rubow (1984) defines biofeedback as "a process of transducing some physiologic variable, transforming the signal to extract useful information, and displaying that information to the subject in a format that will facilitate learning to regulate the physiological variable" (p. 207).

Reducing Tone

At times, the goal of biofeedback is to reduce abnormally high muscle tone. For example, Netsell and Cleeland (1973) presented the case of a 64 year old woman with a 15 year history of parkinsonism who exhibited bilateral lip retraction as the result of bilateral thalamic surgeries six years prior to intervention. Her speech was said to be characteristic of parkinsonism with imprecise consonants, reduced loudness, monopitch, and monoloudness. Intervention involved placement of surface electrodes over the levator labii superioris. The speaker was presented with a tone whose frequency was analogous to the voltages recorded from the electrodes. During each intervention session she performed both nonspeech tasks involving the lip and four speech tasks that did not involve the upper lip. The subject's task was to concentrate on lowering the audible tone, and thus, reducing the hypertonicity in the lip. At the end of 2.5 hours of treatment, the authors report, "the subject was able to modify this (the lip) condition in the direction of normalcy" (p. 138). She demonstrated complete control of the lip in nonspeech activities and some instances of normal lip activity while repeating structured phonetic material not requiring lip movement. Spontaneous speech was still characterized by some excessive contraction.

A case in which biofeedback training not only reduced hemifacial spasm but also had a marked effect on speech production was presented by Rubow, Rosenbek, Collins, and Celesia (1984). Their subject was described as a geriatric individual with an 18 year history of hemifacial spasm characterized by paroxysmal bursts of involuntary tonic or clonic activity. Moderately severe dysarthria was felt to be secondary to the spasm. Training involved biofeedback-assisted relaxation of the frontalis muscle. No speech treatment was undertaken. The authors suggest that when deciding whether to treat speech per se or whether to treat the coexisting abnormal neurological signs, at least two factors must be considered. Treatment focusing on elimination of the underlying neurological problems is likely to be successful only if it is obvious, or at least hypothesized, that it is causing all of the speech symptoms and if the neurological condition is amenable to treatment.

In the cases presented thus far, the biofeedback has focused on reducing tone in specific muscle groups. Finley, Niman, Standley, and Ender (1976) reported the results of a study in which a more general relaxation was sought, using a biofeedback approach in training six athetoid cerebral-palsied patients. Pre- and posttraining measures of speech and motor performance were obtained. Results indicated that the less-impaired subjects showed better "acquisition curves" than more severely impaired subjects. In all but one case, frontalis tension was significantly reduced across sessions. Only the two most severely impaired subjects did not improve on the speech measures.

Strengthening

In the cases presented thus far, the goal of biofeedback was relaxation or reduction of tone either generally or to specific muscle groups. Biofeedback approaches have also been reported in cases where the clinical goal is strengthening. Some of these studies involve the facial musculature, but not specifically speech-related activities. For example, Booker, Rubow, and Coleman (1969) described a biofeedback approach to treat left facial nerve damage. They reported beneficial results both cosmetically and functionally. In other cases, improvement in speech gestures was the goal of treatment. Daniel and Guitar (1978) reported the case of a 25 year old male who had a surgical anastomosis involving the connection of the peripheral portion of cranial nerve VII to the central portion of cranial nerve XII. The goal of their program, which took place five years after surgery, was symmetry in facial gestures for nonspeech and speech activities. They reported substantial increases in muscle action potentials over the course of treatment for both nonspeech and speech gestures.

Both biofeedback to the jaw and lips and strengthening exercises have been recommended for individuals with flaccid dysarthria as the result of involvement of cranial nerves V, VII, and XII. Linebaugh (1983) listed a series of exercises, starting with assistive force as needed to achieve desired movement and advancing to movement against resistance. For the jaw, depression and elevation were recommended. Bilabial closure, rounding retraction, and labiodental approximation were recommended for the lips. Interdental protrusion, retraction, apical elevation, and dorsal elevation were recommended for the tongue. These strengthening exercises may be accompanied by EMG biofeedback.

Historically, the question of when to use strengthening exercises has been controversial. This debate will no doubt continue, especially in light of the lack of clinical studies investigating the impact of strengthening excerises on the overall adequacy of articulatory performance. However, we have found a number of simple guidelines useful in making such clinical management decisions. The first question that we ask is obvious: "Is weakness a problem?"

Weakness is by no means universally present in dysarthria. Many neuromotor disorders are characterized by increased tone and by reduced coordination rather than by weakness. If strength is reduced as compared to normal levels, then the next question is, "Does the weakness interfere with speech function?" The presence of weakness does not necessarily imply a speech disability. Speech is a skilled motor task that is much more demanding in terms of movement precision and coordination than strength. In fact, speech requires only 10 to 20 percent of maximum force of lip movement (Barlow & Abbs, 1983). If weakness is present and it appears to interfere with speech production, then the clinician must ask if there are any contraindications to strengthening exercises. For example, myasthenia gravis is a disorder characterized by progressive weakness following muscular activity. Here, strengthening exercises are obviously contraindicated. In other cases, the natural course of the disorder may make strengthening exercises futile. Such may be the case in degenerative disorders such as ALS. After ruling out cases in which weakness is not a problem or does not interfere with speech and cases in which exercises are contraindicated because of the underlying neuromotor problems or course of the disorder, the clinician is left with a relatively small group of dysarthric speakers for whom strengthening exercises may be appropriate. These individuals typically exhibit flaccid dysarthria with etiologies including such disorders as peripheral nerve damage and brain stem CVAs.

Rosenbek and LaPointe (1985) caution against other abuses of strengthening exercises, including delaying of other intervention approaches until strengthening is "finished," and increasing the strength of certain muscles so they "overwhelm" the efforts of others. Finally, strengthening exercises are only an appropriate management approach for those individuals who are willing to invest the daily time needed for the repetitive drills necessary for increasing strength.

Compensating for the Impairment

Many of the traditional approaches to the treatment of dysarthric individuals have as their goal compensation for a neuromotor impairment that cannot be treated medically or with behavioral approaches such as strengthening exercises. At the center of the compensatory approach to articulation training lies the capability to make adjustments in movement patterns in order to achieve an acceptable speech end-product. Evidence is also accumulating to suggest that dysarthric speakers are able to modify their articulatory productions in response to certain types of feedback. For example, Till and Toye (1986) reported a study in which dysarthric speakers were able to modify acoustic features such as voice onset time after specific feedback indicated that certain sounds were not being understood. Because those changes were made immediately, it is apparent that compensation, rather than a reduction in impairment, was responsible.

Contrastive Production and Intelligibility Drills

A number of training techniques attempt to take advantage of a speaker's ability to modify production depending on the adequacy of the final speech end-product. These approaches do not attempt to train the speaker to change specific movement patterns. Rather, general information about the adequacy of speech is provided. Thus, it is assumed that the speaker will make the necessary changes. A rationale for such an approach is based on the fact that speech, as a motor task, is apparently learned by adjusting the movement patterns based on the success of the perceived output.

De Feo and Shaefer (1983) have provided an excellent example of the compensatory adjustments made by an individual with neurological impairment specific to certain speech components. They presented the case of a young child with Moebius syndrome who was age three years eight months at the time of initial evaluation. Moebius syndrome is characterized by congenital bilateral facial paralysis and abducens palsy. Hypotonicity was noted in the child's cheek and lip musculature. However, sensation of the lip, face, and lingual regions was not impaired. Aside from nerve VII, no other cranial nerves appeared to be involved. An articulatory program was developed in which the child was presented with a correct model of the phoneme he misarticulated and was asked to produce a sound to match that model. Without specific instructions to do so, the child quickly adopted a lingual-dental place of articulation for /p/, /b/, /f/, and /m/. Other compensations developed more slowly. For example, contrastive production drills were used to refine the distinction between bilabial and apical stops. Two compensatory strategies were adopted. One was the insertion of a glottal stop between the target plosive and ensuing vowel. The other was an increase in articulatory force when producing /p/ and /b/ versus /t/ and /d/. In an interesting note, the authors found that they more readily perceived the distinctions if they were not watching the child's face. This impression was confirmed when they compared perceptual judgments of production adequacy made from video/audio presentation with those made from audio presentation only. At the end of one year of treatment, listeners, given an audio presentation, judged as correct 89, 65, and 46 percent of the /m/, /p/, and /b/ productions, respectively. When they judged the video/audio presentation, 54, 44, and 33 percent of the productions were judged to be correct for the same phonemes. Thus, the child appeared to be making acoustically acceptable compensations despite the fact that his movement patterns, as perceived visually by the judges who viewed video tapes, remained nonstandard.

In the case just presented, a child with an impairment restricted to the muscles innervated by a single cranial nerve learned to compensate for that deficit and to produce acceptable sounds. We have found a similiar approach useful with individuals who exhibit more generalized articulatory impairment. Contrastive production drills are tasks in which two sounds are produced in juxtaposition to one another. The speaker is asked to make these sounds as different as possible. For example, the voiced versus voiceless distinction can be practiced with consecutive productions of /bin/ versus /pin/. See Chapter 10 for a more complete description of techniques to aid dysarthric speakers in making voiced versus voiceless consonant distinctions.

Intelligibility drills are slightly different from the contrastive production drills and involve the production of a small set of words similiar except for a single phoneme. The sets may range from two to more than ten words. See Table 12-6 for examples of such word lists. Each word is printed on a card and the cards are shuffled. Unlike contrastive production tasks, the clinician

TABLE 12-6.
Examples of Word Lists for Intelligibility Drills

	Vowels	
mail	hole	feel
Mel	heal	file
mall	hail	foil
mule	hall	fowl
mole	hill	fuel
mile	Hal	fill
mill	who'll	fall
meal	hell	fail
mull	howl	fool
	Initial Consonants	
ban	Paul	beer
pan	ball	tear
tan	tall	dear
Dan	call	gear
can	stall	fear
ran	fall	mere
Stan	mall	near
span	shall	we're
man	small	cheer
fan	hall	shear
	Final Consonants	
lab	map	rub
lack	mat	rut
lag	mad	Russ
lap	Mack	rust
lad	mass	rough
lass	mash	run
last	match	rum
lash	mast	rush
latch	Madge	rug
laugh	ma'am	runs

is naive to the specific sound or word being produced. Thus, instead of making a judgment of "correctness" or "incorrectness," the clinician attempts to identify the utterance being produced.

Intelligibility drills provide a useful framework for treatment of articulation disorders for a number of reasons. First, they do not require specific instructions about how to produce the sound. Rather, they depend on the speaker's ability to compensate for the motor impairment and to find ways to produce a perceptually acceptable sound. In the clinical setting, the clinician rarely has detailed information about movement control and movement patterns of the various articulators. Even if such information were available, it may not make a difference in clinical practice. For example, the speaker simply may not be able to modify a severely impaired lip movement, and instead, may need to compensate for such impairment by making a complex series of adjustments in the movements of other structures. Tasks such as intelligibility drills allow the speaker to attempt compensation in the presence of perhaps the most important kind of feedback—knowledge of whether or not the listener has understood the attempt.

The second feature of intelligibility drills that makes them practical and useful in the clinical setting is that the difficulty of the task can be easily adjusted to meet the needs of the dysarthric speaker. If a target accuracy of 80 to 90 percent is the goal, then the clinician can select phonemes and a list length in order to achieve the target accuracy. Intelligibility drills may be used with the most severely involved speaker as the first practice in speaking. An example of such a speech intervention program is described in Chapter 8.

The third clinical advantage of intelligibility drills is that they allow early training in communication breakdown resolution strategies. Because the drill is based on a "quasi-realistic" communication situation, the speaker learns to provide feedback to the listener about the correctness of the listener's perception. Thus, the dysarthric speaker is active in the breakdown resolution process rather than merely a recipient of the clinician's feedback. When participating in an intelligibility drill, the dysarthric speaker is required to produce the word, watch for a reaction, indicate to the listener the accuracy of the listener's guess, and repeat the word one time if the listener's guess is incorrect. If the listener erroneously guesses the second production, the speaker must resolve the breakdown in some other way. For example, the dysarthric speaker might indicate the correct answer on the alphabet board. Thus, as soon as attempts to speak are begun in the treatment session, dysarthric speakers are practicing the management of their listeners.

The concept of intelligibility drills is not new, and has been extended to sentence productions and to samples of spontaneous speech. For example, Ince and Rosenberg (1973) described a procedure in which two dysarthric speakers were asked to spontaneously produce one sentence at a time. Following the production, the experimenters gave the speakers general feedback by indicating to the speakers whether the production was "clear" or "unclear." Over a period of 38 sessions, the proportion of intelligible sentences increased from 11.8 percent to 100 percent for one speaker and 5 percent to 100 percent for the other. It is clear that such studies need to be replicated with careful descriptions of the dysarthric speakers and perceptual, acoustic, and physiological documentation of changes in speech production over time.

Prosthetic Compensation

In the previous section, techniques for behaviorally training the dysarthric speakers to compensate for their motor impairment were reviewed. At other times in dysarthria treatment, a prosthetic device can be used to compensate for speech component impairment. Use of a palatal lift to compensate for inadequate velopharyngeal function (described in Chapter 11) is perhaps the most common example of prosthetic management. In the oral articulation system, the jaw may be managed prosthetically via a bite block in those individuals in whom jaw control is disproportionally impaired relative to other structures (Netsell, 1985). A bite block is a small, custom-fitted piece of hard, rubber-like material which is held between the upper and lower teeth. Its purpose is to maintain a constant jaw position during speech. Barlow and Abbs (1983) describe the case of a cerebral-palsied individual with and without a bite block. They recorded simultaneous measures of jaw movement, intraoral air pressure, and raw acoustic signal. Their results indicated that the lip movements are much more regular when the jaw is stablized.

The final example of prosthetic management of oral articulation is drawn from the large number of techniques designed to control speaking rate. For certain speakers, rate reduction has the effect of increasing the precision of articulatory movements. A series of prosthetic devices to control speaking rates and improve articulatory precision will be described in Chapter 13. These techniques include pacing and alphabet boards in which the user must point to a different location for each word spoken, thus reducing overall speaking rate. Also included among the prosthetic rate control devices is the Delayed Auditory Feedback Unit, worn while speaking to reduce the excessively rapid rates of selected parkinsonian speakers.

REFERENCES

Ansel, B.M. (1985). *Acoustic predictors of speech intelligibility in cerebral palsied-dysarthric adults.* Unpublished doctoral dissertation, University of Wisconsin, Madison.

Ansel, B.M., & Kent, R.D. (1986, February). *Acoustic predictors of speech intelligibility in cerbral palsied-dysarthric adults.* Paper presented at the third biennial Clinical Dysarthria Conference, Tucson, AZ.

Barlow, S.M., & Abbs, J.H. (1983). Force transducers for the evaluation of labial, lingual, and mandibular function in dysarthria. *Journal of Speech & Hearing Research, 26*, 616–621.

Barlow, S.M., & Abbs, J.H. (1984). Orofacial fine-motor control impairments in congenital spasticity: Evidence against hypertonis-related performance deficits. *Neurology, 34*, 145.

Barlow, S.M., & Abbs, J.H. (1986). Fine force and position control of selected orofacial structures in the upper motor neuron syndrome. *Experimental Neurology, 94*, 699–713.

Booker, H.E., Rubow, R.T., & Coleman, P.J. (1969). Simplified feedback in neuromuscular retraining: An automated approach using eletromyographic signals. *Archives of Physical Medicine & Rehabilitation, 50*, 621–625.

Bryne, M. (1959). Speech and language development of athetoid and spastic children. *Journal of Speech & Hearing Disorders, 24*, 231–240.

Daniel, R., & Guitar, B. (1978). EMG feedback and recovery of facial and speech gestures following neural anastomosis. *Journal of Speech & Hearing Disorders, 43*, 9–20.

Darley, F.L., Aronson, A.E., & Brown, J. (1975). *Motor speech disorders*. Philadelphia: W.B. Saunders.

Darley, F.L., Brown, J.R., & Goldstein, N.P. (1972). Dysarthria in multiple sclerosis. *Journal of Speech & Hearing Research, 15*, 229–245.

De Feo, A., & Sheafer, C. (1983). Bilateral facial paralysis in a preschool child: Oral-facial and articulatory characteristics (A case study). In W.R. Berry (Ed.), *Clinical dysarthria*. Austin, TX: PRO-ED.

Dworkin, J., Aronson, A., & Mulder, D. (1980). Tongue force in normals and dysarthric patients with amyotrophic lateral sclerosis. *Journal of Speech & Hearing Research, 23*, 828–837.

Finley, W. W., Niman, C., Standley J., & Ender P. (1976). Frontal EMG biofeedback training of athetoid cerebral palsy patients: Report of six cases. *Biofeedback Self Regul. 1*, 169–182.

Fisher, H.B., & Logemann. J.A. (1971). *The Fisher-Logemann Test of Articulation Competence*. Boston: Houghton Mifflin Co.

Hardy, J. (1967). Suggestions for physiological research in dysarthria. *Cortex, 3*, 128–156.

Hirose, H., Kiritani, S., Ushijima, T., & Sawashima, M. (1978). Analysis of abnormal articulatory dynamics in two dysarthric patients. *Journal of Speech & Hearing Disorders, 43*, 96.

Hixon, T., & Hardy, J. (1964). Restricted mobility of the speech articulation in cerebral palsy. *Journal of Speech & Hearing Disorders, 29*, 293–306.

Hunker, C., Abbs, J., & Barlow, S. (1982). The relationship between Parkinson rigidity and hypokinesia in the orofacial system: A quantitative analysis. *Neurology, 32*, 749–756.

Johns, D.F., & Darley, F.L. (1970). Phonemic variability in apraxia of speech. *Journal of Speech & Hearing Research, 13*, 556–583.

Ince, L. P., & Rosenberg, D. N. (1973). Modification of articulation in dysarthria. *Archives of Physical Medicine & Rehabilitation, 54*, 233.

Kent, R.D., & Netsell, R. (1975). A case study of an ataxic dysarthric: Cineradiographic and spectrographic observations. *Journal of Speech & Hearing Disorders, 40*, 115–134.

Kent, R., & Netsell, R. (1978). Articulatory abnormalities in athetoid cerebral palsy. *Journal of Speech & Hearing Disorders, 43*, 353–373.

Kent, R., Netsell, R., & Bauer, L.L. (1975). Cineradiographic assessment of articulatory mobility in the dysarthrias. *Journal of Speech & Hearing Disorders, 40*, 467.

Linebaugh, C. (1983). Treatment of flaccid dysarthria. In W. Perkins (Ed.), *Dysarthria and apraxia*. New York: Thieme Stratton.

Logemann, J., & Fisher, H. (1981). Vocal tract control in Parkinson's disease: Phonetic features analysis of misarticulation. *Journal of Speech & Hearing Disorders*, *46*, 348–352.

Logemann, J., Fisher, H., Boshes, B., & Blonsky, B. (1978). Frequency and co-occurrence of vocal tract dysfunctions in speech of a large sample of parkinsonian patients. *Journal of Speech & Hearing Disorders*, *43*, 47–57.

McClean, M.D., Beukelman, D.R., & Yorkston, K.M. (1986, February). Speech-muscle visuomotor tracking in dysarthric and normal speakers. Paper presented at the third biennial Clinical Dysarthria Conference, Tucson, AZ, February.

Neilson, P.D., & O'Dwyer, N.J. (1984). Reproducibility and variability of speech muscle activity in athetoid dysarthria of cerebral palsy. *Journal of Speech & Hearing Research*, *27*, 502–517.

Netsell, R. (1985). Construction and use of a bite-block for use in evaluation and treatment of speech disorders. *Journal of Speech & Hearing Disorders*, *50*, 103–106.

Netsell, R., & Cleeland, C. (1973). Modification of lip hypotonia in dysarthria using EMG feedback. *Journal of Speech & Hearing Disorders*, *38*, 131–140.

Netsell, R., Daniel, B., & Celesia, G. (1975). Acceleration and weakness in Parkinsonian dysarthria. *Journal of Speech & Hearing Disorders*, *40*, 170–178.

O'Dwyer, N.J., Neilson, P.D., Guitar, B.E., Quinn, P.T., & Andrews, G. (1983). Control of upper airway structures during nonspeech tasks in normal and cerebral-palsied subjects: EMG findings. *Journal of Speech & Hearing Research*, *26*, 162–170.

Platt, L., Andrews, G., & Howie, P.M. (1980). Dysarthria of adult cerebral palsy: II. Phonemic analysis of articulation errors. *Journal of Speech & Hearing Research*, *23*, 41–55.

Platt, L., Andrews, G., Young, M., & Quinn, P. (1980). Dysarthria of adult cerebral palsy: 1. Intelligibility and articulatory impairment. *Journal of Speech & Hearing Research*, *23*, 28–40.

Rosenbeck, J.C. (1984). Selected alternatives to articulation training for the dysarthric adult. In H. Winitz (Ed.), *Treating articulation disorders: For clinicians by clinicians*. Austin, TX: PRO-ED.

Rosenbek, J.C., & LaPointe, L.L. (1985). The dysarthrias: Description, diagnosis, and treatment. In D.F. Johns (Ed.), *Clinical management of neurogenic communicative disorders*. Boston: Little, Brown & Co..

Rubow, R. (1984). Role of feedback, reinforcement, and compliance on training and transfer in biofeedback-based rehabilitation of motor speech disorders. In M. R. McNeil, J. C. Rosenbek, & A. E. Aronson (Eds.), *The dysarthrias: Physiology, acoustics, perception, management*. San Diego: College-Hill Press.

Rubow, R., Rosenbek, J., Collins, M., & Celesia, G. (1984). Reduction of hemifacial spasm and dysarthria following EMG feedback. *Journal of Speech & Hearing Disorders*, *49*, 26.

Till, J.A., & Toye, A.R. (1986, February). *Acoustic-phonetic effects of two types of verbal feedback in dysarthric subjects*. Paper presented at the third biennial Clinical Dysarthria Conference, Tucson, AZ..

Weismer, G. (1984a). Acoustic description of dysarthric speech: Perceptual correlates and physiological inference. In J.C. Rosenbek (Ed.), *Current views of dysarthria: Nature, assessment, and treatment; Seminars in Speech and Language*. New York: Thieme-Stratton.

Weismer, G. (1984b). Articulatory characteristics of parkinsonian dysarthria. In M.R. McNeil, J.C. Rosenbek, & A.E. Aronson (Eds.), *The dysarthrias: Physiology, acoustics, perception, management.* San Diego: College-Hill Press.

Yorkston, K.M., Dowden, P.A., Beukelman, D.R., & Traynor, C.D. (1986). *A Phoneme Identification Task as a measure of perceived articulatory adequacy.* Paper presented at the third biennial Clinical Dysarthria Conference, Tucson, AZ.

CHAPTER 13

Rate Control

Clinical Issues: Two dysarthric individuals who differed in etiology and type of dysarthria were scheduled for outpatient evaluations one afternoon when a new student intern had the opportunity to observe. Despite the apparent differences between the two speakers, the general intervention approaches recommended were surprisingly similiar. The first individual was a 70 year old retired executive with parkinson's disease whose speaking rate was excessively rapid (150 percent of a normal rate). The speaking rate interferred with intelligibility, especially when speaking on the telephone. His wife, who had accompanied him to the evaluation, stated, "I tell him to slow down, but he just doesn't remember to do it." The second dysarthric individual was a 25 year old mother who had experienced an episode of anoxia during child birth. Living in a rural area, she had not received speech treatment in the four years since onset. However, she had been practicing, as she put it, "talking as fast as I can," because she was aware that her speaking rate was about half that of normal. Unfortunately, this strategy had not been effective. Reading a short paragraph was an exhausting task in which she would pause only when a breath was mandatory physiologically. Speaking trials at various rates during the evaluation suggested that intelligibility increased and articulatory breakdowns decreased when she slowed her speaking rate. Recommendations for both of these individuals included rate control as part of intervention. For the parkinsonian speaker, a trial with Delayed Auditory Feedback (DAF) was recommended, and for the young ataxic woman, a behavioral rate reduction training program was recommended. The questions asked by the student observing these evaluations were the following:

- *Is rate reduction appropriate for all dysarthric speakers?*
- *If it is not, what factors make an individual a good candidate for rate control?*
- *What techniques are appropriate for those speakers who "can't seem to learn" to slow down voluntarily?*

- *What are the negative consequences of rate reduction and how can they be minimized?*
- *How is an optimum speaking rate selected for a dysarthric individual?*

The instructions to "slow down" or "speak more slowly" have been uttered by many generations of listeners as they attempt to understand dysarthric speech. Rate control is a long-standing strategy in dysarthria treatment for a simple reason—some dysarthric speakers are much easier to understand when they slow their rate of speech. Many clinicians have treated individuals similiar to the speaker whose data appears in Figure 13-1. This figure represents data from an ataxic speaker who read a series of sentences at different rates (Yorkston & Beukelman, 1981b). All recordings were completed during a single session. At his habitual rate (A) of approximately 125 words per minute (wpm), speech intelligibility was low. As he was instructed to slow his rate more and more, intelligibility increased until, at approximately 75 wpm (C), the speaker was over 90 percent intelligible. Without a doubt, this sort of performance change is highly reinforcing for the clinician. Rarely in clinical treatment can such a dramatic change be brought about by manipulating one variable.

Rate control is a frequently employed strategy in treating dysarthric speakers, yet the effects of rate control have only recently begun to receive critical research attention. Our clinical experience has taught us that, although rate control may be beneficial for some speakers, it is not a panacea for the problems faced by all dysarthric speakers. For some speakers, slowing down does not help at all. For others, reducing the speaking rate has some advantages if speakers and their partners are willing to accept the disadvantages. The advantages may include an increase in speech intelligibility; however, the disadvantages frequently involve a reduction in speech naturalness. For still other speakers, only certain rate control techniques are effective and the clinician must carefully choose the technique that is the best compromise between benefits and drawbacks.

Until research provides us with some clearly defined guidelines about when and with whom to use rate control techniques, clinical experience and trials with various techniques and rates must guide our management decisions. Before presenting information regarding rate control for dysarthric speakers, we will review selected literature related to normal speaking rate and how nonimpaired speakers adjust their speaking rates. It is hoped that this information will help to provide a rationale for selection of rate reduction techniques in dysarthria and offer some possible explanations of the effectiveness of rate control for some speakers.

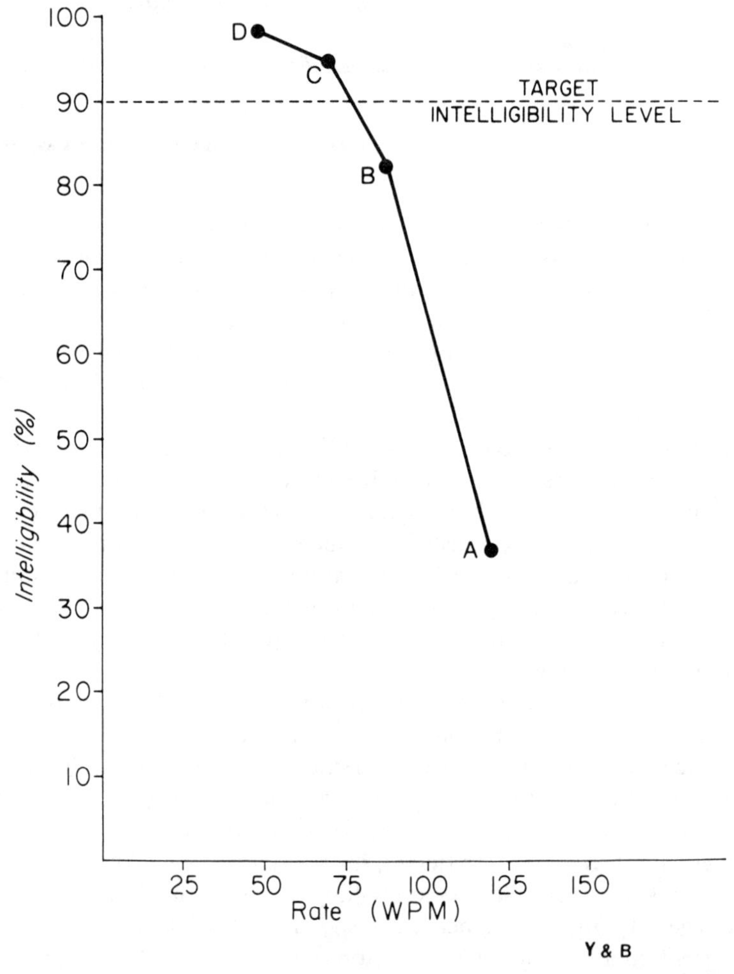

Figure 13-1. Intelligibility scores (percent correct) for sentences read at various speaking rates by an ataxic dysarthric speaker.

NORMAL SPEAKERS

Normal Rates

Perhaps it is best to begin to think about speaking rate and rate control by considering normal speech. Normal speaking rates depend on the task—normal paragraph reading rates range from 160 to 170 wpm (Fairbanks, 1960), and sentence reading rates are approximately 190 wpm (Yorkston & Beukelman, 1981a). Sentence reading rates are somewhat more rapid than paragraph rates because measures based on single sentences do not include intersentence pause times. The normal range of conversational speaking rate varies from 150 wpm to as rapid as 250 wpm (Goldman-Eisler, 1968).

Writers have long cautioned that it is misleading to consider only an overall speaking rate when measuring speaking performance (Kelly & Steer, 1949). Overall speaking time consists of two components—speaking or articulation time and pause time. Of these two components, pause time is the most elastic. Articulatory movement rates, on the other hand, are remarkably constant within a particular individual (Goldman-Eisler, 1961). Although articulatory movement rates may vary from one speaker to another, they generally range from 4.4 to 5.9 syllables per second. Normal speakers only increase articulatory movement rate if the material is highly practiced.

Importance of Pauses

Despite the fact that movement rates are considered stable within an individual, overall speaking rates may vary considerably, depending on the task. This variability is, to a large extent, the result of the changing proportion of pause time to total time in different tasks. Pauses may occupy 30 percent of prose reading and as much as 50 percent of the spontaneous speech in normal individuals (Klatt, 1976). Pauses are not randomly distributed throughout normal speech nor are they tied closely to maximum respiratory potential. In other words, normal speakers do not pause at random locations or simply because they need to take a breath. Instead, pauses are very systematically related to syntactical boundaries. For example, in spontaneous speech we pause at locations related to what have been called "cognitive strides" (Henderson, Goldman-Eisler, & Skarbek, 1966). Thus, pauses give us time to organize and structure what we are about to say.

For the speaker, pauses may serve an organizational function. For the listener, they may serve another function. Pauses chunk utterances into meaningful units. This chunking of information is important for the intelligibility of the message. When speakers do not supply the proper pauses or give the listener durational miscues, intelligibility is reduced. Huggins (1978) refers to this as the "garden path" effect. Suddenly you, the listener, are lost and you have no points of reference to find your way out of the maze.

Pauses also are important for the naturalness of speech. When we speak, we chunk utterances into breath groups which frequently have a falling fundamental frequency pattern. We then impose on that breath group a pattern of stress by making some words or syllables in the utterance more prominent than others. A more detailed discussion of factors related to naturalness appears in Chapter 14.

Comparison to Dysarthric Speakers

In comparing the speaking rates of normal individuals with dysarthric speakers, some facts are obvious. Dysarthric speakers tend to be slower than normal speakers. Of the 212 speakers studied by Darley, Aronson, and Brown

(1975), 170 were said to deviate from normal speaking rates. With all but a subgroup of hypokinetic dysarthric speakers, this deviation represents a trend toward slower than normal speech. Linebaugh and Wolfe (1984) studied the speech of groups of normal, spastic, and ataxic dysarthric individuals. Their results confirmed the clinical impression that dysarthric speakers speak more slowly than normal speakers. Mean syllable durations were 198, 246, and 249 msec for the normal, spastic, and ataxic groups, respectively. Their analysis further concluded that mean syllable durations for the spastic and ataxic groups did not differ from one another. Their hypothesis that the two groups may have different pause times is an important area for future investigation.

Assuming that articulatory movement rates may be physiologically "locked-in" for both normal and dysarthric speakers, pause time becomes critically important when speakers are asked to modify their rates. When normal speakers are asked to speak as rapidly as possible, they can increase their overall rates by approximately 30 percent (Lane & Grosjean, 1973). They do so almost entirely by reducing pause time. It appears that certain dysarthric speakers may adopt this same strategy in an effort to increase their slower than normal overall speaking rate. Thus, they may pause only when physiologically necessary. Unfortunately, this compensatory pattern may be maladaptive, as pauses appear to play such an important role in both speech intelligibility and naturalness. Clearly, further investigation of the role of pauses in the perceived adequacy of dysarthric speech is critical in designing appropriate rate control intervention programs.

CANDIDACY FOR RATE CONTROL

Throughout this chapter a number of case studies will be used to illustrate situations in which rate control has been judged to be effective. Generally, these cases exhibit either ataxic or hypokinetic dysarthria. Rate control might be effective for a number of reasons. Perhaps the most obvious explanation is that rate reduction might improve intelligibility by increasing precision of movement. Slowed rate might give dysarthric speakers better opportunity to move through the full articulatory range and thus, to achieve targets more adequately (Hardy, 1984). Slower speaking rates may prevent a phenomenon that Daniloff (1973) calls "undershoot," where at fast rates, a signal for one speech gesture arrives at the periphery before a preceding gesture is complete. The result is that gestures may be aborted before their completion.

Slowed rate might increase the ability of dysarthric speakers to coordinate the various speech components. Improper timing of the various speech subsystems is a characteristic deficit in ataxic speakers (Kent, Netsell, & Bauer, 1975). Many types of intercomponent coordination are necessary for adequate speech. For example, respiratory efforts must be precisely timed with phonatory efforts, voicing must be properly timed with oral articulatory gestures, and velopharyngeal closure must be timed to correspond with voicing and oral gestures.

Rate control might improve intelligibility because of its effect on respiratory patterning. Selected rate control techniques enable certain speakers to produce more appropriate breath group units and to intersperse pauses at appropriate junctures. Appropriate phrasing may chunk the dysarthric utterance into appropriate syntactic units, and thus, increase the redundancy of the information provided to the listener. Another explanation of the effect of rate control may also relate to the listener. The extra processing time provided by the slowed rates may give the listener the opportunity to "fill in the gaps" when attempting to interpret a distorted signal. Finally, rate control techniques may pace certain speakers and keep speech moving forward. This may be particularly important for speakers with hypokinetic dysarthria. Clearly, the list of speculations could go on.

At first glance, encouraging speakers who already speak more slowly than normal to reduce their speaking rates still further may seem counterproductive. However, readers are reminded that a frequent goal with dysarthic speakers is not "normalcy" but compensated intelligibility. Their physiological impairment may necessitate a slower than normal rate. The critical question in assessing the appropriateness of a dysarthric speaker's rate is not "How does it compare to normal?" but rather "Can speaking performance be improved (be made more intelligible and/or more natural) by modifying the rate?" Candidacy for rate control must be determined empirically because we cannot consistently predict who will benefit from a reduced rate and who will not.

SELECTING THE APPROPRIATE TECHNIQUE

Together with the question of candidacy for rate control is the selection of the most appropriate rate control technique. Again, management decisions must be based on clinical trials. We evaluate rate control techniques by examining the following issues.

Effectiveness

The first question that must be answered is obvious: "Does the technique actually elicit the desired speaking rate?" In a sense, all of the other questions become meaningless if the technique does not produce the desired rate or does not maintain that rate for a period of time. On the surface, this question is relatively easy to answer. Overall speaking rates are obtained for habitual speech and for speech controlled by the selected technique. However, knowing the overall speaking rate is not sufficient, and other factors must be considered. For example, pause time and distribution of pauses appears to be important for both the intelligibility and the naturalness of normal speech. Consider the parkinsonian individual using a pacing board whose articulatory rate is very rapid but whose pauses are interspersed between every word. This speaker's overall rate may be identical to that of a speaker with a much slower articulatory rate who pauses only at phrasal boundaries. Despite similar overall speaking rates, these two individuals manage the durational aspects of speech quite differently. Because pause time and the distribution of pauses may have an important impact on not only intelligibility but also on the perceived naturalness of speech, it is essential to consider these durational aspects of speech. Measures of pause time and articulation time may be obtained instrumentally. However, for clinical purposes, it is usually adequate to make perceptual judgments by listening to the sample and estimating the frequency and distribution of pauses during the sample.

In summary, in order to evaluate the effectiveness of a rate control technique, changes in the overall speaking rate must be documented. Additional considerations include the changes that occur in pause time and articulation time and the distribution of pauses throughout the utterance. Knowing as precisely as possible how the rate is being slowed may allow a better understanding of the consequences of the technique.

Training Requirements

The second question important in selecting a particular rate control technique is, "Are the training requirements of the technique reasonable, considering the speaker's communication needs and availability of training time?" Some rate control techniques, particularly the rigid rate control technique described later and techniques such as Delayed Auditory Feedback (DAF), require very little training. In effect, they are prosthetic devices. When they are removed, speakers are expected to return to their habitual speaking rates. Effective prosthetic techniques are acceptable in certain cases, but they clearly are a compromise and often are not as desirable as an independent, client controlled speaking rate. Prosthetic devices typically are considered when they are the only rate control technique that is effective.

Selection of many of the rate control techniques, particularly those that attempt to preserve prosody, require commitment to an intensive, and perhaps, extended period of training. Training to control rate independently is not a quick process. As will be apparent in the discussion of rate control drills that follow, independent control of rate requires many hours of practice.

Consequences

The third and final question to ask when evaluating a rate control technique is, "What are the consequences of slowing this speaker's rate?" Because research has provided so few predictors of success or failure of particular rate control techniques, evaluation of any technique must rely on a trial examination of its consequences. Of primary concern are the consequences in two overall aspects of speech—intelligibility and naturalness. Each of these areas will be discussed in greater detail later as individual cases are described. Briefly, however, rate control is typically considerd only for those individuals who are not completely understandable. Improvement in speech intelligibility is the primary goal. If intelligibility does not improve, rate control may not be appropriate for that individual, and other management approaches must be considered.

Rate control may also affect speech naturalness. Intelligibility is expected to improve with rate control; however, just the opposite is true with speech naturalness. Many rate control techniques interfere with the speaker's ability to produce natural speech. At times, the negative consequences of rate control are acceptable because of the associated improvement in intelligibility. Slight reduction in naturalness may be an acceptable compromise in order to achieve increases in intelligibility. Not all rate control techniques adversely affect naturalness to the same degree. Therefore, the naturalness of speech produced under a given rate control technique must be carefully considered. The clinician usually assesses the naturalness of speech under a specific rate control strategy by asking such questions as:

- Does the overall naturalness of speech decrease using this technique?
- Does this rate control technique negatively affect the speaker's ability to produce breath groups that are closely associated with the meaning of the utterance?
- Is the speaker able to signal stress on the most prominent words of the utterance within the breath group?

A more detailed discussion of the assessment of naturalness appears in Chapter 14.

RIGID RATE CONTROL TECHNIQUES

The following section reviews some of the rate control techniques that have been reported in the clinical and research literature. We will highlight the advantages and disadvantages of each and describe with brief case studies the types of speakers for whom these techniques have been successful. The discussion will be organized according to the amount of control needed to achieve the desired rate. Few dysarthric speakers can reduce their speaking rate and maintain a slowed rate after simply being instructed to "slow down"—training and practice are needed for nearly everyone. The technique selected depends on how rigidly the speaker's rate must be controlled in order to maintain the desired target speaking rate. A general word of caution is warranted: the more rigid the control technique, the more unnatural the resulting speech. Rigid rate control techniques include those that impose a one-word-at-a-time style upon the speaker. These techniques are usually reserved for the most severely involved and often involve some sort of external pacing.

Pacing Boards

Helm (1979) presented a case study of a parkinsonian speaker who was thought to be demented but instead was severely palilalic, in that words or phrases were repeated several times with increasing rate. Palilalia has been compared to the festinating gait pattern in some parkinsonian speakers. Helm introduced a pacing board in order to impose the necessary "stop/go" control over speech production, thus bringing an automatic act under voluntary control. The pacing board is a simple device consisting of a series of colored slots separated by ridges (Figure 13-2). The speaker is instructed to touch one slot per word. This technique meters speech and separates each word of the utterance.

Alphabet Board Supplementation

Another rigid rate control technique is the alphabet board supplementation approach described by Beukelman and Yorkston (1978). The speaker is instructed to identify the first letter of each word on an alphabet board or augmentative communication device as the word is spoken. See Chapter 8 for more details about the board and issues of partner training.

The alphabet board supplementation approach not only forces speakers into a slowed rate as they locate and point to the letters of the alphabet, but also provides their listeners with extra information in the form of the first

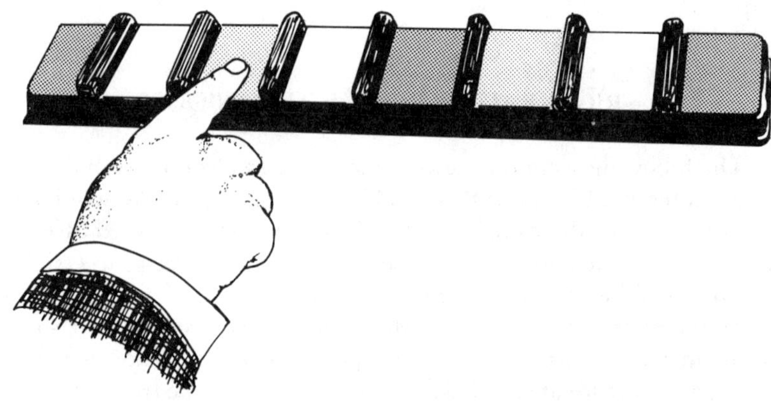

Figure 13-2. A pacing board.

letter of each word. With some speakers, intelligibility increases depend on the listener's ability to read the letter. For other speakers, the slowed speaking rate alone appears to the major contributing factor to improved intelligibility.

Case Presentation

The following case illustrates the clinical application of rigid rate control techniques. Of particular interest here is the compromise between perceived benefits and drawbacks. Amy was 25 years old when she participated in a job sampling program through our Rehabilitation Medicine Department. Her duties included work as a cashier in a small shop, and thus, involved extensive public contact. Understandable speech was mandatory. She came to us after many years of speech treatment during her school-age years. With the encouragement of her vocational counselor, she indicated that she was willing to give speech treatment "one last try."

Her medical history was sketchy. Birth was normal, but early neurologic degeneration followed, which was soon stablized. Amy's diagnosis was cerebral palsy with dystonic posturing. Her speech was characterized by rapid rate, rushes of speech, monoloudness, reduced loudness levels, monopitch, little articulatory excursion, and reduced stress patterning. Speech intelligibility measures confirmed her reports that listeners frequently asked her to repeat. Single word intelligibility was 76 percent; and sentence intelligibility was 24 percent at her habitual rate of 145 wpm (Yorkston & Beukelman, 1981a). The large discrepancy between single word and sentence intelligibility suggested that rate control might be an appropriate strategy. At Amy's level of severity, sentences should be more intelligible than single words because sentences provide contextual cues that a single word production task does not provide.

The clinician who served Amy chose a rigid rate control technique as a trial for a number of reasons. Extended periods of training with other rate control techniques had not been successful, Amy could master the rigid rate control technique with little training, and time was limited to the six week period of job sampling. The clinician first chose a finger tapping method that required that Amy touch her thumb to each finger in succession in a metered fashion as she produced each word of an utterance. Her clinician chose this particular technique because Amy had sufficient fine motor control in her hands to accomplish the maneuver, and this technique did not require her to carry a device such as a pacing or an alphabet board. By the end of the evaluation session, Amy had learned the technique and sentence intelligibility measures were obtained once again. Figure 13-3 contains measures of speech intelligibility and speaking rate for both habitual and slowed sentence production. A review of the figure indicates that by slowing her rate from 145 to 70 wpm using finger tapping, her sentence intelligibility improved from 24 percent to 68 percent.

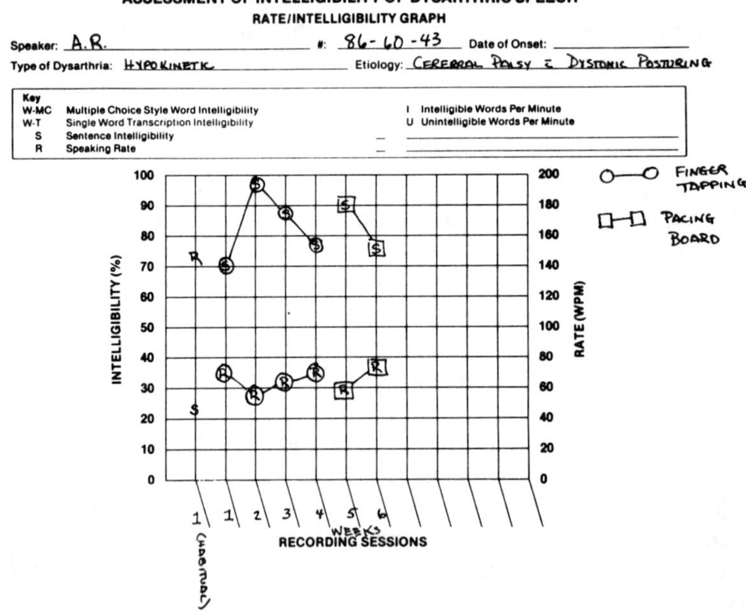

Figure 13-3. Speech intelligibility and rate measures for Amy when using various rigid rate control techniques.

Encouraged by these results, the clinician scheduled Amy for a once a week training session, hoping to stabilize her performance with the finger tapping technique. By the end of the first training session following the evaluation, Amy's sentence intelligibility had increased to 95 percent. Unfortunately, during the second training session, intelligibility fell to 85 percent. When another 10 percent decrease in intelligibility was observed during the third training session, her clinician began to realize that finger tapping was no longer a powerful enough pacing technique for Amy. As she became increasingly practiced with the simple motor activity of finger tapping, the activity became more and more automatic. By the end of the third training session, the clinician felt that a more powerful pacing technique was needed and she introduced the small pacing board described earlier in the work of Helm (1979). It took only a few minutes to train Amy to use the new system. During the fourth training session, intelligibility was again measured, and this time Amy paced herself with the board. Figure 13-3 contains sentence intelligibility and speaking rate measures that had been obtained during the initial evaluation and during each of the successive training sessions. Introduction of the new pacing board improved her intelligibility from 75 percent to 90 percent. Note the reciprocal relationship between Amy's speaking rate and intelligibility. As her rate increased, her intelligibility systematically decreased. Further, with practice, those pacing systems that involved simple repetitive movement appeared to lose their effectiveness over time. Unfortunately, use of the pacing board became as automatic as the finger tapping pacing method had become. After a relatively short time, it no longer appeared to pace her speech adequately.

The pacing board also had another important drawback, at least in Amy's opinion. She found the board cosmetically unacceptable. In fact, she called it "just another badge of disability," this despite the clinician's endorsement and long discussion of the importance of understandable speech. As a final resort, the clinician introduced the alphabet board. Although the alphabet board was clearly no more cosmetically acceptable than the pacing board, the motor activity required to point to the letters on the board is not routine or repetitive, and thus, cannot become automatic as the two other pacing techniques had become. With the alphabet board, Amy was nearly 100 percent understandable—when she would use it. It quickly became apparent to the clinician that Amy's dislike of the board would frequently result in her "forgetting" to use it when she was on the job. With some discussion, a compromise was reached. Amy would use the alphabet board at home and with friends. When she was on the job, rate control techniques were rotated, so that every third day she was able to use the preferred finger tapping technique. This compromise was one attempt to minimize the "overlearning" that reduced the effectiveness of the repetitive pacing techniques.

Advantages and Disadvantages of Rigid Techniques

As with many management decisions involving dysarthric speakers, the selection of a rigid rate control technique represents a compromise between the advantages and disadvantages. On the positive side, a number of advantages of the rigid rate control techniques are apparent. First, these techniques often are effective in slowing a speaker's rate when other techniques fail. Second, speech intelligibility increases for certain speakers as a consequence of the slowed rates. The alphabet board supplementation system goes one step beyond other rigid rate control techniques by providing listeners with extra information in the form of the first letter of every word. This extra information often further increases intelligibility. Third, most of the rigid rate control techniques are not highly technical and therefore are inexpensive. Fourth, the rigid rate control techniques require little training of the user. Finally, these techniques allow for continual practice of slowed rate. Individuals are able to leave the therapy room and continue to use their system for all of their daily communication.

Despite their major advantages, rigid rate control techniques are not without their drawbacks. In fact, the drawbacks often are considered so important that rigid rate control techniques may justifiably be used only as the last resort when nothing else is effective. First, rigid rate control techniques disrupt the naturalness of speech. By encouraging a one-word-at-a-time style with pauses between each word, they disrupt the breath group units that are important in normal prosody. Rigid rate control techniques also may be perceived as being unnatural because they encourage a disproportionate amount of pause time. Many severely involved parkinsonian speakers using rigid rate control techniques do not prolong articulation time, rather, they merely expand their pause time. Second, many of the rigid rate control techniques rely on a device that many users find cosmetically unacceptable. For others, the advantage of communication without frequent breakdowns is so appealing that the need for a device is accepted willingly. Finally, adaptation to the rate control technique may be a problem. This is especially true when the rate control technique depends on a simple movement that may easily be overlearned. Once the movement is overlearned, the technique may no longer serve as an effective pacer.

TECHNIQUES THAT PRESERVE PROSODY

The following is a series of rate control techniques that do not impose the one-word-at-a-time speaking style. Thus, these techniques are not as disruptive to speech naturalness as the rigid rate control techniques. Because, for the most part, the following techniques depend on speaker training rather than on a device that imposes the desired rate, additional demands are placed on the speaker. The speaker must demonstrate learning ability and must devote time in order to master the new motor skill.

Oscilloscopic Feedback

Berry and Goshorn (1983) presented the case study of an individual who had severe ataxic dysarthria secondary to several cerebrovascular episodes six months prior to treatment. These authors hypothesized that their patient was "overdriving" his poorly controlled speech mechanism by speaking too rapidly and too loudly. They developed a training program in which he received visual feedback from the intensity-by-time tracing on an oscilloscopic screen. The clinician modeled the sentence on the top half of the screen. The dysarthric speaker was instructed to (1) "fill up the screen," that is, increase the overall duration of his utterance to the target duration, and (2) keep his loudness level below a preset line.

Berry and Goshorn measured intelligibility using sentences from the SPIN list (Kalikow, Steven, & Elliot, 1977). Audio-recorded sentences produced by the dysarthric speaker were played for a judge who attempted to transcribe the last word of the sentence. Some of the sentence-final words were highly probable, whereas others were considered low-probability completions of the sentence. Results of a five week training period indicated that the patient was able to slow his speaking rate. An increase in intelligibility was associated with this decrease in rate.

Of particular interest in this case was how the speaker adjusted his rate. When given no instructions other than to slow down and prolong the entire utterance (fill the screen), he developed a very interesting strategy of durational adjustments. The average duration of key words (words in the sentence final position) did not change from pre- to posttreatment recording. Instead, he systematically prolonged the pauses prior to key words in the posttreatment condition. Further, he appeared to pause longer prior to words that were unlikely to occur in that sentence (low probability words) than prior to high probability words. This clinical finding illustrates the importance of strategically placed pauses to improve intelligibility and suggests that increasing word duration may not be the only goal of rate control programs. This case also illustrates another important advantage of the less rigid rate control techniques. Techniques that do not impose rigid timing on speakers allow them to develop their own compensatory strategies. Often these strategies are both effective and subtle.

Rhythmic Cueing

The Technique

In an effort to move away from rigid pacing techniques, we began to use a training technique called *rhythmic cueing* (Yorkston & Beukelman, 1981b). The technique is a simple one. The clinican signals the desired speaking rate by pointing to the words of a passage in a rhythmic fashion. The clinician gives more time to prominent words and intersperses pauses where appropriate. This technique must, of course, be used with printed passages. However, one disadvantage of the use of printed material is the difficulty in precisely cueing the desired speaking rate. Usually, the clinician simply estimates appropriate rates when using the technique with printed material.

Computerization

Recently, the rhythmic cueing technique has been computerized (Beukelman, 1983). Passages have been entered into the computer along with timing information that approximates the rhythmic durational relationships between words in normal speech. The clinician then enters a target rate and the passage appears on the computer screen with a cursor cueing that target rate. The computerization of the rhythmic cueing technique has two advantages over the printed material. First, precise rates can be selected, and second, speakers can practice independently once a set of practice materials and the appropriate rates have been established by the clinician. Typically, many hours of practice are necessary to establish a new optimum speaking rate.

Case Presentation

The following case illustrates the use of rhythmic cueing as a training technique. Donna was a 24 year old woman with a 10 year history of Friedreich's ataxia. At the time of our evaluation, she was wheelchair dependent and exhibited such severe ataxia in her upper extremities that the use of a typewriter or pointing to letters on an alphabet board was not possible. Although her speech was severely dysarthric, she spoke as her sole means of communication. During our evaluation, speech intelligibility and rate were measured (Yorkston, Beukelman, & Traynor, 1984). At her habitual rate, Donna spoke at 57 wpm with a sentence intelligibility score of 23 percent. A similar series of sentences were computer-presented using a rhythmic cueing technique. The rate of the second sample was slowed to 45 wpm or approximately 80 percent of her habitual rate. When her rate was reduced in this manner, intelligibility increased to 45 percent.

Although we are typically cautious about embarking on an extended period of training in rate control with an individual who is suffering from a degenerative disorder such as Friedreich's ataxia, we chose to initiate treatment because Donna did not have the hand function to benefit from any of the rigid pacing techniques; all of which required manipulation of a device. She practiced for 30 minutes each day for six weeks, reading sentences of varying lengths presented to her by the computer in a rhythmic manner at 45 wpm. At the end of this training period, the pacing was removed and a third sentence sample was recorded and scored for intelligibility. Results of this posttreatment sample (See Table 13-1), indicated that Donna was now speaking at an habitual rate of 48 wpm with a sentence intelligibility score of 52 percent.

TABLE 13.1.
Sentence intelligibility measures (Yorkston, Beukelman, & Traynor, 1984) obtained for Donna.

	PRETREATMENT		POSTTREATMENT
	Unpaced	**Paced**	**Unpaced**
Rate WPM	73	44	46
Intelligibility (%)	23	46	52
Rate of intelligible speech (IWPM)	16	18	23

From Yorkston, K.M., Beukelman, D.R., & Traynor, C.D. (1984). *Computerized assessment of intelligibility of dysarthric speech*. Tigard, OR: C.C. Publications.

In an effort to understand more completely the changes that are brought about by rate control techniques, we further analyzed the samples produced by Donna. Acoustic analysis revealed that although pauses represented only 23 percent of the total sample during the pretreatment habitual condition, this percentage increased to 40 percent and 41 percent during the pretreatment paced condition and the posttreatment habitual condition, respectively. Six months after our intervention, this young woman continued to speak at a rate that approximated the target rate during training. She resolved communication breakdowns by verbally indicating the first letter of each word that her listener did not understand.

"Backdoor" Approaches to Rate Control

A number of rate control techniques come under the general heading of "backdoor" approaches because, although they have the effect of reducing rate, rate control is not their primary focus. One illustration of such a case was presented by Simmons (1983), who described the management of a 26 year old, closed-head-injured patient with ataxic dysarthria. Treatment focused on improving the naturalness of his speech. Initial acoustic analysis suggested that the speaker's perceived monotony was related to flat fundamental frequency contours and lack of high frequency energy. Listeners also perceived his speech to be "excess and equal." This characteristic was attributed to his slowed rate as compared to normal and essentially equal syllable durations. Simmons outlined a four-phase treatment program that included, as a first phase, training loudness and pitch variation and, as a second phase, altered word and sentence stress patterns. Acoustic analysis was carried out after each treatment phase. Results of the analysis after the first and second phases of treatment suggested that the most striking changes were brought about in the time dimension, despite the fact that rate control was not the goal of intervention. This led Simmons to suggest that "target behaviors were not independent; working on a specific aspect of speech, such as intonation or pitch variation, caused changes in other areas, such as time and articulation" (p. 290).

Another backdoor approach to rate control training is appropriate phrasing and breath patterning. Chunking utterances into meaningful units based on breath groups has been shown to be important for the intelligibility of normal speech. Dysarthric speakers frequently fail to do this. The relationship between speaking rate and respiratory control is clinically important. Hardy (1984) discussed rate control in developmentally dysarthric individuals with compromised respiratory support. He suggested that although one might predict that speakers would produce fewer units on a single breath if rates were reduced, this is not necessarily the case. Decreasing speaking rates prolonged the phonated elements of speech more than the nonphonated elements. Because the laryngeal valving of the phonated elements in some speakers tends to be more aerodynamically efficient than the valving for the nonphonated elements, rate reduction may not negatively affect respiratory support. Also, it should be noted again that some rate control techniques, particularly the ones that impose rigid rate control, may disrupt respiratory patterning for speech. Other rate control techniques, especially those that encourage appropriate phrasing, may improve speech-related respiratory function.

Delayed Auditory Feedback (DAF)

Research Findings

DAF is an intervention technique that has been used with a number of different communication disorders, most notably in the area of stuttering (Soderberg, 1969). Curlee and Perkins (1969) studied the effects of DAF on a group of stutterers and found that DAF reduced the stutterers' rate of speech and frequency of stuttering. Trials of DAF use have been reported with neurogenically involved populations, including aphasic subjects (Stanton, 1958), patients with left or right hemisphere lesions (Vrtunski, Mack, Boller, & Kim, 1976), and a group of dysarthric speakers of varying types (Singh & Schlanger, 1969). These studies generally report mixed results with large variability in effect from patient to patient. Although a number of the studies of the effects of DAF included subject groups that were heterogeneous, other studies restricted themselves to a more homogeneous population. Downie, Low, and Lindsay (1981) tested DAF with 11 parkinsonian patients. They reported "dramatic improvement in intelligibility" in two of the patients. These patients were described as having a "festinating" type of speech.

Hansen and Metter (1980) reported the use of a small, solid state, battery-operated DAF unit, similiar to the one that appears in Figure 13-4 with two

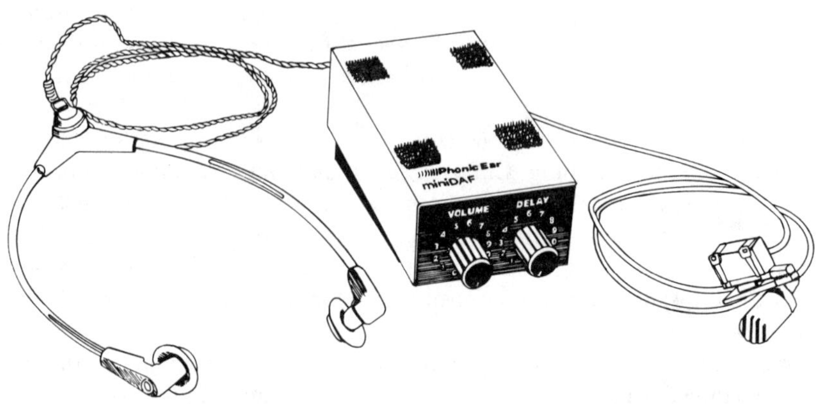

Figure 13-4. Portable DAF Unit (MiniDAF, Phonic Ear, Mill Valley CA).

patients with supranuclear palsy and hypokinetic dysarthria. With the delay at 100 msec, speech was slowed, vocal intensity increased, and speech intelligibility improved.

Hansen and Metter (1983) reported a DAF application with two speakers with Parkinson's disease. For both of these speakers, the intervention had an impact on speech performance, including improvement in intelligibility and an increase in intensity. Measures of these changes are summarized in Table 13-2. Hansen and Metter suggest that, when using DAF, both speakers increased their physiological effort.

A question that logically follows from the positive case reports of Hansen and Metter relates to how universally helpful DAF is for dysarthric speakers. Both clinical experience and a review of the literature suggest that it is only effective in selected cases of hypokinetic dysarthia. Specific data related to the proportion of the population benefiting from DAF are not yet available. However, Hansen, Metter, and Riege (1984) presented a continuation of their work in this area. They presented an acoustic profile of a typical candidate who benefited from DAF. Acoustic features of this speech included:

- duration and articulation time both more than 2.5 standard deviations below normal
- pause time, number of pauses, and mean length of pauses approximately at a normal level of performance
- percent of voicing 2.0 standard deviations above normal

Thus, their patient's speech was excessively rapid and voicing was consistently present throughout speech. When speaking with DAF, the following acoustic

TABLE 13-2.
A Summary of Changes Seen in Parkinson Subjects A and B with and without DAF

	Subject A	**Subject B**
Reduction in Speaking Rate	255 to 139 wpm	184 to 122 wpm reading 242 to 161 wpm conversation
Increased Speech Intelligibility	5.0 to 2.0 (7-pt. scale)	increased or same
Increased Speech Intensity	66 to 72 dB SPL	77 to 79 dB SPL reading 78 to 71 dB SPL conversation
Improved Phrasing	yes	

From Hanson, W., & Metter, E. (1983). DAF speech rate modification in Parkinson's disease: A report of two cases. In W. Berry (Ed.), *Clinical dysarthria*. San Diego: College-Hill Press.

features of this individual's speech moved toward normal: duration, articulation time, fundamental frequency variability, mean intensity, and intensity variability.

Case Presentation

Clinical trials remain critical in assessing the benefits and drawbacks of any of the rate control techniques that attempt to preserve prosody. To illustrate this point, we will present the case of a 72 year old man with a 10 year history of Parkinson's disease. A number of different rate control strategies were tried. Habitually, his rate, as measured on a sentence production task (Yorkston, Beukelman, & Traynor, 1984), was excessively rapid at 262 wpm. This rate represents 138 percent of normal rate and is over 3.0 standard deviations above the mean of normal male speakers. At this rapid rate, speech intelligibility was 67 percent. The first rate control technique evaluated was rhythmic cueing. Initially, we were interested in the question "Does reducing this speaker's rate improve intelligibility?" A computerized pacing program was used in conjunction with the intelligibility measurement task to answer this question. When sentences were presented at 127 wpm, approximately 60 percent of his habitual rate, he spoke at 137 wpm. At this slowed rate he was 94 percent intelligible. Judges who rated speech naturalness felt that the slowed rate was more natural than the excessively rapid speech.

The initial trial with pacing had indicated that slowing his rate had beneficial consequences for both intelligibility and naturalness. Our next question was "How do we translate the result of this clinical trial, which was carried out under highly controlled conditions, into a training program that will slow his rate in real communication situations?" Three options were considered. The first was the training program described earlier for Donna. Choosing this alternative would mean an extended period of training and practice, using the computer to slow his rate. We did not choose this alternative because the patient demonstrated only limited awareness of his rapid rate and there seemed to be no carryover from the reading of computer-presented paced passages to unpaced reading or conversation. The second alternative would also require a period of training, but on a task that the speaker appeared to be able to learn more quickly. This training would involve one of the "backdoor" approaches to rate control and would involve the speaker learning to pause at appropriate phrasing boundaries and thereby chunking his speech into syntactically appropriate, but short, breath groups. The third alternative for this speaker would be use of a DAF system. We chose to begin our exploration of rate control strategies with the DAF because, if effective, it would require the least amount of training. Results of these trials will be illustrated with a variety of measures in order to describe as fully as possible the impact of DAF on this speaker.

As with the evaluation of any rate control technique, our first question, "Does DAF control rate at the target level?" concerned the effectiveness of

DAF. To answer this question, the speaker was recorded as he read passages with the sidetone of the DAF unit set at a number of different levels. Figure 13-5 illustrates the results we obtained. This figure displays the sidetone setting of the DAF versus the speaking rate (in syllables per minute) that was produced at each sidetone. Examination of the figure suggests that a reduction in speaking rate occurred when the delay was increased from a normal sidetone (no delay) to a 100 msec delay. An additional reduction occurred when the delay was increased from a 100 to a 150 msec delay. No additional reduction in rate occurred as the sidetone delay was increased from 150 to 200 msec. This information not only confirmed the effectiveness of DAF on this task, but also allowed the selection of a sidetone delay setting that produced the greatest effect in terms of rate control.

Our next question was "What are the consequences of DAF?" Of course, our hope was that the reduced rate brought about by DAF would result in

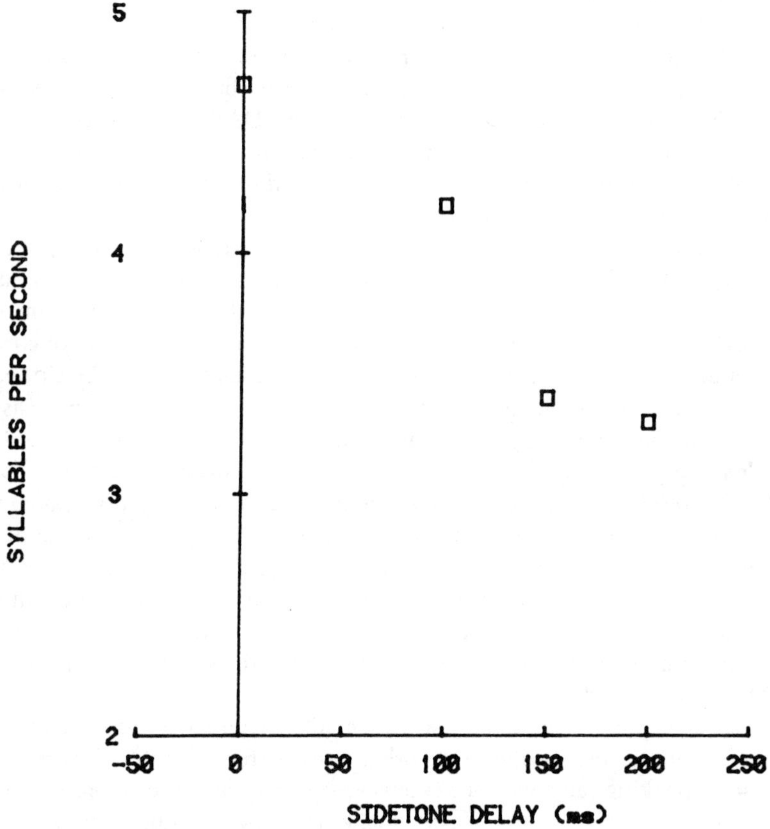

Figure 13-5. Speaking rates (syllables per minute) for a parkinsonian speaker at 0, 500, 130, 150, and 200 msec sidetone delays.

an increase in intelligibility. This proved to be the case. Speech intelligibility was measured as the speaker read sentences at a DAF sidetone delay of 150 msec. This DAF setting produced a speaking rate of 135 wpm and an intelligibility score of 97 percent. Thus, DAF produced both a higher intelligibility score and a more rapid rate than either of the other rate control strategies—computerized rhythmic cueing or insertion of pauses at the appropriate locations related to breath groups.

Although increased intelligibility is certainly important when evaluating the consequence of rate control, the effect of rate control on the naturalness of our patient's speech was also of concern. Perceptually, reducing speaking rate with DAF appeared to improve the naturalness. The rapid rushes of speech that were present during habitual speech were gone, and the pattern of breath groups and intonation contours was preserved. In order to acoustically document these changes, a short segment embedded in a paragraph read by the speaker was selected for further measurement. The fundamental frequency and intensity contours were analyzed for the habitual reading and for a sidetone delayed condition (150 msec). Fundamental frequency and intensity by time plots for these segments appear in Figure 13-6. A review of this figure reveals that the speaker does not intersperse pauses in the DAF-slowed speech. Further, fundamental freqency excursion on the DAF-slowed speech was slightly greater than for habitual speech. Generally, the acoustic measures suggest that the speaker increased overall speaking time, and at the same time, maintained natural prosodic patterns.

Further acoustic analysis was performed on another short sample of habitual and DAF-slowed speech. In this analysis, consonant and vowel-nasal segment duration were obtained from an acoustic analysis for two parkinsonian speakers. Table 13-3 contains the percentage change in duration of consonant and vowel-nasal segments for the habitual and three DAF-slowed conditions. For Speaker 1, the speaker we have been discussing in this case presentation, consonant and vowel-nasal segments were slowed in a roughly equivalent proportion under the 150 and 200 msec delay conditions. For Speaker 2, however, the vowel-nasal segments were increased proportionally more than the consonant segments. Thus, there appear to be individual differences among speakers in the effect of DAF on segment duration. However, in both speakers DAF had the effect of increasing total articulation time rather than simply increasing pause duration. The increase in articulation time rather than pause time may be an important contributor to perceived naturalness of DAF slowed speech.

When considering the data just presented, DAF appears to have many advantages for selected speakers over other rate control strategies. DAF effectively slow speaking rates without extensive training, improves intelligibility while maintaining a somewhat faster speaking rate than other rate control techniques, and it preserves, and may even improve, the overall naturalness of speech. However, in order to clinically measure intelligibility and to compare

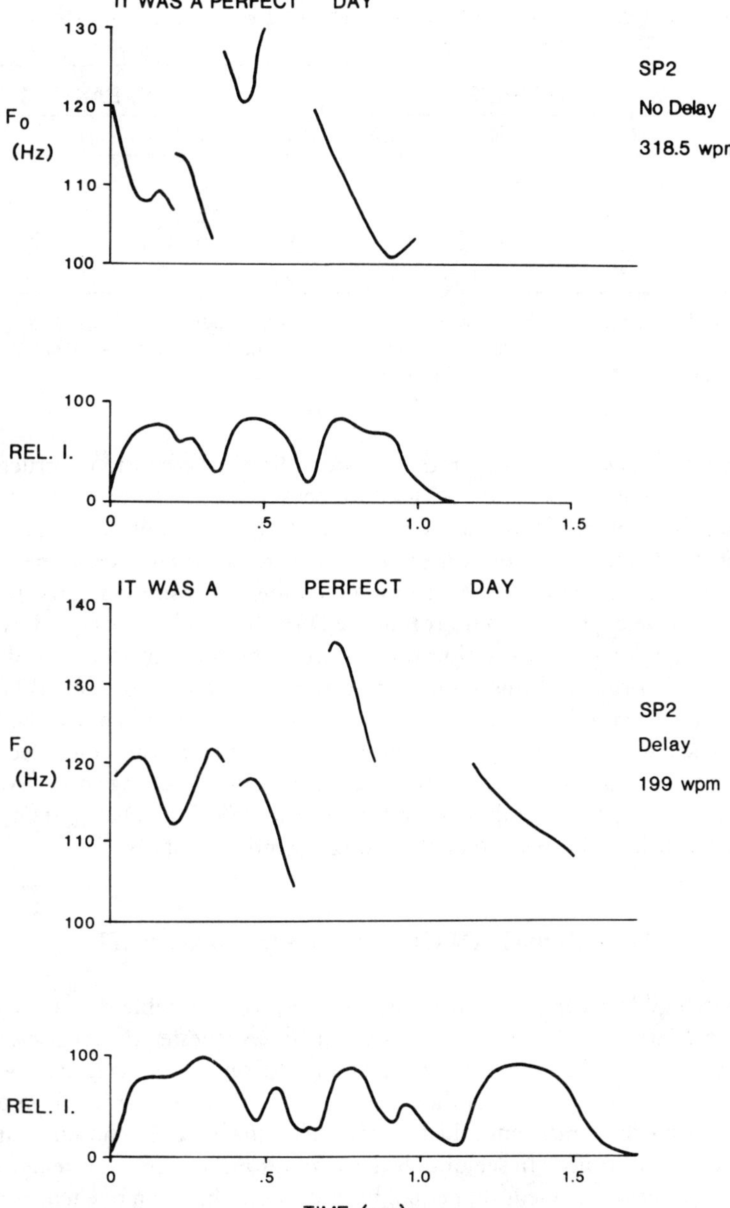

Figure 13-6. Fundamental frequency-by-time and intensiy-by-time tracings of habitual and DAF-slowed speech of a parkinsonian speaker.

TABLE 13-3.
Percent Changes in Consonant and Vowel-Nasal Durations for Two Parkinsonian Speakers at Three DAF-Slowed Speaking Rates

msec	SPEAKER 1			SPEAKER 2		
delay	C	V–N	Total	C	V–N	Total
50				8	46	28
100	–10	9	1	16	108	65
150	45	39	40	29	110	72
200	29	34	31			

From Beukelman, D.R., Yorkston, K.M., & McClean, M.D. (1984). *The effects of rate control on dysarthric speech.* Miniseminar presentation at the annual convention of the American Speech-Language-Hearing Association, San Francisco, CA.

acoustically speech samples produced under different conditions, structured samples must be used. In this case, our speaker was asked to read material that had been prepared for him. Unfortunately, the DAF unit did not control his rate as effectively during conversation. This reduction in effectiveness may have been due, in part, to the telegraphic nature of his sponanteous speech. Utterances were typically so short that the DAF effect did not occur. However, DAF pacing during conversation was judged to be superior to unpaced productions. In order to bring conversation under more control with DAF, we attempted to train this speaker in strategies that we felt would allow the DAF unit to be a more effective pacer of his speech. These strategies included producing the initial word of an utterance with relatively strong intensity, not attempting to speak rapidly in an effort to "overdrive" the DAF system, and speaking in full phrases rather than single word utterances.

SELECTING AN OPTIMUM SPEAKING RATE

Intelligible speech at normal rates is rarely an attainable goal for dysarthric speakers. Throughout this chapter, we have suggested that the selection of rate control techniques often reflects a compromise between the positive and negative consequences of those techniques. Likewise, the selection of an optimum speaking rate, once the training technique has been chosen, requires a clinical compromise. In seeking the best compromise between intelligibility and naturalness, it is clear that equal weight cannot be given to each. If there is a choice between intelligibility and naturalness, intelligibility must be the deciding variable. Relatively natural but unintelligible speech is not acceptable. When speech intelligibility reaches an acceptable range (over 90 percent), we find ourselves compromising slightly in terms of intelligibility in order to achieve naturalness.

Data presented at the beginning of this chapter illustrated the case of an ataxic dysarthric speaker who clearly benefited from rate control. A review of that data (Figure 13-1) reveals that the highest intelligibility score for this speaker was obtained at a rate of approximately 50 wpm. Because the speaker felt, and the clinician agreed, that this rate was too disruptive of naturalness, a slightly more rapid rate was selected as a target during training. A rate of approximately 70 wpm was selected because, at that rate, the speaker was over 90 percent intelligible and was able to achieve at least some degree of natural breath patterning and stressing within breath group units.

Many of the dysarthric speakers we serve clinically are not neurologically stable. The course for some is improving, for others it is degenerative. Since

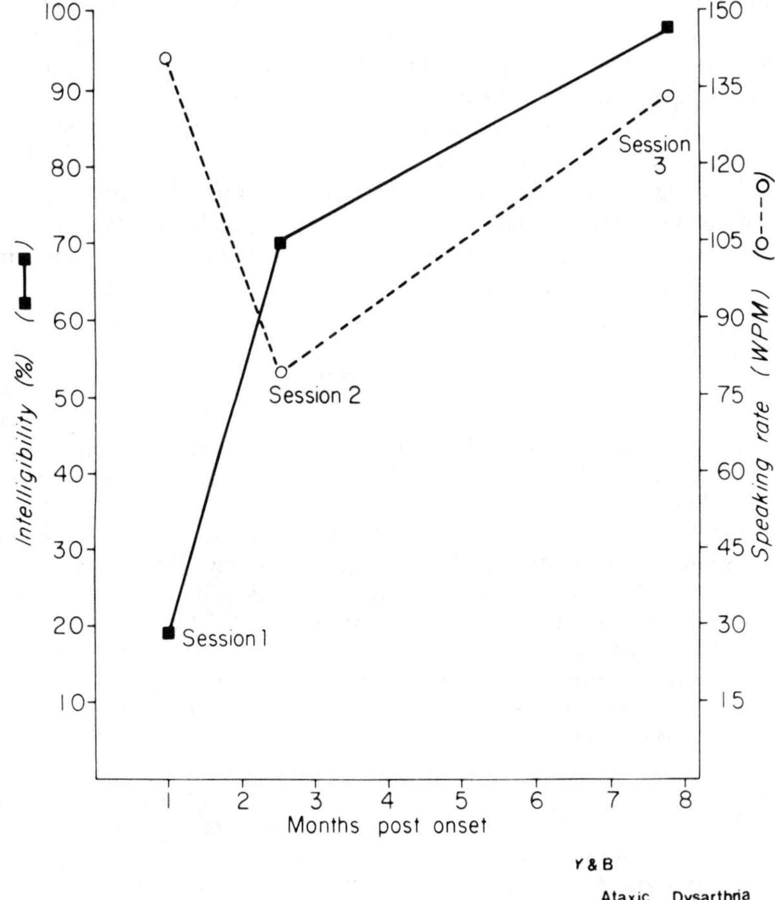

Figure 13-7. Sentence intelligibility and speaking rate obtained over a period of recovery for an ataxic dysarthric speaker.

our goal is to maximize speech performance regardless of the course of the disorder, the selection of an optimum rate and rate control technique must be reevaluated periodically. Figure 13-7 contains data illustrating the recovery pattern of a head-injured ataxic dysarthria speaker (Yorkston & Beukelman, 1981b). At one month postonset, when the patient was speaking at 137 wpm, intelligibility was low, approximately 20 percent. At that point, a training program utilizing rhythmic cueing was initiated. By the second recording session, this patient had reduced his rate to 80 wpm with an accompanying increase in intelligibility to approximately 70 percent. As the speaker continued to improve, his target speaking rate was systematically increased. By eight months post onset, he was nearly completely intelligible at a speaking rate of over 130 wpm. Thus, the target speaking rate must continue to change as long as the speaker is able to maintain an acceptable level of intelligibility. Once intelligibility has been achieved at a particular rate, treatment can appropriately focus on increasing the rate and naturalness of speech.

The speaker just presented was recovering from head injury. However, management frequently involves individuals with degenerative disorders such as Parkinson's disease. For these individuals, optimum speaking rates and rate control strategies also need to be periodically reevaluated. More rigid rate control techniques are selected as the severity of the speech disability increases. As a consequence of the more rigid rate control techniques, target speaking rates are progressively slowed.

REFERENCES

Berry, W.R., & Goshorn, E.L. (1983). Immediate visual feedback in the treatment of ataxic dysarthria: A case study. In W.R. Berry (Ed.), *Clinical Dysarthria*. Austin, TX: PRO-ED.

Beukelman, D.R. (1983). *The effects of rate control on dysarthric speech.* Grant funded by National Institute of Neurological & Communicative Disorders & Stroke.

Beukelman, D.R. & Yorkston, K.M. (1978). Communication options for patients with brain stem lesions. *Archives of Physical Medicine & Rehabilitation, 59*, 337–340.

Beukelman, D.R., Yorkston, K.M., & McClean, M.D. (1984). *The effects of rate control on dysarthric speech.* A miniseminar presentation at the annual convention of the American Speech-Language-Hearing Association, San Fransisco.

Curlee, R., & Perkins, W. (1969). Conversational rate control therapy for stuttering. *Journal of Speech & Hearing Disorders, 34*, 245–250.

Daniloff, R.G. (1973). Normal articulation process. In F.D. Minifie, T.J. Hixon, & F. Williams (Eds.), *Normal aspects of speech, hearing and language.* Englewood Cliffs, NJ: Prentice-Hall, Inc.

Darley, F., Aronson, A., & Brown, J. (1975). *Motor speech disorders.* Philadelphia: W.B. Saunders.

Downie, A.W., Low, J.M., & Lindsay, D.D. (1981). Speech disorders in parkinsonism. Usefulness of delayed auditory feedback in selected cases. *British Journal of*

Disorders of Communication, *16*, 135–139.

Fairbanks, G. (1960). *Voice and articulation drillbook* (2nd ed.). New York: Harper & Brothers.

Goldman-Eisler, F. (1961). The significance of changes in the rate of articulation. *Language & Speech, 4*, 171.

Goldman-Eisler, F. (1968). *Psycholinguistics: Experiments in spontaneous speech.* New York: Academic Press.

Hanson, W., & Metter, E. (1983). DAF speech rate modification in parkinson's disease: A report of two cases. In W. Berry (Ed.), *Clinical dysarthria*. Austin, TX: PRO-ED.

Hanson, W., & Metter, E. (1983). DAF speech rate modification in parkinson's disease: A report of two cases. In W. Berry (Ed.), *Clinical dysarthria*. San Diego: College-Hill Press.

Hanson, W., Metter, E., & Riege, W.H. (1984). *Variability in the Parkinson disease.* Paper presented at the Annual Convention of the American Speech-Language-Hearing Association, San Fransisco, CA.

Hardy, J.C. (1984). *Cerebral palsy.* Englewood Cliffs, NJ: Prentice Hall, Inc.

Helm, N.A. (1979). Management of palilalia with a pacing board. *Journal of Speech & Hearing Disorders, 44*, 350–353.

Henderson, A., Goldman-Eisler, F., & Skarbek, A. (1966). Sequential temporal patterns in spontaneous speech. *Language and Speech, 9*, 207–216.

Huggins, A.W.E. (1978). Speech timing and intelligibility. In J. Requin (Ed.), *Attention and performance VII*. Hillside NJ: Lawrence Erlbaum Associates.

Kalikow, D., Steven, K., & Elliot, L. (1977). Development of a test of speech intelligibility in noise using sentence material with controlled predictability. *Journal of the Acoustic Society of America*, *61*, 1337–1351.

Kent, R., Netsell, R., & Bauer, L.L. (1975). Cineradiographic assessment of articulatory mobility in the dysarthrias. *Journal of Speech & Hearing Disorders, 40*, 467.

Kelly, J., & Steer, M. (1949). Revised concept of rate. *Journal of Speech & Hearing Disorders, 14*, 222–226.

Klatt, D.H. (1976). Linguistic uses of segmental duration in English: Acoustic and perceptual evidence. *Journal of the Acoustic Society of America, 59*, 1208–1221.

Lane, H., & Grosjean, F. (1973). Perception of reading rate by listeners and speakers. *Journal of Experimental Psychology, 97*, 141–147.

Linebaugh, C.W., & Wolfe, V.E. (1984). Relationship between articulation rate, intelligibility, and naturalness in spastic and ataxic speakers. In M.R. McNeil, J.C. Rosenbek, & A.E. Aronson (Eds.), *The dysarthrias: Physiology-acoustics-perception-management*. San Diego: College-Hill Press.

Simmons, N.N. (1983). Acoustic analysis of ataxic dysarthria: An approach to monitoring treatment. In W.R. Berry (Ed.), *Clinical Dysarthria*. Austin, TX: PRO-ED.

Singh, S., & Schlanger, B.B. (1969). Effects of delayed sidetone on the speech of aphasic, dysarthric, and mentally retarded subjects. *Language & Speech, 12*, 167.

Soderberg, G. (1969), Delayed auditory feedback and the speech of stutterers: A review of studies. *Journal of Speech & Hearing Disorders, 34*, 20–29.

Stanton, J.B. (1958). The effects of DAF on the speech of aphasic patients. *Scot. Med. J., 3*, 378–384.

Vrtunski, P.B., Mack, J.L., Boller F., & Kim, Y. (1976). Response to delayed auditory feedback in patients with hemispheric lesions. *Cortex, 12*, 395–404.

Yorkston, K.M., & Beukelman, D.R. (1981a). *Assessment of intelligibility of dysarthric speech.* Austin, TX: PRO-ED.

Yorkston, K.M., & Beukelman, D.R. (1981b). Ataxic dysarthria: Treatment sequences based on intelligibility and prosodic considerations. *Journal of Speech & Hearing Disorders, 46*, 398–404.

Yorkston, K.M., Beukelman, D.R., & Traynor, C.D. (1984). *Computerized assessment of intelligibility of dysarthric speech.* Austin, TX: PRO-ED.

CHAPTER 14

Maximizing Speech Naturalness

Clinical Issues: At times, the physician who authorizes our state's Medicaid funding for speech treatment asks us for a second opinion regarding the appropriateness of treatment. On one occasion, we were asked to review the case of a young dysarthric woman. The speaker was a 25 year old former elementary school teacher who was three years post onset of ataxic dysarthria resulting from an episode of anoxia in a motor vehicle accident. She had received extensive speech treatment from the time she aroused from a coma with severely dysarthric speech until one year postonset when her speech was described as slow but intelligible. The first phase of treatment had involved attempts to control her excessively rapid speaking rate. Initially, only rigid means of rate control were effective because of cognitive limitation that prevented her from monitoring her speech adequately. Later, less rigid rate control techniques became effective. These were accompanied by practice on emphatic stressing tasks, monitoring voice loudness, and appropriate phrasing of connected speech. Her current vocational goal was to work part time in a day care center. One of the tasks she was expected to perform at the center was oral reading to the children. Despite the fact that the last speech evaluation had indicated that her speech was over 95 percent intelligible, her speech clinician had requested a four week period of treatment, specifically focusing on the prosodic aspects of speech. The physician who was considering authorization of this treatment had a number of questions:

- *What is prosody and why is it important to dysarthric speakers?*
- *Is it standard practice (i.e., appropriate) to continue to treat a dysarthric speaker after intelligibility has been achieved?*

- *What intervention sequences are appropriate for those dysarthric speakers who are intelligible but handicapped by speech that does not sound natural?*

Treatment of prosodic deficits in dysarthria is a clinically important but poorly understood topic. Thus far in this text, techniques for increasing articulatory precision and intelligibility have been considered and clinical reports presented which suggest that speech treatment for selected dysarthric individuals has the impact of reducing these aspects of disability. In contrast with these areas of management, clinical researchers have only recently begun to focus on the prosodic aspects of dysarthria. Rosenbek and LaPointe (1985) suggested that it is a mistake to consider prosody the "formal wear" of speech and to attend to it only after all other aspects of treatment have been completed.

Although documentation of the prosodic aspects of dysarthric speech is only beginning (Barnes, 1983; Caligiuri & Murry, 1983; Murry, 1983; Simmons, 1983), we believe that attention to prosody is important at all severity levels. For individuals who are not understandable, attention to prosodic features such as stress patterning may improve intelligibility. For the less severely involved, attention to prosody may improve the naturalness of speech and thus be important in reducing the handicap.

TERMINOLOGY

Individuals from such widely differing disciplines as linguistics, poetry analysis, neurology, and speech/language pathology have been interested in the study of speech prosody. Perhaps because of the varying interests of these professionals, terminology associated with prosody may be confusing. Therefore, we will begin this chapter by providing some definitions related to prosody and dysarthria.

Prosody

The term *prosody* is taken from the Greek and literally means "to add song." Thus, prosody refers, in part, to the melodic aspects of speech that signal linguistic and emotional features. Prosody includes a number of features that extend across a series of sound segments and are usually referred to as suprasegmentals. These include stress patterning, intonation, and rate-rhythm. Despite the rather poetic origin of the term, prosody is now considered a linguistic phenomenon. The prosodic code, although it is much less fully understood than the phonemic code, carries its own meaning. Prosodic features indicate to the listener whether an utterance is a statement or a question, which words in the utterance are the most important, and what the mood of the speaker may be. Because prosodic features also chunk or break the utterance into small units, they no doubt contribute to the listener's ability to identify the speech sound segments and therefore, to understand speech. In short, prosody, which is characterized by a series of suprasegmental features, carries unique information and plays an important role in the perception of segmental information.

Correlates of Prosody

Stress Patterning

The prosodic features of stress patterning, intonation, and rate-rhythm have perceptual, acoustic, and physiological correlates. These are listed in Table 14-1. Stress patterning, when measured perceptually, indicates the level of prominence of one syllable or word in an utterance in comparison to the rest of the utterance. Stress patterning can be measured acoustically by analyzing adjustments made in fundamental frequency, intensity, and duration throughout the course of an utterance. The roles of these variables in coding syllable prominence in normal speech are reported elsewhere (Fry, 1955; Lehiste, 1970; Lieberman, 1960, 1967; Morton & Jassem, 1965; O'Shaughnessy, 1979). Generally, syllables that are stressed within an utterance are longer in duration and higher in fundamental frequency and voice intensity than unstressed syllables within the same utterance. However, the relationship between these features and perceived stress is not simple. For example,

TABLE 14-1.
Correlates of Prosodic Features

Prosodic Features	Perceptual	Acoustic	Physiological
Stress Patterning	prominence	fundamental frequency intensity duration	effort
Intonation	pitch	fundamental frequency	respiratory-vocal fold activity
Rate-Rhythm	perceived speaking	segment duration	movement rates

some prosodic features serve a number of functions in addition to signaling prominence. Fundamental frequency shifts and syllable lengthening may serve as boundary features. In many instances, an unstressed syllable in the final position of a sentence may be of greater duration than stressed syllables occurring elsewhere within the utterance. Physiologically, syllable stress reflects heightened effort compared to other syllables within an utterance. However, it is extremely difficult to measure subtle changes in physiologic effort against a background of speech movement. The physiology of the production of stressed syllables is not well understood in either normal or dysarthric speakers.

Intonation

According to Netsell (1973), intonation "is the perception of changes in fundamental frequency of vocal fold vibration during speech production." Thus, perceptually, intonation is an indicator of changes in pitch; acoustically, it is an indicator of changes in fundamental frequency; and physiologically, it is the result of respiratory and vocal fold action. There is an average variation in pitch or fundamental frequency for a particular speaker. Intonational contours within a breath group signal such features as declarative or interrogative forms. In English, the simple declarative utterance has a rise-fall intonational pattern. According to the breath group theory of intonation (Lieberman, 1967), fundamental frequency is reset to the higher level after each inhalation.

Rate-Rhythm

Netsell (1973) defined rhythm as the "perception of the time program applied to the phonetic events of the speaker." Thus, perceptually, rhythm is a timing pattern; acoustically, it is relative segmental and pause durations; and physiologically, it is an indicator of movement rates and patterns. Nestell suggested that phrases have the rhythm they do in English because of the "stress-timed" nature of the language. A more detailed discussion of speaking rate and the durational adjustments in normal and dysarthric speech is found in Chapter 13.

Naturalness

Naturalness, as the term is used here, is a perceptually derived, overall description of prosodic adequacy. Speech is natural if it conforms to the listener's standards of rate, rhythm, intonation, and stress patterning, and if it conforms to the syntactic structure of the utterance being produced. It is considered unnatural or bizarre if it deviates from the expected or is unconventional in terms of these prosodic features. Bizarreness is one of the two overall speech dimensions examined in the Mayo Clinic studies (Darley, Aronson, & Brown, 1975).

PROSODY IN DYSARTHRIA

Perceptual Characteristics

Prosodic deficits are common in dysarthric speech. A number of the speech dimensions studied by Darley, Aronson, and Brown (1969 a, b; 1975) relate to prosody. Those that relate to stress patterning, intonation, and rate-rhythm are included in Table 14-2.

Prosodic disturbances occurred as a characteristic of all the dyarthrias studied by the Mayo group. For example, the speech dimensions monopitch and monoloudness were ranked in the 10 most deviant speech dimensions for all of the disorders studied and in the five most deviant dimensions along with reduced stress in parkinsonism and pseudobulbar palsy. The dimension of excess and equal stress was the second most deviant speech dimension in cerebellar lesions after the dimension of imprecise consonants. The dimensions of prolonged intervals, variable rates and monopitch were among the five most deviant speech dimensions in chorea. Darley and colleagues (1969b) identified two general types of prosodic disruption: one was the excessiveness seen in cerebellar lesions and the other was the reduced prosody characterized by monopitch and monoloudness in parkinsonism.

TABLE 14-2.
Speech Dimensions from the Mayo Study That Relate to Various Aspects of Prosody

Stress Patterning	Intonation	Rate-Rhythm
Monoloudness	Pitch level	Rate
Monopitch	Monopitch	Increased rate in segments
Excessive loudness variation	Short phrases	Increased overall rate
Loudness decay		Variable rate
Alternating loudness		Prolonged intervals
Reduced stress		Inappropriate silences
Excess & equal stress		Short rushes of speech

Acoustic Characteristics

Prosodic disturbances in dysarthria have also been studied using acoustic analysis techniques. Kent and Rosenbek (1982) identified *dysprosody* (distorted prosody) in five ataxic and seven apraxic speakers and *aprosody* (lack of normal prosody) in 20 parkinsonian and three right-hemisphere-damaged individuals. The dysprosody seen in ataxia and apraxia may be characterized by:

1. A "sweeping" pattern (exaggerated sweeping in fundamental frequency accompanied by generally longer syllable durations)
2. A "dissociated" pattern (a regularity of intrasyllabic features of duration, fundamental frequency contour, and intensity with syllables being separated by large but constant intervals)
3. A "segregated" pattern (some prosodic cohesion is maintained across syllables)

They suggested that the similarities found in ataxic dysarthria and apraxia may reflect "compensations made in response to an impairment of speech production." The fused pattern seen in parkinsonism is characterized by a "syllable chain that is flattened or indistinct." Kent and Rosenbek listed the following features of a fused pattern:

1. Small and gradual fundamental frequency variation across syllables
2. Small and gradual intensity variations between syllables
3. Continuous voicing
4. Limited variation in syllable durations,
5. Syllable reduction
6. Indistinct syllable boundaries because of faulty consonant articulation
7. Nasalization spread over several consecutive syllables (p. 283)

Contributors to Bizarreness

Monotony

Dysarthric speech can be unnatural or bizarre for a number of reasons that usually involve complex and incompletely understood interactions between prosodic features. For example, monotony, a frequent contributor to the bizarreness of dysarthric speech, may be the result of an excessively even rhythmic patterning of syllables, an evenness of stress patterning, a minimizing of intonation contours, or a combination of all of these features. In parkinsonism, monotony takes the form of monopitch and monoloudness, or the minimization of prosody in which no syllable stands out as stressed. In ataxic dysarthria, monotony takes the form of an excess and equal pattern. Each syllable is produced with such effort that none stands out from the others. Monotony can also be the result of "mono-patterning." In one of the cases presented later in this chapter, short and regular breath groups each with a simple falling intonational contour leads to the perception of monotony.

Syntactic Mismatches

Dysarthric speech also can be bizarre because the prosodic features do not coincide with the syntactic structure of the utterance. For example, a dysarthric speaker, who is physiologically limited to a small number of words per breath group, may inhale at syntactically inappropriate locations. Breathing every third or fourth word without regard to the syntactic structure of the utterance not only contributes to the monotony of speech but may also be perceived as unnatural because prosodic and syntactic features no longer overlap. Normal speakers have sufficient respiratory support to breathe only at syntactically appropriate boundaries so that prosodic features reinforce syntactic structures.

Inconsistency Across Features

Dysarthric speech may also be perceived as bizarre if prosodic features are in conflict with one another. For example, stress is signaled in normal speakers by a complex and subtle manipulation of fundamental frequency, duration, and intensity. Although normal speakers send consistent signals, dysarthric speakers may produce utterances with peak fundamental frequency on one syllable, peak intensity on another, and maximum duration on still another. The net result is perceptually confusing and unnatural.

ASSESSMENT AND INTERVENTION

Assessment and intervention for the prosodic aspects of speech are in many ways similar to the decison-making processes for other aspects of dysarthria. They involve gathering information and using that information to make decisions about whom to treat, what tasks to use, and how to sequence the intervention program. However, working in the prosody or naturalness domain is slightly different from some other aspects of dysarthria treatment, because as yet, there is no standard assessment protocol yielding "objective" data upon which to base decisions. Instead, assessment involves a series of questions. By answering these questions in a sequential fashion, the clinician describes the disability and identifies an appropriate starting place for intervention. Answering these questions more often than not involves perceptual judgments by the clinician. In some cases, acoustic analysis is also useful in obtaining detailed information. The following sequence may serve as a guideline for management of the prosodic aspects of dysarthria.

Speaker's Understanding of the Task

The first phase in assessment of the prosodic aspects of dysarthric speech is to confirm the speaker's understanding of the task. Because prosodic patterning is used to signal meaning, clinicians need to confirm the dysarthric speaker's cognitive and language skills. This can be done either by reviewing available neuropsychological and language testing results or by confirming the speaker's understanding of the tasks used to sample speech prosody. For example, when assessing stress patterning, an emphatic stressing task is often employed. For normal individuals, the task is cognitively simple. The speaker is asked to read a written sentence aloud, and then to read it in response to questions that are designed to elicit particular stressing patterns. Table 14-3 contains some examples of stimulus and response utterances designed to sample emphatic stress patterning. These particular sentences were selected for ease of acoustic analysis, that is, consecutive phonemes are readily segmentable from the raw acoustic waveforms. After each sentence is recorded, the speaker is asked, "What word did you wish to make the most important in that sentence?" If the speaker does not correctly identify the word that should be targeted for primary stress, the clinician stops there, at least for the moment, and either trains the recognition task or explores the use of other cognitively simpler stress patterning tasks.

Habitual and Maximum Breath Group Length

As described earlier, the breath group theory of intonation suggests that words are grouped into units based on breath groups. The breath group is marked for intonation and stress. Because analysis of intonation and stress

TABLE 14-3.
Examples of Clinicians' Questions and Dysarthric Speakers' Response Designed to Sample Emphatic Stress Patterning

Stimulus	Response
To whom should I show the snow?	Show SAM some snow.
Should I show Sam all the snow?	Show Sam SOME snow.
What should I show Sam?	Show Sam some SNOW.
What should I do with the applesauce?	SAVE some applesauce.
Should I save all of the applesauce?	Save SOME applesauce.
Should I save the applebread?	Save some appleSAUCE.

patterning involves comparison within and not across breath group units, breath groups must be identified. The importance of breath groups can be illustrated by comparing an emphatically stressed sentence produced by a normal speaker and one produced by a dysarthric speaker. Figure 14-1 contains a fundamental frequency and intensity-by-time plot of the sentence "Show SAM some snow" as produced by a normal speaker. Note that the fundamental frequency contour is represented by the dashed line. A line of declination has been drawn from the peak fundamental frequency of the first syllable of this declarative sentence to the peak fundamental frequency of the final syllable. Note the generally falling fundamental frequency pattern, except for the word that receives the primary stress. Cooper and Sorenson (1981) suggest that there is a generally falling fundamental frequency pattern within a breath group unit in declarative sentences. Fundamental frequency is reset after a breath group to the higher level. In normal speakers, stressed syllables consistently fall above this line of declination for emphatically stressed utterances such as those in Table 14-2. Thus, the fundamental frequency of the stressed

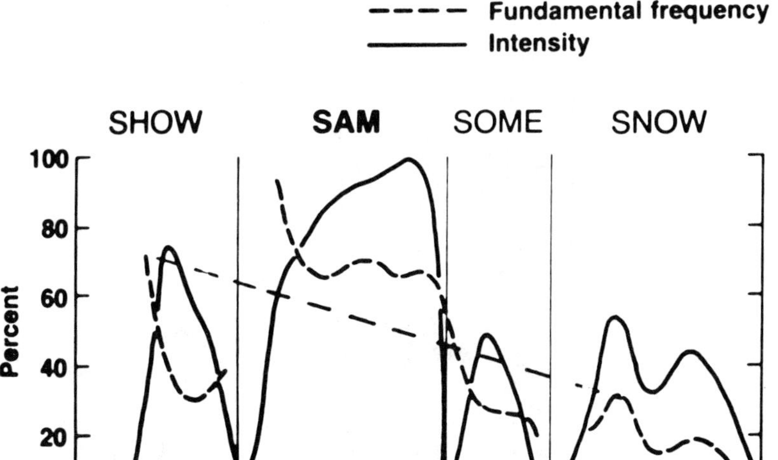

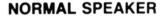

Figure 14-1. A fundamental frequency and intensity-by-time tracing for a normal speaker producing the emphatically stressed sentence "Show SAM some snow." A line of declination is drawn from the fundamental frequency peak of the first syllable to the peak of the final syllable.

syllable may not be the highest in the sentence, but it tends to be higher than the line of declination. The fundamental frequency contour characterized by this "high—to—low—then—reset" pattern is based on the breath group unit.

Many severely dysarthric speakers produce breath groups that are extremely restricted in length. In fact, some of the most severely dysarthric speakers produce only one or two words per breath. Other dysarthric speakers, although they appear to have the physiological potential of producing longer breath groups, treat each word as if it were a breath group. This is the case for an ataxic dysarthric speaker whose sentence production is illustrated in Figure 14-2. Note that there is a generally falling fundamental frequency pattern for each syllable, and the fundamental frequency is reset at the beginning of each syllable. This case appears to be an example of the "dissociated" prosodic pattern described by Kent and Rosenbek (1982). Because this speaker had the underlying motor control to produce much longer breath groups, a

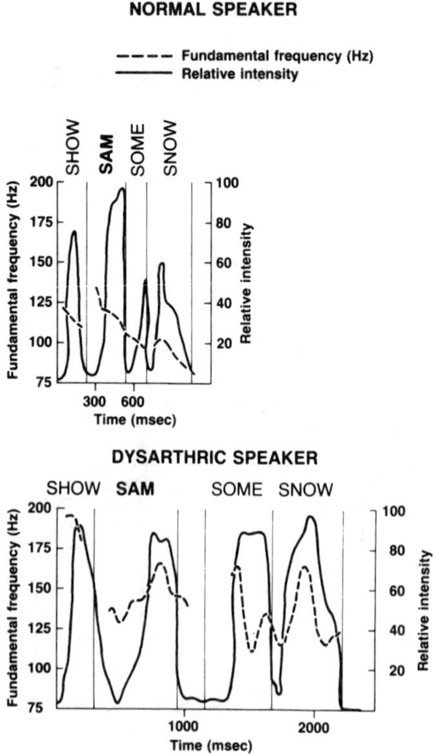

Figure 14-2. A fundamental frequency and intensity-by-time tracing for an ataxic dysarthric speaker producing the emphatically stressed sentence "Show SAM some snow." Also included for comparison is an acoustic analysis of a normal production.

treatment program was developed to encourage him to extend his breath group, and thus, to make the entire sentence an intonational unit.

Other speakers exhibit such poor physiological support that they can produce only a syllable or two per breath group. With these speakers, a different approach to assessment is appropriate. Stimulus material should be shortened so that the utterances are within the speaker's breath group capacity. At the same time, the clinician may wish to work on the underlying respiratory/phonatory control in order for the speaker to produce longer breath group units. To summarize briefly, the breath group may be considered the unit of prosody. Therefore, the breath groups that speakers are producing, or are able to produce, must be identified in order to adequately understand prosodic patterning.

Perceptual Assessment of Accuracy and Naturalness

Once the speaker's cognitive understanding of the task has been established and materials appropriate for the speaker's breath group have been selected, then the "successfulness" of prosodic patterning can be assessed. When assessing stress patterning, the term *targeted stress* refers to the syllable where the speaker intends to place primary stress, and the term *perceived stress* to the syllable that the listener judges to be the most prominent. The distinction is an important one clinically. If the speaker is not successful in achieving stress on the targeted syllable, then the first treatment task must be to increase the ability to signal stress.

Failure to signal locus of stress accurately may be the result of two types of errors. The first error is to send the listener no signals. In this case, speakers are not signaling prominence with any of the suprasegmental features—intensity, duration, or fundamental frequency. Such is the case in the sample presented in Figure 14-2. Note that none of the acoustic features give a clear indication of prominence.

The second error that frequently results in a failure to signal locus of stress is the sending of misleading acoustic signals. Such is typically the case in ataxic speakers. Figure 14-3 contains the acoustic information from such a "confusing" sample. Note that duration is longest on the word "Sam," relative intensity is greatest on the word "snow," and fundamental frequency is highest on the word "show." In effect, the listener is forced to choose between a number of conficting signals. Most judges indicate that primary stress is on the syllable "snow," however, agreement is not unanimous.

If the speaker is able to accurately signal stress on the targeted word or syllable, the clinician next considers questions related to the naturalness of the production. A speaker may successfully signal stress at the appropriate locus yet may be perceived to be highly unnatural. Figure 14-4 contains acoustic information from a production in which the ataxic dysarthric speaker understands the task and is able to produce the entire utterance in one breath

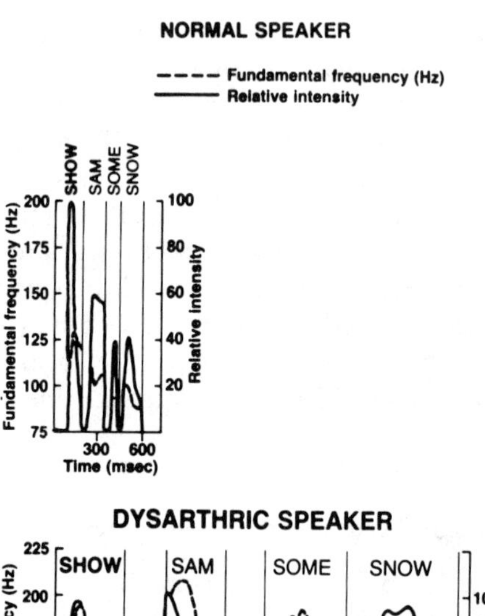

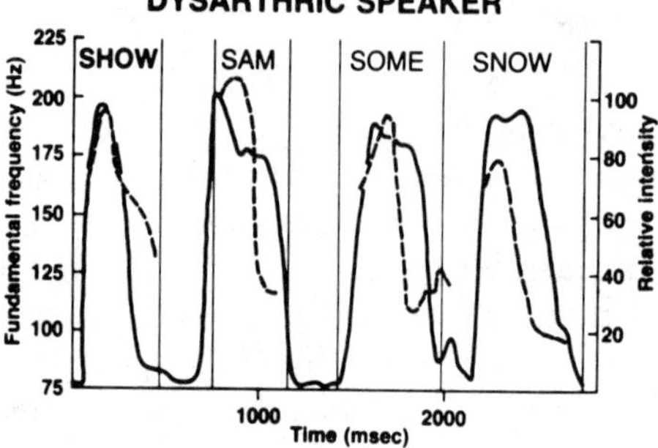

Figure 14-3. A fundamental frequency and intensity-by-time tracing for an ataxic dysarthric speaker producing the emphatically stressed sentence "SHOW Sam some snow." Perceptual judgments indicate that listeners usually perceive stress on the final syllable of the utterance rather than on the target syllable.

group, and where judges unanimously agree about the locus of stress. However, judges all rate these productions to be highly unnatural. The goal in training is to maximize both the naturalness and accuracy of the prosodic pattern.

Acoustic Analysis of Habitual Prosodic Patterning

Although naturalness is a perceptually derived phenomenon, perceptual measures of naturalness may be supplemented with acoustic information. Instrumentation is becoming available in more and more clinical settings. This instrumentation allows the clinician to display fundamental frequency and intensity by time contours on an oscilloscopic screen or on a computer monitor. If perceptual judgments indicate how successful the speaker has been in signaling stress, then acoustic analysis gives some insights into how speakers are achieving the perceptual results. Fundamental frequency and intensity

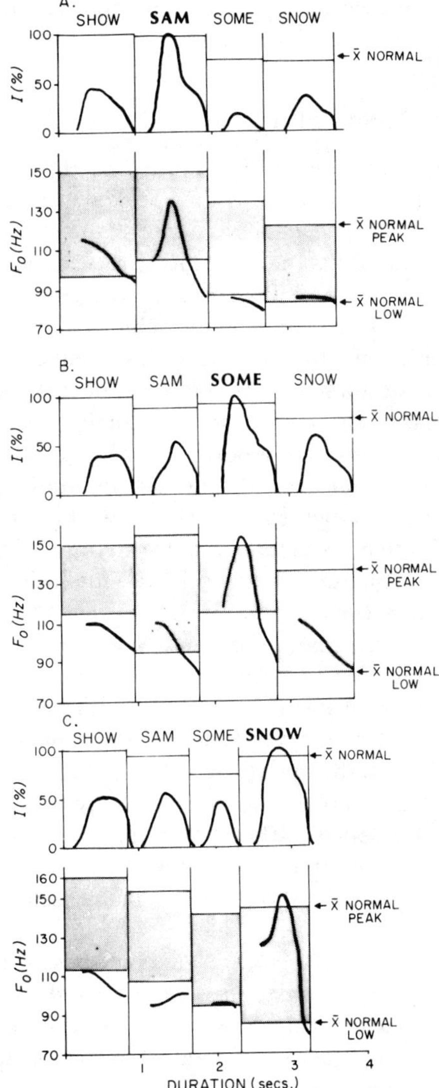

Figure 14-4. Intensity and fundamental frequency-by-time tracings of three emphatically stressed sentences produced by an ataxic dysarthric speaker. Stress patterning on these sentences was judged to be accurate but highly unnatural (From Yorkston, Beukelman, Minifie, & Sapir, 1984).

contours indicate what suprasegmental features or strategies are being used to signal stress. Information about suprasegmental features often helps to explain the perceived lack of naturalness.

Analysis of Modified Prosodic Patterning

The next step in intervention is to ask the dysarthric speaker to modify his or her production. For example, if the speaker were using exaggerated shifts in fundamental frequency and intensity to signal stress, the instructions might be to use only durational adjustments (prolongations of the stressed syllable or pauses) to signal stress. Perceptual assessment techniques are used to indicate whether or not the speaker was achieving stress on the targeted syllable and whether or not the new strategies produced a more natural-sounding result. Acoustic analysis is used to document the features that have been changed. Thus, the sequence of training usually involves the following steps. First, the speaker is asked to modify his or her production in an effort to signal targeted stress. Initially, specific instructions are not provided regarding which parameter to change. By experience, we have realized that such instructions can yield attempts that are quite unnatural. Finally, the features associated with the most natural productions are identified and the speaker is trained to consistently use those features.

In this sequence of training, a "normal" model is rarely used because suprasegmental features used by normal speakers are complex, subtle, and require a high level of motor control. Normal performance simply may not be possible for the dysarthric speaker. Rather than normalcy, our goal is "the best possible speech," given the dysarthric individual's motor control deficits. Again, as in many other treatment approaches in dysarthria, the speaker is asked to compensate for deficits rather than to produce normal speech. The following are some examples of modifications or compensatory adjustments we have asked dysarthric speakers to make in an effort to maximize the naturalness of their speech.

For individuals with insufficient prosodic patterns, general instructions such as "make the target word stronger," "emphasize the target word," "use extra force on the target word" may have the desired consequence of bringing into play one or more of the suprasegmental features that signal stress to the listener. For those individuals with prosodic excess, treatment may involve reducing the number of suprasegmental features that signal stress. Ataxic dysarthric speakers are encouraged to use durational adjustments as their primary means of signaling stress. Speakers learn to prolong stressed syllables and insert pausing at appropriate locations. Instructions to signal stress using only durational adjustments have a number of benefits. First, the control and coordination to simultaneously modify three suprasegmental features is often well beyond the capabilities of the more severely involved ataxic speakers. Reducing the task to a single stressing feature has the effect of simplifying the speaking task. Syllable prolongation is an adjustment that is usually within the capability of the speakers. Second, exaggerated durational adjustments tend to be perceived as less bizarre than exaggerations of either intensity or fundamental frequency. We have found that fundamental frequency and intensity adjustments do not disappear when the ataxic individuals are given the instructions not to use them as stress signalers. Rather, both contours may become more natural as they are deemphasized.

Comparisons Across Breath Groups

Thus far, prosody has been perceptually and acoustically assessed within the breath group unit. The final phase of assessment involves identifying abnormalities of prosodic patterning across breath groups. Monotony is a feature that often reduces the speech naturalness of those dysarthric individuals whose speech is intelligible but not normal. Monopitch and monoloudness both rank among the 10 most deviant dimensions in all of the seven diagnostic groups in the Mayo study (Darley et al., 1975). Both of these features rank within the five most deviant speech dimensions in parkinsonism and pseudobulbar palsy.

Recent studies have suggested that the perception of monotony may be more complex than simply reduced ranges of fundamental frequency and relative intensity. Solomon, Ludolph, and Thomson (1984) acoustically analyzed the fundamental frequency of speech samples of individuals who were judged to exhibit monopitch using the perceptual methods of Darley and colleagues. Solomon and his colleagues found that the range of fundamental frequency excursion was not reduced as compared to normal. This suggests that other factors contributed to the perception of monopitch.

In addition to being a phenomenon that occurs within a breath group, the perception of monotony also may be the result of excessive uniformity across breath group units. For normal speakers, the breath group unit is regulated to a large extent by the syntactic demands of the utterance being produced. In Chapter 9, data were presented that illustrated the variability of breath group length as normal individuals read a passage. Although the average number of words per breath group was just less than 10 words, these speakers frequently produced breath groups of only four words. At other times they spoke nearly 20 words before taking a breath. These data suggest that normal individuals vary their breath group durations depending on the material they are reading. Further, their breath group duration is not restricted by the limits of their physiological support. Dysarthric speakers are quite different.

Bellair, Yorkston, and Beukelman (1986) present the case of a 20 year old male who suffered a closed head injury in a motor vehicle accident. His speech was intelligible at a speaking rate of 90 words per minute (wpm), but was judged to be quite monotonous. He was able to signal stress within breath groups accurately and without exaggerating any of the suprasegmental features of fundamental frequency, relative intensity, or duration. However, when prosodic patterning across breath groups was analyzed, an explanation of the monotony was found. The speaker produced breath groups that were both shorter than normal and more regular, nearly every pause in the paragraph production contained an inhalation, and the sample was characterized by a restricted fundamental frequency range. Because the speaker appeared to have the physiological support to produce more extended breath groups, a training

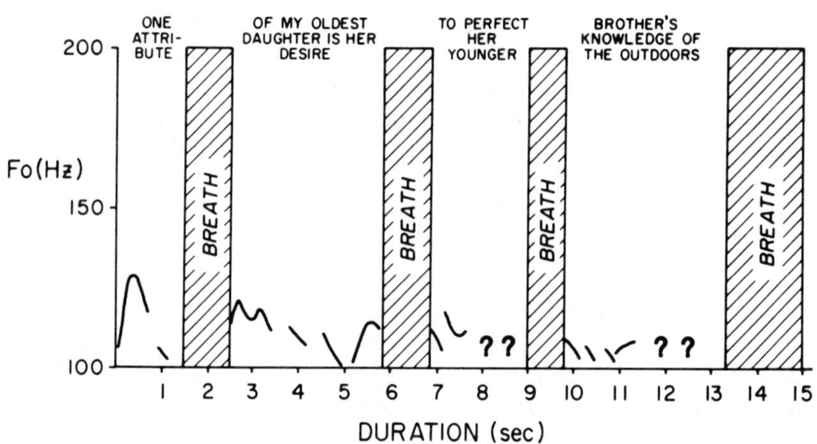

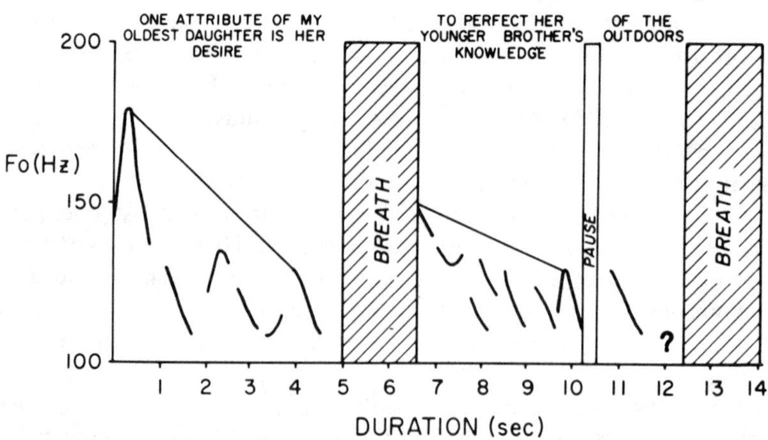

Figure 14-5. Fundamental frequency-by-time tracings from reading samples obtained pre- and posttreatment (From Bellaire, Yorkston, and Beukelman, 1986).

program was undertaken in which he was asked to increase the number of words per breath and to increase the frequency of pause without inhalation. Data obtained at the end of treatment suggested he had learned to do what was asked of him. Mean words per breath groups increased from 5.1 to 9.8, and his speech was judged to be more natural. Figure 14-5 contains fundamental frequency-by-time tracings for a portion of a paragraph read pre- and posttreatment. Note that in the posttreatment sample, breath group lengths were extended and fundamental frequency excursions were greater than in the pretreatment tracings. This case illustrates the point that the perception of monotony may arise from a number of sources. It may be the result of monoloudness and monopitch within a breath group, or it may be the result of "monopatterning" across breath groups. Breath groups of equal length add to the perception of monopitch because of the repetitive fundamental frequency pattern that they create.

Generalization to Spontaneous Speech

The final phase of intervention for individuals with prosodic disruption involves generalization of the strategies learned during highly structured tasks to spontaneous speech. This may be accomplished using a series of steps in which feedback provided to the speaker is gradually faded and practice materials are made more complex. An intermediate step between reading of sentence and paragraph material and spontaneous speech is the creation of short dialogues or scripts of conversations between the dysarthric individual and the clinician. During the generalization phase, speakers are also taught to critique their own productions. Initially, they may learn to judge the adequacy of their performance as they review an audio- or video-tape. Later, they are encouraged to monitor speech in an ongoing fashion.

REFERENCES

Barnes, G. (1983). Suprasegmental and prosodic considerations in motor speech disorders. In W.R. Berry (Ed.), *Clinical dysarthria*. Austin, TX: PRO-ED.

Bellaire, K., Yorkston, K.M., & Beukelman, D.R. (1986). Modification of breath patterning to increase naturalness of a mildly dysarthric speaker. *Journal of Communication Disorders*, *19*, 271–280.

Caligiuri, M.P., & Murry, T. (1983). The use of visual feedback to enhance prosodic control dysarthria. In W.R. Berry (Ed.), *Clinical dysarthria*. Austin, TX: PRO-ED.

Cooper, W.E., & Sorenson, L. (1981). *Fundamental frequency in sentence production*. New York: Springer-Verlag.

Darley, F.L., Aronson, A.E., & Brown, J.R. (1969a). Clusters of deviant speech dimensions in the dysarthrias. *Journal of Speech & Hearing Research*, *12*, 462–469.

Darley, F.L., Aronson, A.E., & Brown, J.R. (1969b). Differential diagnostic patterns of dysarthria. *Journal of Speech & Hearing Research*, 12, 246–269.

Darley, F.L., Aronson, A.E., & Brown, J.R. (1975). *Motor speech disorders.* Philadelphia: Saunders.

Fry, D. (1955). Duration and intensity as physical correlates of linguistic stress. *Journal of the Acoustic Society of America*, 27, 765–768.

Kent, R., & Rosenbek, J. (1982). Prosodic disturbance and neurogenic lesion. *Brain & Language*, 15, 259–291.

Lehiste, I.P. (1970). *Suprasegmentals.* Cambridge: MIT Press.

Lieberman, P. (1960). Some acoustic correlates of word stress in American English. *Journal of the Acoustical Society of America*, 32, 451–454.

Lieberman, P. (1967). *Intonation, perception and language.* Cambridge, Mass: MIT Press.

Morton, J., & Jassem, W. (1965). Acoustic correlates of stress. *Language & Speech*, 8, 159–181.

Murry, T. (1983). The production of stress in three types of dysarthric speech. In W.R. Berry (Ed.), *Clinical dysarthria*. Austin, TX: PRO-ED.

Netsell, R. (1973). Speech physiology. In F.D. Minifie, T.J. Hixon, & F. Williams (Eds.), *Normal aspects of speech, hearing and language.* Englewood Cliff, NJ: Prentice Hall.

O'Shaughnessy, D. (1979). Linguistic features in fundamental frequency patterns. *Journal of Phonetics*, 7, 119–145.

Rosenbek, J., & LaPointe, L.L. (1985). The dysarthrias: Description, diagnosis, and treatment. In D.F. Johns, (Ed.), *Clinical management of neurogenic communicative disorders*. Boston: Little Brown.

Simmons, N.N. (1983). Acoustic analysis of ataxic dysarthric. An approach to monitoring treatment. In W. Berry (Ed.), *Clinical dysarthria*. Austin, TX: PRO-ED.

Solomon, J.R., Ludolph, L.B., & Thomson, F.E. (1984). *How "mono" is monopitch? An acoustic analysis of Motor Speech Disorders tapes.* Paper presented at the Second Biennial Clinical Dysarthria Conference, Tucson, AZ.

Yorkston, K.M., Beukelman, D.R., Minifie, F.D., & Sapir, S. (1984). Assessment of stress patterning. In M.R. McNeil, J.C. Rosenbek & A.E. Aronson (Eds.), *The dysarthrias: Physiology, acoustics, perception, management.* San Diego: College-Hill Press.

Subject Index

Author Index